HUMAN FERTILITY AND REPRODUCTION

THE OOCYTE, THE EMBRYO, AND THE UTERUS

ANNALS OF THE NEW YORK ACADEMY OF SCIENCES

Volume 943

HUMAN FERTILITY AND REPRODUCTION

THE OOCYTE, THE EMBRYO, AND THE UTERUS

Edited by Carlo Bulletti, Dominique de Ziegler, Seth Guller, and Mortimer Levitz

The New York Academy of Sciences
New York, New York
2001

Library of Congress Cataloging-in-Publication Data

Human fertility and reproduction: the oocyte, the embryo, and the uterus/ edited by Carlo Bulletti ...[et al.]
   p. ; cm. — (Annals of the New York Academy of Sciences, ISSN 0077-8923; v.943)
Includes bibliographical references and indexes.
ISBN 1-57331-332-7 (cloth : alk. paper) — ISB N1-57331-333-5 (paper : alk. paper)
  1. Human reproductive technology—Congresses. 2.Human reproduction—Congresses.
3. Fertility, Human—Congresses. 4. Infertility—Congresses. 5.
Uterus–Physiology—Congresses. I. Bulletti, Carlo. II. International Conference on the
Uterus (4th : 2000 New York, N.Y. III. Series.
  [DNLM: 1. Reproduction Techniques–Contresses. 2. Fertility– Congresses. 3.
Infertility—therapy—Congresses. 4. Preganancy Complications—therpy—Congresses. 5.
Reproduction—physiology—Congresses. 6. Uterus–physiology—Congresses. WQ 208
H918 2001]
RG133.5 .H856 2001
500 s—dc21
[618.1'7806]   2001042767

GYAT / BMP
Printed in the United States of America
ISBN 1-57331-332-7 (cloth)
ISBN 1-57331-333-5 (paper)
ISSN 0077-8923

ANNALS OF THE NEW YORK ACADEMY OF SCIENCES
Volume 943
September 2001

HUMAN FERTILITY AND REPRODUCTION

THE OOCYTE, THE EMBRYO, AND THE UTERUS

Editors
CARLO BULLETTI, DOMINIQUE DE ZIEGLER, SETH GULLER, AND
MORTIMER LEVITZ

This volume is the result of a conference entitled **Human Fertility and Reproduction: The Oocyte, the Embryo, and the Uterus: The 4th International Conference on the Uterus**, organized by New York University School of Medicine Department of Obstetrics and Gynecology and The First Institute of Obstetrics and Gynecology and Physiopathology of Reproduction of the University of Bologna and Hospital of Rimini, Italy, and held on October 2–4, 2000 in New York City.

CONTENTS

Financial assistance was received from:

Major Sponsor

- ORGANON ITALIA

Sponsors

- BEAUFOUR IPSEN PHARMA
- OLYMPUS ITALIA S.p.I.
- SCHERING AG
- SIEMENS AG
- ITALIA FARMACEUTICI S.p.A.
- WYETH-AYERST LABORATORIES
- ZACCANTI

Preface

CARLO BULLETTI,[a] DOMINIQUE DE ZIEGLER,[b] SETH GULLER,[c] AND
MORTIMER LEVITZ[c]

[a]First Institute of Obstetrics and Gynecology, University of Bologna, Bologna, Italy

[b]Columbia Laboratories, 75008 Paris, France

[c]Department of Obstetrics and Gynecology, New York University School of Medicine,
New York, New York 10016, USA

Proceedings contained within this volume of the *Annals of the New York Academy of Sciences* comprise lectures presented at the conference entitled "Human Fertility and Reproduction: The Oocyte, the Embryo, and the Uterus" and held at New York University School of Medicine on October 2 through 4, 2000. From its inception, this conference was an international collaboration made possible through the combined efforts of the New York University Post-Graduate Medical School and the First Institute of Obstetrics and Gynecology and Physiopathology of Reproduction of the University of Bologna and Hospital of Rimini, Italy. This represents the fourth volume of a renowned series of conferences on this topic. The goal of this conference was to present in a single venue comprehensive information concerning recent developments in reproductive biology and their impact on human fertility and sterility. To accomplish this, internationally recognized leaders in both clinical and basic science aspects of human reproduction presented their work. At the conclusion of the meeting, participants had a clearer understanding of how underlying mechanisms of uterine/ovarian function regulate human reproduction. In addition, this volume concludes with papers dealing with ethical issues confronting investigators in modern reproductive medicine.

This conference was the fourth in a series spanning 10 years that was initiated in 1990 with the convening of the First International Conference on the Primate Endometrium at the Mount Sinai School of Medicine in New York City. This first meeting was convened largely through the efforts of Dr. Erlio Gurpide, who realized the importance and need for a comprehensive conference on the uterus. The Second International Conference on the Uterus was held in Bologna in 1993, and the Third International Conference on the Uterus: Endometrium and Myometrium was held at New York University School of Medicine in 1996.

We gratefully acknowledge the efforts of several colleagues who enhanced the quality of this meeting by chairing sessions and promoting energetic discussions following the presentation of lectures. In addition, we recognize and appreciate the effort and encouragement of Dr. C. Flamigni and Dr. C.J. Lockwood, chairmen of the Departments of Obstetrics and Gynecology at The University of Bologna and the New York University School of Medicine, respectively.

In addition, we would like to thank the New York Academy of Sciences for publishing the proceedings of this meeting and for continuing our now long-standing relationship. In particular, we acknowledge the efforts of Linda Hotchkiss Mehta and Angela Fink, associate editors of the *Annals*, who delivered these papers to the press in an efficient and timely manner.

❦

A final note: we would like to acknowledge the efforts of Dr. Mortimer Levitz, our co-editor and colleague. In this, his 80th year, he maintains an unrivaled level of enthusiasm and energy. We salute his dedication in the editing of this volume and recognize his ongoing and lifelong contributions to science.

— C.B., D. DE Z. & S.G.

Embryo Effects in Human Implantation

Embryonic Regulation of Endometrial Molecules in Human Implantation

CARLOS SIMÓN,[a] FRANCISCO DOMINGUEZ,[a,b] JOSÉ REMOHÍ,[a] AND ANTONIO PELLICER[a]

[a]Fundación Instituto Valenciano de Infertilidad para el Estudio de la Reproducción Humana (FIVIER), 46020 Valencia, Spain

[b]Department of Obstetrics and Gynecology, School of Medicine, University of Valencia, Valencia, Spain

ABSTRACT: Embryonic implantation requires coordinated development of the blastocyst and the maternal endometrium. Considerable advances have been made in the understanding of the cell biology of human embryo and maternal endometrium as separate entities. Nevertheless, communication between them and their reciprocal effects on each other constitute an exciting and as-yet unsolved problem in reproductive medicine. Cross-talk among the embryo, endometrium, and the corpus luteum are known to occur in ruminants and primates; more specifically, endometrial–embryonic interactions have been reported in rodents and primates. Here, we present updated information in humans on the embryonic regulation of endometrial epithelial molecules such as chemokines, adhesion molecules, antiadhesion molecules, and leptin during the apposition and adhesion phases of human implantation. Also the embryonic induction of apoptosis in endometrial epithelial cells as a mechanism for crossing the epithelial barrier will be described.

KEYWORDS: embryonic implantation; endometrial epithelial cell chemokines; antiadhesion molecules; adhesion molecules; leptin; endometrial epithelial cell apoptosis

INTRODUCTION

The implantation process requires a receptive endometrium, a functionally normal embryo at the blastocyst stage, and a dialogue, or cross-communication, between the maternal and embryonic tissues. Embryonic implantation, the process by which the human embryo orients, attaches, and finally invades the underlying maternal endometrial tissue, is very complex. During apposition a human blastocyst finds a place to implant, as it is guided to a specific area in the maternal endometrium. In the adhesion phase, which occurs between days 6 and 7 after ovulation within the so-called "implantation window," direct contact occurs between endometrial epithelium (EE) and the trophoectoderm (TE). The last phase is the invasion of the embry-

Address for correspondence: Carlos Simón, Instituto Valenciano de Infertilidad (IVI), Guardia Civil 23, 46020, Valencia, Spain. Voice: 34-963624399; fax: 34-3694735.
csimon@interbook.net

onic trophoblast, which traverses the basal membrane and reaches the endometrial stroma up to the uterine vessels.

In addition to hormonal regulation, increasing evidence demonstrates that embryonic regulation also has a significant impact by inducing reciprocal embryo–uterine interactions that change throughout the implantation process. During apposition, this dialogue is mediated by soluble proteins produced and received in a bidirectional fashion, whereas in the adhesion phase this interaction requires direct contact and seems to be mediated by membrane-bound factors.

In order to understand embryonic regulation of the implantation process and the molecular mechanisms involved, several aspects of the process must be considered. Chemokines are the first wave of molecules produced locally by the endometrium that recruit leukocytes to the implantation site. These chemokines also induce a second wave of cytokines, such as leukemia inhibitor factor (LIF), interleukin-1 (IL-1), heparin–binding epidermal growth factor (HB-EGF), and others, which by binding to their receptors may induce molecular changes in the expression pattern of adhesion and antiadhesion molecules. The implanting blastocyst must break the natural barrier that it may encounter at the epithelial glycocalix, which is composed of antiadhesion molecules, mainly MUC-1. Then the embryo has to activate endometrial epithelial adhesion molecules to create binding bonds between trophoectoderm and endometrial epithelial cells (EECs). Leptin, a molecule initially found to be involved with food intake and energy balance, has recently been discovered to be involved in the regulation of reproductive function. Here, we present data demonstrating its presence and regulation at the human embryonic–endometrial interface. A crucial question concerns how the implanting blastocyst is able to break the epithelial barrier; this process can be explained by the blastocyst's induction of apoptosis in human EECs.

In this review, we summarize our current knowledge of the embryonic regulation of the EEC chemokines, antiadhesion and adhesion molecules, leptin, and the induction of EEC apoptosis during the apposition and adhesion phases of human implantation.

IN VITRO MODEL FOR APPOSITION AND ADHESION PHASES

For the apposition phase, we developed, on the basis of our previous work,[1] an in vitro model to study interactions between the human embryo and EECs.[2] This model has resulted in a clinical program in which embryos are cocultured with EECs until the blastocyst stage and then are transferred back to the mother.[3] Embryos were obtained after ovarian superovulation and insemination, employing routine in vitro fertilization (IVF) or intracytoplasmic sperm injection (ICSI) procedures. EECs were isolated from luteal phase endometria and cultured until confluence. Individual human embryos were cocultured with EECs for 5 days (from day 2 until day 6 of embryonic development). After embryo transfer, EEC wells were divided according to the embryonic status: EECs with embryos that had reached the blastocyst stage, EECs with arrested embryos, and EECs without embryos (FIG. 1).

For the adhesion studies, a three-dimensional culture was prepared. Epithelial and stromal cells were obtained from endometrial biopsies and processed as described above, but with slight modifications. Epithelial cells were grown polarized

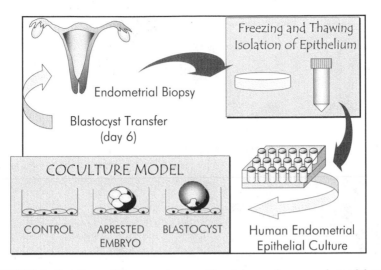

FIGURE 1. Coculture of human embryos with autologous human endometrial epithelial cells. Endometrial biopsy samples are taken in the cycle before patients undergo assisted reproduction and are frozen immediately. In the treatment cycle, the biopsy sample is thawed and processed to obtain the epithelial fraction, seeded, and cultured until confluence. Embryos are co-cultured under these conditions, and blastocysts are transferred to the patients on day 6. (From Simón *et al.*[3] Reproduced with permission.)

on inserts with extracellular matrix (ECM-gel, Sigma), and stromal cells were seeded on plastic culture dishes beneath them. Spare blastocysts were cultured on these endometrial epithelial cells. We let the blastocysts attach to the epithelial surface. After 48–72 hr, cells were fixed (4% PFA in PBS, 30 min, 4°C), permeabilized (0.2% Triton X-100 in PBS, 5 min, 4°C), and washed with PBS. Attached blastocysts were immunologically localized with an anti-β-hCG mouse monoclonal antibody from Sigma (1/50, 90 min, RT) and a rabbit anti-mouse biotin-conjugated secondary antibody from Dako (1/400, 60 min, 37°C)[4] (FIG. 2).

EMBRYONIC REGULATION OF EEC CHEMOKINES

Chemokines (or chemoattractant cytokines) are a newly identified family of small polypeptides (70–80 amino acids) that specialize in the attraction of specific leukocytes. In reproductive biology these molecules and related cells have been implicated in ovulation, menstruation, parturition, and embryo implantation as well as with pathological processes such as preterm delivery, endometriosis, ovarian hyperstimulation syndrome, and HIV infection.[5] Traditionally, chemokines are classified into two groups, based on the position of the first two of four consecutive cysteine residues, the α or CXC chemokines and the β or CC chemokines. Interleukin-8 (IL-8) (α-chemokine) is a potent chemoattractant and activator for neutrophils[6] and T-lymphocytes.[7] IL-8 is produced by a variety of cell types: monocytes, fibroblasts, lym-

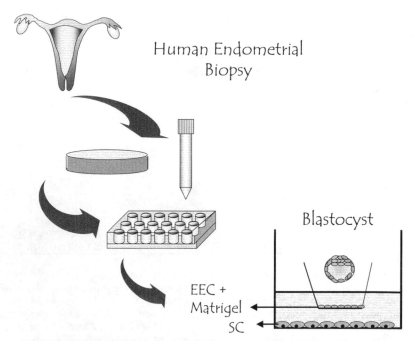

FIGURE 2. Epithelial and stromal cells were obtained from endometrial biopsies. Epithelial cells were grown polarized on inserts with extracellular matrix (ECM-gel, Sigma), and stromal cells were seeded on plastic culture dishes beneath them. Spare blastocysts were cultured on these endometrial epithelial cells.

phocytes, and epithelial and endothelial cells.[8] It has been detected in the human reproductive tract at the cervix,[9] placenta,[10] chorio-decidua,[11] and endometrium.[12] Monocyte chemoattractant protein (MCP-1), although it belongs to the β-chemokine subfamily, is a closely related protein and a potent chemoattractant and activator for monocytes, macrophages, T-cells, basophils, mast cells, and natural killer cells. MCP-1 is secreted by a number of cell types, such as endothelial cells,[13] fibroblasts,[14] monocytes, and lymphocytes.[15] It has been detected in normal endometrium[16] and endometrial cells.[17] The β-chemokine RANTES (regulated upon activation normal T cell expressed and secreted) is a chemoattractant for monocytes, eosinophils, and basophils and is localized in eutopic endometrium and ectopic endometriosis implants.[18]

During implantation, there is specific leukocyte subset infiltration into the endometrium from blood vessels and neighboring tissues.[19] The accumulation of leukocytes in the endometrial stroma is associated with hormones, and progesterone-mediated decidualization.[20] The cyclical pattern of leukocyte presence is suggestive of steroid control, but the fact that they do not possess either estrogen or progesterone receptors implies that this regulation is exerted indirectly.[21] Overall, the leukocyte migration is a multistep process involving the expression of adhesion molecules, their ligands, and additionally the synthesis and secretion of specific chemotactic agents.[22]

Northern Blot IL-8

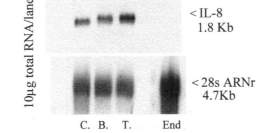

A   10µg total RNA/lane

< IL-8
1.8 Kb

< 28s ARNr
4.7Kb

C. B. T.   End

B   ## Densitometric analysis

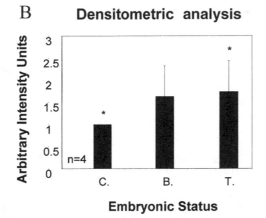

Arbitrary Intensity Units

n=4

C.   B.   T.

Embryonic Status

FIGURE 3. (**A**) Northern blot analysis of IL-8 mRNA in the three groups: C, control; B, blocked blastocysts; T, transferred blastocysts; End, endometrial biopsy control. (**B**) Densitometric analisys of the results, expressed as arbitrary intensity units (AIU ± SEM) compared with the control (EECs without blastocysts). Student's *t* test statistical analyses were performed.

We have investigated the hormonal regulation *in vivo* of endometrial chemokines IL-8, MCP-1, and RANTES and their specific receptors (CXCR1, CCR2B, and CCR5) at the protein immunoreactive level within the human endometrium[23] and the embryonic regulation of endometrial epithelial chemokines in the apposition phase. Immunohistochemical localization demonstrated that IL-8, MCP-1, and the three receptors were mainly expressed in glandular and luminal epithelium and endothelial cells; whereas RANTES staining was localized mainly in stromal and perivascular cells of blood vessels. Northern blot analysis was not sensitive enough to detect IL-8 and MCP-1 mRNA in total endometrial RNA. These mRNAs were easily detected in total RNA from EEC cultures (FIG. 3). Flow cytometry measurements of IL-8 and MCP-1 in EEC cultures confirmed the intracellular expression of these endometrial epithelial chemokines. Unlike these molecules, RANTES mRNA was detected in the whole endometrial RNA extract, but was absent in EEC cultures. These findings confirm previous reports on the endometrial expression of chemokines within the human endometrium.[12,16,24,25] After previous estradiol priming, progesterone up-regulates EEC IL-8 and MCP-1 mRNA in the prereceptive (day 18) and receptive (day 21) periods of the secretory phase of the menstrual cycle. These data are consistent with previous findings using a model of progesterone withdrawal and maintenance in vivo[26] and with results from normal menstrual cycles.[27] Nevertheless, stromal RANTES is not regulated in vivo by steroid hormones (FIG. 3).

The human embryo does not secrete IL-8, MCP-1, nor RANTES. The secretion of IL-8 and MCP-1 by cultured EECs was not under direct steroid control. These findings indicate that in vivo steroid regulation of IL-8 and MCP-1 expression at peptide level by EECs without the presence of an implanting embryo might be through an indirect mechanism, which could imply stromal or other endometrial cell factors.[28] In the apposition phase, however, the blastocyst upregulates EEC IL-8 at the protein level and mRNA and not EEC MCP-1 nor RANTES, suggesting that embryonic regulation of synthesis and secretion of IL-8 might be done directly throughout the EECs. Nevertheless, the results of the embryonic regulation of endometrial chemokines should be interpreted with the limitations of an in vitro model of coculture of EECs and human embryos. These data corroborate the evidence that in addition to the precise temporal pattern of chemokine production driven by ovarian steroids,[29,30] the human blastocyst participates in the modulation and release of chemokines during the apposition phase and in the leukocyte recruitment that occurs within the endometrium.

EMBRYONIC REGULATION OF ANTIADHESION AND ADHESION MOLECULES IN EECs

Antiadhesion molecules are present in the glycocalix of the epithelium and are the first barrier that the human embryo may encounter. Mucins are a family of highly glycosylated, high-molecular-mass (250–500 kDa) glycoproteins present on the surface of human epithelial cells. The most studied mucin is MUC1. The locus of the MUC1 gene is on band 21 of the long arm of chromosome 1 (1q21). MUC1 has the features of an integral membrane protein, with a carboxy-terminal region containing degenerate tandem repeats, a transmembrane domain (hydrophobic) of 31 amino acids, and a 69 amino acid cytoplasmic tail. MUC1 has been detected in the endometrium: Its expression varies throughout the menstrual cycle, and variations are found among different species.[31] In humans, MUC1 mRNA increases from the proliferative to the secretory phase in endometrial tissue, decreasing in the late secretory phase.[32] In patients with hormonal replacement therapy (HRT), no variation was observed with higher doses or time of exposure to E_2; however, when progesterone is administered, MUC1 increases in the luminal compared to glandular epithelial cells.[33] The concentration of secretory MUC1 in timed uterine flushings indicates that MUC1 concentrations increase in the luteal phase: concentrations from flushings performed before LH+7 were higher than those taken after LH+7.[34] The possible substrate candidates for MUC1 binding include selectins, which bind sialyl-lewis X and sialyl-lewis A carbohydrate antigens,[35] or intercellular adhesion molecules

(ICAM-1), which recognize a core protein epitope of the extracellular domain of MUC1. Whether these molecules are present on the trophoblast is still unknown. Recently, paracrine downregulation of endometrial MUC-1 expression by the embryo has been reported in rabbits,[36] a species in which the hormonal regulation of MUC1 is very similar to that in humans, suggesting that only healthy embryos have the ability to decrease MUC1 expression.

In the apposition phase in humans, EEC MUC1 is upregulated by the human blastocyst.[37] MUC1 mRNA increased in EECs in blastocysts compared to controls when studied by Northern blot analysis with a specific MUC1 cDNA probe. MUC1 protein was upregulated by the presence of the embryo when measured by flow cytometry using CT-1, BC-2, and HMFG-1 antibodies with or without sialidase (FIG. 4). These results suggest that the presence of a human embryo can increase the presence of MUC1 in the plasma membrane of EECs during the apposition phase. Given that progesterone upregulates endometrial MUC1 during the implantation window and the human blastocyst induces an increase of this molecule in EECs, it is controversial as to whether this molecule is a true antiadhesion molecule or serves as the first site of attachment for the embryo to the apical epithelial surface.

Using the *in vitro* model for embryonic adhesion, we have shown that cultured epithelial cells beneath and immediately adjacent to the attached embryo lacked detectable MUC-1 reactivity, with a progressive increase in signaling from cells farther away in the epithelial layer.[37] Cytokeratin labeling further demonstrates the presence of epithelial cells that did not show MUC1 expression at the implantation site. These results demonstrate a coordinated hormonal and embryonic regulation of EEC MUC1. Progesterone combined with estradiol priming induces an upregulation of MUC1 at the receptive endometrium. During the apposition phase, the presence of a human embryo increases EEC MUC1. In the adhesion phase, however, the embryo induces a paracrine cleavage of EEC MUC1 at the implantation site. These findings strongly suggest that MUC1 may act as an endometrial antiadhesive molecule that has to be locally removed by the human blastocyst in the adhesion phase.

Integrins[38,39] are transmembrane heterodimers that contain one α and one non-covalently associated β subunit. Several extracellular matrix (ECM) proteins including fibronectin, vitronectin, and collagen type IV possess the sequence RGD (Arg-Gly-Arg) for integrin binding, although there are other target sequences for integrin interaction.[39] Endometrial integrins are hormonally regulated.[40] Integrins α4 and α1 are progesterone-driven; they appear when progesterone production starts and endometrial progesterone receptors (PRs) are at their peak.[41,42] In contrast, β3 integrins appear when progesterone production is maximal and endometrial PRs are lowest. Integrin knockout studies reveal that in β1-null mice (−/−), embryos develop normally to the blastocyst stage but fail to implant.[43,44] However, no implantation-related phenotypes have been observed in knockouts lacking α4,[45] α5,[46] α6,[47] or αvβ3.[48]

Our group has examined the embryonic regulation of β3, α4, and α1 integrins in human EECs at the protein level in the apposition phase and analyzed putative embryonic factors responsible for such a regulation.[2] Our results demonstrate the selective effect of a developing human embryo on EEC expression of β3 that is maximal when a human blastocyst instead of an arrested embryo is considered. Furthermore, the embryonic IL-1 system seems to be involved in the EEC β3 upregulation. There-

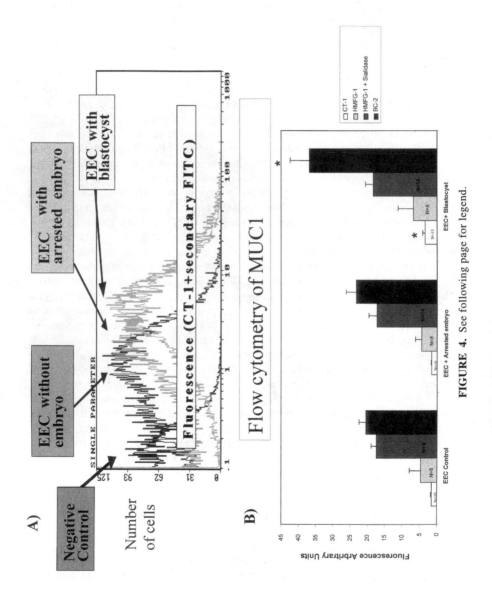

FIGURE 4. See following page for legend.

fore, after breaking the glycocalix barrier, the embryo could induce a favorable epithelial integrin pattern for its implantation, reinforcing the concept of precise paracrine cross-talk between blastocyst and endometrial epithelium.

Other adhesion molecules must be also considered as candidate ligands for embryo attachment: for example, osteopontin, which is expressed in the uterine epithelium[49] and promotes adhesion mediated by integrins of the aαv family and laminin, which is also present at the external surface of trophoectoderm.[50] Also, in human embryos there are cell-adhesion molecules such as ICAM-1, NCAM, and VCAM-1 that are present in early preimplantation stages of development but not yet studied on blastocysts. CD44 is present at the blastocyst stage; in contrast it is absent from the first-trimester trophoblast.[51] CD44 can recognize polyanionic glycans including hyaluronan and chondroitin sulfate, abundant on the endometrial apical epithelium, suggesting another possible mode of interaction between the two surfaces.

EXPRESSION OF LEPTIN AND LEPTIN RECEPTOR IN HUMAN ENDOMETRIUM

Leptin, or the OB gene product, is a small pleiotropic peptide of 146 amino acid residues (16 kDa) first found to be secreted by adipose tissue, and its secretion is tightly linked to food consumption and energy balance.[52,53] More recently, investigations have implicated leptin in the regulation of reproductive function.[54,55,56] The ob/ob mutant female mouse is characterized by obesity and sterility as a result of the synthesis of a nonactive, truncated version of leptin.[57] Fertility in these animals can be restored by exogenous leptin treatment but not by food restriction, suggesting that leptin is required for normal reproductive function.[58] Moreover, impaired reproductive function of ob/ob male mice can be corrected only with leptin treatment.[59]

In addition to adipose tissue, leptin has been found to be secreted by a variety of reproductive tract tissues including placenta.[60,61] *In vitro* cultures of cytotrophoblastic cells secreted leptin, and this secretion is regulated by interleukin-1 (IL-1) and estradiol.[62] Leptin protein and leptin mRNA has also been detected in human ovary[63,64] and is coexpressed in a polarized manner with STAT3 protein in oocytes and embryos at all stages of development[65] as well as in mammary glands.[66]

The long form of the leptin receptor (OB-R) with complete signaling capabilities predominates at the hypothalamus, anterior pituitary, and several other areas of the brain.[67,68] OB-R mRNA has also been detected in granulosa and theca cells of the ovary.[63,64] OB-R is also expressed in hepatic and adrenal cells.[69,70] A soluble form of the leptin receptor has also been reported to exist in humans.[71,72]

FIGURE 4. (A) Representative cytofluorometric analysis of EECs stained against MUC1 using CT-1 as primary antibody (Ab). In this graphic, the number of cells is represented against fluorescence in a logarithmic scale. (B) Data for the experiments with each antibody were combined and expressed as the mean ± SEM of the luminous intensity of cells expressed as fluorescence arbitrary units (FAU). Asterisks (*) denote a significant increase ($p < 0.05$) of intensity from cells in contact with blastocyst versus control cells. N indicates the number of wells studied in each category. When the secondary Abs were used alone, no appreciable fluorescence was detected.

Embryonic implantation is a crucial event in the human reproductive process, and leptin has been linked to reproductive function and to the inflammatory response. Gonzalez et al.[73] have described for the first time the expression of leptin and leptin receptor (long form) in the secretory endometrium. They have further found that leptin secretion is regulated in EECs by the human embryo during the apposition phase. Leptin and leptin receptor mRNA and protein were identified in secretory endometrium and in EECs cocultured with human embryos by RT-PCR and immunoblot, respectively. We also report that individual human blastocysts and EECs secrete leptin. The concentration of immunoactive leptin secreted by competent blastocysts was significantly higher than that from arrested blastocysts cultured alone. In contrast, the concentration of leptin secreted from cocultures of arrested blastocysts with EECs was significantly higher than that from cocultures of competent blastocysts with EECs. These findings suggest that the endometrium is a target tissue for circulating leptin and in addition is a site of local production. Expression of components of the leptin signaling system in the endometrium and EECs and regulation of leptin secretion by EECs due to the presence of the human embryo implicate the leptin system in the process of human implantation.

APOPTOSIS

Apoptosis, the highly orchestrated form of programmed cell death in which cells neatly commit suicide without triggering an inflammatory response in the tissue, is becoming a relevant event in reproductive physiology.[74] Programmed cell death is implicated in gonadal function,[75] human endometrial physiology,[76] preimplantation embryo development,[77] embryonic implantation,[78] and placenta formation.[79]

In the human endometrium, proliferation and apoptosis appear at opposing poles of the menstrual cycle, working as a homeostatic mechanism. The proliferative phase is characterized by a low number of apoptotic cells, whereas in the secretory phase the number increases significantly, peaking in the menstrual phase.[80,81] The majority of the apoptotic cells are present in the epithelial compartment; the endometrial stroma is less affected.[82] The artificial withdrawal of ovarian hormones is also followed by apoptosis of uterine epithelial cells; in fact, the predominant type of cell death observed in the endometrial epithelium is apoptosis (97.5%) as opposed to necrosis (2.5%).[83] At the molecular level, Fas (also called CD 95) and Fas-L (CD 95L) are co-expressed on the surface of human glandular endometrium[84] throughout the menstrual cycle.[85] The implanting blastocyst has to appose and adhere to the endometrial epithelium and subsequently invade it. Locally regulated uterine epithelial apoptosis induced by the embryo is a crucial step in the epithelial invasion in rodents. To address the physiological relevance of this process in humans, Galan et al.[4] have investigated the effect of single human blastocysts on the regulation of apoptosis in cultured human endometrial epithelial cells (hEECs) in the apposition and adhesion phases of implantation. In the apposition phase, the presence of a human blastocyst induces a reduction of EEC apoptotic cells (35.2%) compared to EECs cultured without blastocysts (48.8%) ($p < 0.05$). Interestingly, EEC monolayers cultured in the presence of an embryo arrested during their development also have a decreased number of apoptotic cells (39.2%) compared to EECs without embryos

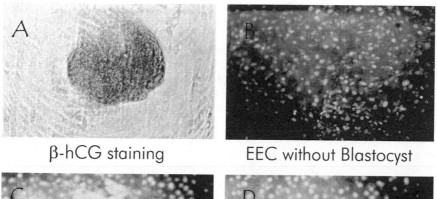

FIGURE 5. Double labeling (β-hCG and TUNEL) at the attachment site. (A) β-hCG staining of the implanting human blastocyst. (B) TUNEL staining in the control EEC monolayer without blastocysts. (C, D) An implantation site with apoptotic cells around the embryo and live cells away from it (×200).

(48.8%), suggesting the existence of an antiapoptotic effect exerted by soluble factors secreted by the human embryo, even if only for a few days.

When the human blastocyst adheres to the hEEC monolayer, however, it induces a paracrine apoptotic reaction. Unlike the apposition phase, when a human blastocyst adheres to polarized human EECs, we found a massive induction of apoptosis in EECs beneath and around the embryo attachment site compared to cells away from the blastocyst and control cultures (FIG. 5). This embryonic proapoptotic effect seems to be mediated by direct contact between the trophoectoderm of the blastocyst and EECs.

Confocal microscopy studies revealed the presence of Fas in the polarized EEC monolayer located at the apical cell surface. To quantify the percentage of EEC Fas-positive cells, flow cytometry was performed on EEC monolayers during the apposition phase, revealing that 60% of cells contained Fas, the death receptor, regardless of the presence or absence of human blastocyst. Finally, the Fas ligand was searched for in the human ($n = 6$) and mouse blastocysts ($n = 20$) using an anti-human antibody. Immunostaining for Fas ligand was present in the trophoectoderm of the spare human blastocysts and mouse blastocyst. Neutralizing adhesion assays revealed that the Fas/Fas-L death system may be an important mechanism to cross the epithelial barrier, which is crucial for embryonic adhesion. Neutralization experiments were performed blocking Fas with anti-Fas antibody at the endometrial–embryonic interface. Embryonic adhesion and outgrowth (rupture of the epithelial monolayer) were significantly reduced in EECs cultured in the presence of anti-Fas compared to those EECs cultured in the absence of anti-Fas (40% versus 82.8%, respectively).

In summary, a coordinated regulation of embryonic induction of EEC apoptosis, crucial for the embryo to breach the epithelial barrier as a basic physiological mechanism, has been described in human embryonic implantation. Furthermore, it has been demonstrated that the Fas/Fas-L death system mediates this mechanism, at least in part, and its manipulation may have potential clinical implications at interception.

REFERENCES

1. DE LOS SANTOS, M.J., A. MERCADER, A. FRANCÉS, et al. 1996. Role of endometrial factors in regulating secretion of components of the immunoreactive human embryonic interleukin-1 system during embryonic development. Biol. Reprod. **54:** 563–574.
2. SIMÓN, C., M.J. GIMENO, A. MERCADER, et al. 1997. Embryonic regulation of integrins β3, α4 and α1 in human endometrial epithelial cells in vitro. J. Clin. Endocrinol. Metab. **82:** 2607–2616.
3. SIMÓN, C., A. MERCADER, J. GARCIA VELASCO, et al. 1999. Co-culture of human embryos with autologous human endometrial epithelial cells in patients with repeated implantation failures. J. Clin. Endocrinol. Metab. **84:** 2638–2646.
4. GALAN, A., E. O'CONNOR, D. VALBUENA, et al. 2000. The human blastocyst regulates endometrial epithelial apoptosis in embryonic adhesion. Biol. Reprod. **63:** 430–439.
5. SIMÓN, C., P. CABALLERO-CAMPO, J.A. GARCÍA-VELASCO & A. PELLICER. 1998. Potential implications of chemokines in reproductive function: an attractive idea. J. Reprod. Immunol. **38:** 169–193.
6. MUKEIDA, N., M. SHIROO & K. MATSUSHIMA. 1989. Genomic structure of the human monocyte derived neutrophil chemotactic factor IL-8. J. Immunol. **143:** 1366–1371.
7. LARSEN, C., A. ANDERSON, E. AELLA, et al. 1989. The neutrophil-activating protein (NAP-1) is also chemotactic for T lymphocytes. Science **243:** 1469–1466.
8. BAGGIOLINI, M. & A. DAHINDEN. 1994. CC Chemokines in allergic inflammation. Immunol. Today **15:** 127–133.
9. BARCLAY, C.G., J.E. BRENNARD, R.W. KELLY & A.A. CALDER.. 1993. Interleukin-8 production by human cervix. Am. J. Obstet. Gynecol. **169:** 625–632.
10. SAITO, S., T. KASAHARA, S. SAKAKURA, et al. 1994. Detection and localization of interleukin-8 mRNA and protein in human placenta and decidual tissues. J. Reprod. Immuol. **27:** 161–172.
11. DUDLEY, D.J., M.S. TRANTMAN & M.D. MITCHEL. 1993. Inflammatory mediators regulate interleukin-8 production by cultured gestational tissues: evidence for a cytokine network at the chorio-decidual interface. J. Clin. Endocrinol. Metab. **76:** 404–410.
12. ARICI, A., J.R. HEAD, P.C. MACDONALD & M.L. CASEY. 1993. Regulation of interleukin-8 gene expression in human endometrial cells in culture. Mol. Cell. Endocrinol. **94:** 195–204.
13. SICA, A., J.M. WANG, F. COLOTTA, et al. 1990. Monocyte chemotactic and activating factor gene expression induced in endothelial cells by interleukin-1 (IL-1) and tumor necrosis factor (TNF-α). J. Immunol. **144:** 3034–3038.
14. YOSHIMURA T. & E.J. LEONARD. 1990. Secretion by human fibroblasts of monocyte chemoattractant protein-1, the product of the gene JE. J. Immunol. **144:** 2377–2383.
15. YOSHIMURA, T., N. YUHKI & S. MOORE. 1989. Human monocyte chemoattractant protein 1 (MCP-1): full-length cDNA cloning, expression in mitogestimulated blood mononuclear leukocytes and sequence similarity to mouse competence gene. JE. FEBS Lett. **244:** 487–493.

16. ARICI, A., P.C. McDONALD & M.L. CASEY. 1995. Regulation of monocyte chemotactic protein-1 gene expression in human endometrial cells in cultures. Mol. Cell. Endocrinol. **107:** 189–197.
17. AKOUM, A., A. LEMAY, S. McCOLL, *et al.* 1996. Elevated concentration and biologic activity of monocyte chemotactic protein-1 in the fluid of patients with endometriosis. Fertil. Steril. **66:** 17–23.
18. HORNUNG, D., I.P. RYAN, V.A. CHAO, *et al.* 1997. Immunolocalization and regulation of the chemokine RANTES in human endometrial and endometriosis tissues and cells. J. Clin. Endocrinol. **82:** 1621–1628.
19. BULMER, J.N. & P.M. JOHNSON. 1985. Immunohistological characterization of the decidual leukocytic infiltrate related to endometrial gland epithelium in early human pregnancy. Immunology **55:** 35–44.
20. BULMER, J.N., L. MORRISON, M. LONGFELLOW, *et al.* 1991. Granulated lymphocytes in human endometrium: histochemical and immunohistochemical studies. Hum. Reprod. **6:** 761–768.
21. KING, A., L. GARDNER & Y.W. LOKE. 1996. Evaluation of oestrogen and progesterone receptors expression in uterine mucosal lymphocytes. Hum. Reprod. **11:** 1079–1082.
22. DEL POZO, M.A., C. CABAÑAS, M.C. MONTOYA, *et al.* 1997. ICAMs redistributed by chemokines to cellular uropods as a mechanism for recruitment of T-lymphocytes. J. Cell. Biol. **137:** 1–16.
23. DOMINGUEZ, F., P. CABALLERO-CAMPO, A. PELLICER & C. SIMÓN. 2000. Hormonal end embryonic regulation of chemokines IL-8, MCP-1, RANTES and their receptors CXCRI, CCR2B and CCR5 in human endometrium. J. Soc. Gynecol. Invest. (Suppl.) **7(1):** 213.
24. CRITCHLEY, H.O.D., R.W. KELLY & J. KOOY. 1994. Perivascular localization of interleukin-8 in human endometrium: a preliminary report. Hum. Reprod. **8:** 1406–1409.
25. JONES, R.L., R.W. KELLY & H.O.D. CRITCHLEY. 1997. Chemokines and cyclooxygenase-2 expression in human endometrium coincides with leukocyte accumulation. Hum. Reprod. **12:** 1300–1306.
26. CRITCHLEY, H.O.D., R.L. JONES, R.G. LEA, *et al.* 1999. Role of inflammatory mediators in human endometrium during progesterone withdrawal and early pregnancy. J. Clin. Endocrinol. Metab. **84:** 240–248.
27. GARCIA-VELASCO, J.A. & A. ARICI. 1999. Interleukin-8 expression in endothelial stromal cells is regulated by integrin-dependent cell adhesion. Mol. Hum. Reprod. **5:** 1135–1140.
28. KING, A., L. GARDNER & Y.W. LOKE. 1996. Evaluation of oestrogen and progesterone receptotrs expression in uterine mucosal lymphocytes. Hum. Reprod. **11:** 1079–1082.
29. ROBERTSON, S.A., G. MAYRHOFER & R.F. SEAMARK. 1996. Ovarian steroid hormones regulate granulocyte-macrophage colony-stimulating factor synthesis by uterine epithelial cells in the mouse. Biol. Reprod. **54:** 183–196.
30. CRITCHLEY, H.O.D., R.W. KELLY, R.G. LEA, *et al.* 1996. Sex steriod regulation of leukocyte traffic in human decidua. Hum. Reprod. **11:** 2257–2262.
31. MESEGUER, M., A. PELLICER & C. SIMÓN. 1998. MUC1 and endometrial receptivity. Mol. Hum. Reprod. **4:** 1089–1098.
32. HEY, N.A., R.A. GRAHAM, M.W. SEIF & J.D. APLIN. 1994. The polymorphic epithelial mucin MUC1 is regulated with maximal expression in the implantation phase. J. Clin. Endocrinol. Metab. **78:** 337–342.
33. MESEGUER, M., P. GAITAN, A. MERCADER, *et al.* 1998. Hormonal regulation in vivo of MUC1 in mock cycles from patients undergoing oocyte donation. Hum. Reprod. **13:** 121–122.
34. HEY, N.A., T.C. LI, P.L. DEVINE, *et al.* 1995. MUC1 in secretory phase endometrium: expression in precisely dated biopsies and flushings from normal and recurrent miscarriage patients. Hum. Reprod. **10:** 2655–2662.
35. HEY, N.A. & J.D. APLIN. 1996. Syalil-Lewis x and Syalil-Lewis a are associated with MUC1 in human endometrium. Glycoconj. J. **13:** 769–779.

36. HOFFMAN, L.H., G.E. OLSON, D.D. CARSON, et al. 1998. Progesterone and implanting blastocyst regulate MUC1 expression in rabbit uterine epithelium. Endocrinology 139: 266–271.
37. MESEGUER, M., J. APLIN, P. CABALLERO-CAMPO, et al. 2001. Human endometrial Mucin MUC1 is up-regulated by progesterone and down-regulated in vitro by the human blastocyst. Biol. Reprod. 64(2): 590–601.
38. HYNES, R.O. 1992. Integrins: versatility, modulation, and signalling in cell adhesion. Cell 69: 11–25.
39. RUOSLAHTI, E. 1996. RGD and other recognition sequences for integrins. Annu. Rev. Cell. Dev. Biol. 12: 697–715.
40. LOPATA, A. 1996. Blastocyst–endometrial interaction: an appraisal of some old and new ideas. Mol. Hum. Reprod. 7: 519–525.
41. LESSEY, B.A., I. YEH, A.J. CASTELBAUM, et al. 1996. Endometrial progesterone receptors and markers of uterine receptivity in the window of implantation. Fertil. Steril. 65: 477–483.
42. INGAMELLS, S., I.G. CAMPBELL, F.W. ANTHONY, et al. 1996. Endometrial progesterone receptor expression during the human menstrual cycle. J. Reprod. Fertil. 106: 33–38.
43. FASSLER, R. & M. MEYER. 1995. Consequences of lack of β1 integrin gene expression in mice. Genes Dev. 9: 1876–1908.
44. STEPHENS, L.E., A.E. SUTHERLAND, I.V. KLIMANSKAYA, et al. 1995. Deletion of β1 integrins in mice results in inner cell mass failure and peri-implantation lethality. Genes Dev. 9: 1883–1895.
45. YANG, J.T., H. RAYBURN & R.O. HYNES. 1995. Cell adhesion events mediated by α4 integrins are essential in placental and cardiac development. Development 121: 549–560.
46. YANG, J.T., H. RAYBURN. & R.O. HYNES. 1993. Embryonic mesodermal defects in α5 integrin-deficient mice. Development 119: 1093–1105.
47. GIMOND, C., C. BAUDOIN, R. VAN DER NEUT, et al. 1998. Cre-loxP-mediated inactivation of the alpha6A integrin splice variant in vivo: evidence for a specific functional role of alpha6A in lymphocyte migration but not in heart development. J. Cell Biol. 143: 253–266.
48. HODIVALA-DILKE, K.M., K.P. MCHUGH, D.A. TSAKIRIS, et al. 1999. Beta3-integrin-deficient mice are a model for Glanzmann thrombasthenia showing placental defects and reduced survival. J. Clin. Invest. 103: 229–238.
49. BROWN, L.F., B. BERSE, L. VAN DE WATER, et al. 1992. Expression and distribution of osteopontin in human tissues: widespread association with luminal epithelial surfaces. Mol. Biol. Cell 3: 1169–1180.
50. CARSON, D.D., J.P. TANG & J. JULIAN. 1993. Heparan sulfate proteoglycan (perlecan) expression by mouse embryos during acquisition of attachment competence. Dev. Biol. 155: 97–106.
51. CAMPBELL, S., H.R. SWANN, M.W. SEIF, et al. 1992. Cell adhesion molecules on the oocyte and preimplantation human embryo. Mol. Hum. Reprod. 1: 1571–1576.
52. HOUSEKNECHT, K.L., C.A. BAILE, R.L. MATTERI & M.E. SPURLOCK. 1998. The biology of leptin: a review. J. Anim. Sci. 76: 1405–1420.
53. MILLER, K.K., M.S. PARULEKAR, E. SCHOENFELD, et al. 1998. Decreased leptin levels in normal weight women with hypothalamic amenorrhea: the effects of body composition and nutritional intake. J. Clin. Endocrinol. Metab. 83: 2309–2310.
54. FINN, P.D., M.J. CUNNINGHAM, K.Y. PAU, et al. 1998. The stimulatory effect of leptin on the neuroendocrine reproductive axis in the monkey. Endocrinology 139: 4652–4662.
55. TATARANNI, P.A., M.B. MONROE, C.A. DUECK, et al. 1997. Adiposity, plasma leptin concentration and reproductive function in active and sedentary females. Int. J. Obs. Relat. Metab. Disord. 21: 818–821.
56. CLARKE, I.J. & B.A. HENRY. 1999. Leptin and reproduction. Rev. Reprod. 4: 48–55.
57. ZHANG, Y., R. PROENCA, M. MAFFEI, et al. 1994. Positional cloning of the mouse obese gene and its human homologue. Nature 372: 425–432.

58. CHEHAB, F., M. LOM & R. LU. 1996. Correction of the sterility defect in homozygous obese female mice by treatment with the human recombinant leptin. Nature Genet. **12:** 318–320.
59. MOUNZIH, K., R. LU & F.F. CHEHAB. 1997. Leptin treatment rescues the sterility of genetically obese ob/ob males. Endocrinology **138:** 1190–1193.
60. MASUZAKI, H., Y. OGAWA, N. SAGAWA, *et al.* 1997. Nonadipose tissue production of leptin: leptin as a novel placenta-derived hormone in humans. Nat. Med. **3:** 1029–1033.
61. SENARIS, R., T. GARCIA-CABALLERO, X. CASABIELL, *et al.* 1997. Synthesis of leptin in human placenta. Endocrinology **138:** 4501–4504.
62. CHARDONNES, D., P. CAMEO, M.L. AUBERT, *et al.* 1999. Modulation of human cytotrophoblastic leptin secretion by interleukin-1β and 17β-estradiol, and its effect on human chorionic gonadotropin secretion. Mol. Hum. Reprod. **5:** 1077–1082.
63. KARLSSON, C., K. LINDELL, E. SVENSSON, *et al.* 1997. Expression of functional leptin receptors in human ovary. J. Clin. Endocrinol. Metab. **82:** 4144–4148.
64. CIOFFI, J.A., J. VAN BLERKOM, M. ANTCZAK, *et al.* 1997. The expression of leptin and its receptors in pre-ovulatory human follicles. Mol. Hum. Reprod. **3:** 467–472.
65. ANTCZAK, M. & J.V. VAN BLERKOM. 1997. Oocyte influences on early development: the regulatory proteins leptin and STAT3 are polarized in mouse and human oocytes and differentially distributed within the cells of the preimplantatation stage embryo. Mol. Hum. Reprod. **2:** 1067–1086.
66. SMITH-KIRWIN, S.M., D.M. O'CONNOR, J. JOHNSTON, *et al.* 1998. Leptin expression in human mammary epithelial cells and breast milk. J. Clin. Endocrinol. Metab. **83:** 1810–1812.
67. CAMPFIELD, L.A., F.J. SMITH & P. BURN. 1996. The OB protein (leptin) pathway—a link between adipose tissue mass and central neural networks. Horm. Metab. Res. **28:** 619–632.
68. MAGNI, P., R. VETTOR, C. PAGANO, *et al.* 1999. Expression of a leptin receptor in immortalized gonadotrophin-releasing hormone-secreting neurons. Endocrinology **140:** 1581–1585.
69. WANG, Y., K.K. KUROPATWINSKI, D.W. WHITE, *et al.* 1997. Leptin receptor action in hepatic cells. J. Biol. Chem. **272:** 16216–16223.
70. GLASOW, A., A. HAIDA, U. HILBERS, *et al.* 1998. Expression of ob receptor in normal human adrenals: differential regulation of adrenocortical and adrenomedullary function by leptin. J. Clin. Endocrinol. Metab. **83:** 4459–4466.
71. LIU, C., X.J. LIU, G. BARRY, *et al.* 1997. Expression and characterization of a putative high affinity human soluble leptin receptor. Endocrinology **138:** 3548–3554.
72. LEWANDOWSKI, K., R. HORN & C.J. O'CALLAGHAN. 1999. Free leptin, bound leptin, and soluble leptin receptor in normal and diabetic pregnancies. J. Clin. Endocrinol. Metab. **84:** 300–306.
73. GONZALEZ, R., P. CABALLERO, M. JASPER, *et al.* 2000. Leptin and leptin receptor are expressed in the human endometrium and endometrial leptin secretion is regulated by the human blastocyst. J. Clin. Endocrinol. Metab. **85:** 4883–4888.
74. TILLY, J.L., J.F. STRAUSS III & M. TENNISWOOD. 1997. Cell Death in the Reproductive Physiology. Serono Symposia USA. Springer-Verlag. Norwell, MA. pp. 1–7.
75. PIQUETTE, G.N., J.L. TILLY, L.E. PRICHARD, *et al.* 1994. Detection of apoptosis in human and rat ovarian follicles. J. Soc. Gynecol. Invest. **1:** 297–301.
76. TABIBZADEH, S. 1995. Signals and molecular pathways involved in apoptosis, with special emphasis on human endometrium. Hum. Reprod. Update **1:** 303–323.
77. JURISICOVA, A., S. VARMUZA & R.F. CASPER. 1995. Involvement of programmed cell death in preimplantation embryo demise. Hum. Reprod. Update **1:** 558–566.
78. PARR, E.L., H.N. TUNG & M.B. PARR. 1987. Apoptosis as the mode of uterine epithelial cell death during embryo implantation in mice and rats. Biol. Reprod. **36:** 211–225.
79. WELSH, A.O. & A.C. ENDERS. 1993. Chorioallontoic placenta formation in the rat. III. Granulated cells invade the uterine luminal epithelium at the time of epithelial cell death. Biol. Reprod. **49:** 38–57.

80. TAO, X.J., K.I. TILLY, D.V. MARAVEI, *et al.* 1997. Differential expression of members of the *bcl*-2 gene family in proliferative and secretory human endometrium: glandular epithelial cell apoptosis is associated with increased expression of bax. J. Clin. Endocrinol. Metab. **82:** 2739–2746.

81. TOKI, T., A. MORI, M. SHIMIZU, *et al.* 1998. Localization of apoptotic cells within the human endometrium and correlation between apoptosis and p21 expression. Mol. Hum. Reprod. **4:** 1157–1164.

82. RANGO, U., I. CLASSEN-LINKE, C.A. KRUSCHE & H. BEIER. 1998. The receptive endometrium is characterized by apoptosis in the glands. Hum. Reprod. **13:** 3177–3189.

83. NAWAZ, S., M.P. LYNCH, P. GALAND & L.E. GERSCHENSON. 1987. Hormonal regulation of cell death in rabbit uterine epithelium. Am. J. Pathol. **127:** 51–59.

84. YAMASHITA, H., Y. OTSUKI, K. MATSUMOTO, *et al.* 1999. Fas ligand, Fas antigen and Bcl-2 expression in human endometrium during the menstrual cycle. Mol. Hum. Reprod. **5:** 358–364.

85. WATANABE, H., H. KANZAKI, S. NARUKAWA, *et al.* 1997. Bcl-2 and Fas expression in eutopic human endometrium during the menstrual cycle in relation to endometrial cell apoptosis. Am. J. Obstet. Gynecol. **176:** 360–368.

Maternal–Embryonic Cross-Talk

JOSEPH A. HILL

Division of Reproductive Medicine, Department of Obstetrics and Gynecology, Brigham and Women's Hospital, Harvard Medical School, Boston, Massachusetts 02115, USA

ABSTRACT: The human menstrual cycle evolved to prepare the uterus for blastocyst implantation, which is fundamentally under the control of gonadal steroids. Ovarian hormones induce marked morphological, physiological, and biochemical changes within reproductive tissues. These changes in turn induce alterations in the biosynthetic activity and release of a myriad of locally produced proteins into the microenvironment of the reproductive tract. These same factors may be further modified by proteins secreted by the developing embryo and accompanying cumulus cells in intimate contact with reproductive epithelium in a network signaling process. Communication is not one-way, but rather maternal–embryonic cross-talk may occur as maternal proteins are secreted into the microenvironment of the oviduct and uterus, facilitating fertilization and early embryo development and serving as homing beacons for blastocyst nidation. The communicating language facilitating this dialogue includes cytokines, growth factors, angiogenic factors, apoptotic factors, adhesion molecules, and, potentially, homeotic genes.

KEYWORDS: implantation; cytokines; growth factors; adhesion molecules; blastocyst; embryo

INTRODUCTION

The human menstrual cycle evolved to prepare the uterus for pregnancy. Implantation is among the pivotal events leading to our species' perpetuation and is ultimately under the control of gonadotropins and gonadal steroids. This statement is an oversimplification, as a myriad of biologic proteins are fundamentally involved. Over the past decade, much attention has been given to studying the molecular and cellular processes involved in implantation. In this review the basic fundamental processes involved in embryo implantation and evidence for maternal–embryonic cross-talk will be presented.

A receptive window for implantation occurs in the uterus between postovulatory days 5 and 7 of a normal 28-day menstrual cycle.[1] This is marked by both cellular and biochemical changes within the endometrium. These changes, brought on by gonadal steroids, may also be facilitated by other biologic molecules secreted by the embryo and the reproductive tissues themselves in a communicative, interconnected network referred to as maternal–embryonic cross-talk.

Address for correspondence: Joseph A. Hill, M.D., Department of Obstetrics and Gynecology, Brigham and Women's Hospital, 75 Francis Street, Boston, MA 02115. Voice: 617-732-4648; fax: 617-566-7752.

jahill@partners.org

The communicating language facilitating this dialogue includes such proteins as the following: (1) cytokines, encompassing interleukins (IL-1–18 at present), colony-stimulating factors (CSFs), interferons (IFNs), tumor necrosis factors (TNFs), and chemokines; (2) growth factors, including fibroblast growth factor (FGF), keratinocyte growth factor (KGF), hepatocyte growth factor (HGF), epithelial growth factor (EGF), leukemia-inhibiting factor (LIF), insulin growth factor (IGF), IGF-binding protein (IGFBP), and the transforming growth factor (TGF) superfamily including activin and inhibin; (3) angiogenic factors such as vascular endothelial growth factor (VEGF), platelet-activating factor (PAF), platelet-derived growth factor (PDGF), and angiopoietin; (4) adhesion molecules such as integrins and their modifiers; (5) apoptotic factors; and, potentially, (6) homeotic (HOXA) genes. These factors—ligands, receptors, and their modifiers—work in concert, serving paracrine, autocrine, and juxtacrine functions via membrane-associated and soluble extracellular ligand-binding components enabling hatched blastocyst implantation into the gonadal steroid–prepared endometrium.

Many of the cytokines and growth factors were originally isolated from supernatants prepared from activated white blood cells; however, they are now known to be secreted by a wide variety of cells and tissues including endocrinologically responsive tissues within the reproductive tract. Inherent among these factors is the fact that their effects are redundant, pleuripotent, and pleiotropic, which should not be surprising from a teleologic perspective.

Implantation fundamentally involves four basic steps: (1) *placement* of the blastocyst into the uterine cavity; (2) *attachment* of the hatched blastocyst onto endometrial surface epithelium; (3) *invasion* of the trophoblast into subepithelial cell layers; and (4) *growth* of trophoblast tissues forming the placenta. These basic steps are fundamental to all implantations, whether they involve the hatched blastocyst onto endometrium, metastatic carcinoma, or endometrial implantation in ectopic locations as occurs in endometriosis. Investigating the basic processes involved in implantation events would thus be important in understanding tumor biology and gynecologic disorders such as endometriosis, unexplained infertility, recurrent pregnancy loss, intrauterine growth restriction, preeclampsia, and other placental growth abnormalities such as molar gestations, choriocarcinoma, and placenta accreta, percreta, and increta.

PLACEMENT

Placement of the blastocyst in the uterine cavity is the first step in human nidation. This fundamental process is dependent on an ordered sequence of events, including gamete maturation, fertilization, early embryo cleavage, and entry through the uterotubal ostia. These events are influenced by a myriad of communicating signals under gonadotropin and gonadal steroid regulation involving a complex neuroendocrine–ovarian interaction influenced by cytokines such as IL-1, Il-6, and IL-8 and growth factors such as EGF, FGF, VEGF, PAF, and PDGF.[2–4]

Fertilization and early embryo cleavage occur naturally in the fallopian tube. Whether this structure is more than just a passive conduit facilitating embryo placement is unknown, although tubal epithelium is capable of cytokine and growth factor secretion,[5,6] most prominently of TGF-β1 and LIF, which are proposed to be involved in a maternal–embryonic dialogue.[7,8] The three-day transient time of the early embryo through the human fallopian tube may facilitate maternal–embryonic recognition.

The mammalian embryo expresses many cytokine and growth factor ligands and receptors.[9,10] How and when these factors become expressed is unknown, although many are expressed in zygotes and oocytes. Cumulus cells accompanying the ovulated oocytes are also capable of secreting many cytokines and growth factors, an ability that may be important in oocyte nourishment and facilitate embryo cleavage following fertilization. IL-1, LIF, TGF, and other factors secreted by the developing embryo may feed back to the fallopian tube in the endometrium, facilitating the expression and secretion of other soluble and cell-associated cytokines and growth factors and providing another opportunity for maternal–embryonic recognition.

Concomitant with embryo development in the fallopian tube, the endometrium during the secretory phase of the menstrual cycle is undergoing profound cellular and molecular changes under the control of progesterone, which is itself modulated by cytokines, growth factors, and other intraovarian molecules.[11,12]

White blood cells are recruited to the human endometrium following ovulation in response to progesterone or other chemotactic factors mediated by progesterone since lymphocytes lack progesterone receptors themselves.[13] Once in the endometrium, these cells are capable of proliferation and cytokine secretion.[14–16] CD3, T-lymphocytes, of both CD4 and CD8 types comprise approximately 45% of the leukocyte population in proliferative endometrium. During the secretory phase, these cells reduce to approximately 10%, being replaced by a unique population of CD56 natural killer (NK)-like cells.[17] These CD56-positive cells comprise over 90% of the leukocyte population at the time of implantation and in early pregnancy. There are very few CD68 macrophages and no antibody-secreting plasma cells in human endometrium in the absence of infection.

The precise function of CD56 cells in the developing decidua is unknown, although they have been proposed to be important in implantation and pregnancy maintenance.[18] The mechanism is unclear; however, recognition by NK cells and their receptors and receptor inhibitors of HLA class I molecules, specifically HLA-G on trophoblasts, has been proposed to protect the implanting blastocyst from NK cell lysis.[19,20] Dysregulation of these potentially important events may be involved in either failed implantation or pregnancy failure.

Decidual cytokine levels have been characterized primarily at the mRNA level. Among the many genes upregulated during the implantation window, the most prominent include IL-1, CSF, LIF, EGF, and TBF-β.[21] The secretion of these factors can be modified by gonadal steroids and the blastocyst itself. The blastocyst expresses receptors for these same factors, providing a communicative link from maternal tissue to embryo.

IL-1 has been proposed to be involved in implantation, because IL-1 receptor antagonist can block implantation in mice.[22] IL-1 is not required for implantation, however, as mice missing the IL-1 gene nevertheless successfully reproduce.[23]

The presence of TGF-β in reproductive tissues may facilitate blastocyst development. Blastocysts also secrete TGF-β and may be a feature of higher quality embryos.[24,25] The presence of TGF-β in the developing decidua may also serve an immunomodulating role downregulating maternal immunity and potentially facilitating pregnancy.[26]

LIF is also produced and secreted by human endometrium and blastocysts.[27,28] LIF, like TGF-β, may enhance blastocyst development,[29] although this is controversial.[30] Maximum endometrial expression of LIF coincides with implantation, as does LIF receptor expression on hatched blastocysts.[31] Genetically altered mice deficient in LIF have defective implantation,[32] indicating that LIF is a primary factor for implantation. LIF has also been shown to modulate trophoblast differentiation[33] and to facilitate adhesion.[34]

The EGF family of genes are also maximally expressed in human endometrium during the implantation window. The blastocyst also expresses EGF receptors at this same time, providing the necessary anatomic link for interaction.[16]

Entry of the human embryo into the uterus is thought to occur three days before implantation. Why this occurs is unknown; however, the embryo has been proposed to use cytokine/growth factors as "homing beacons" for attachment. The epithelial cell surface mucin MUC-1 is present in endometrial epithelial cells and is secreted into the glandular lumen.[35] MUC-1 mRNA and protein increase after ovulation and may have the potential to either facilitate or hinder adhesion. Inhibition may occur through steric hindrance of receptor-mediated, cell-to-cell attachment, whereas the specific glycan recognition structures displayed by MUC-1 could potentially facilitate blastocyst attachment.[36] The embryo itself has been speculated to be involved in signaling the endometrium to modify mucin expression.[36] MUC-1 has also been implicated in influencing embryo selection for implantation.[37]

The implantation window on the cellular level is characterized by the formation of pinopodes, which are smooth, apical membrane projections of endometrial epithelium.[38] The function of these pinopodes remains speculative, although they may be involved in the expression and secretion of factors important for implantation.

ATTACHMENT

Attachment of the hatched blastocyst onto endometrial surface epithelium is dependent on adhesion molecule expression. These molecules include members of the immunoglobulin superfamily and the selectin family of adhesion proteins. Other adhesion molecules potentially involved include integrin subunits of both alpha (collagen and laminin) and beta (fibronectin and vitronectin) forms. At least 10 integrin subunits have been described in human endometrium.[39] The α9β1 integrin is expressed throughout the menstrual cycle but is only expressed in endometrial glandular epithelium during the mid to late secretory phase corresponding to the implantation window.[40] The αvβ3 integrin has also been implicated in implantation, since maximal expression is observed during the implantation window.[41]

Trophoblast cells themselves may also alter their integrin profiles during implantation.[39] Trophin and tastin are detected in both endometrial epithelium and trophoblast, forming a cell-adhesion molecular complex that may also be involved in attachment.[42] Bystin, a cytoplasmic protein, interacts with trophin, lastin, and cytokeratin and may be involved in trophin-mediated cell adhesion facilitating implantation.[43]

Complement and complement receptors are implicated in maternal–embryonic recognition, since both the blastocyst and endometrial surface epithelium express receptors for complement.[44,45] Complement has also been described in the endometrial cavity, where it may be either locally produced or derived as a transludate from the peripheral circulation.[46] Complement may be involved in initial blastocyst attachment by binding to its receptors, both on the blastocyst and surface epithelium. In pathologic conditions such as may accompany infection or in some cases of endometriosis,[46] excess complement may saturate all available receptors, disallowing attachment.

INVASION

Following attachment, invasion must occur for successful implantation. Invasion requires enzymatic digestion of the extracellular matrix while simultaneously controlling hemostasis and neoangiogenesis within decidual tissues. These enzymatic processes involve proteinases, metalloproteinases, collagenases, gelatinases, stromelysins, metallolastases, and urokinase. Plasminogen activators, including tissue plasmin activator and urokinase plasmin activator, are upregulated to control hemostasis brought about by remodeling of the extracellular matrix.[16,47]

Both LIF and EGF can regulate urokinase plasmin activator and metalloproteinase-9 activity,[48] which may facilitate trophoblast invasion. Certain integrins may also be involved in trophoblast invasion. The $\alpha5\beta1$ integrin has been proposed to control the rate of blastocyst migration and trophoblast invasion into the decidua.[49]

GROWTH

Trophoblast growth must occur concomitantly with invasion for successful implantation and placental development. Growth is dependent on both enabling and limiting factors. One key feature is vascular development within the developing placenta and decidua. This generally occurs in two defined stages. The first is vasculogenesis, involving a primitive vascular network followed by angiogenesis with the formation of a microcirculation.

Vascular endothelial growth factor (VEGF), platelet-derived growth factor (PDGF), platelet-activating factor (PAF), and angiopoietins are critical for the earliest stages of vascular development.[50] Hepatocyte growth factor (HGF) produced by mesechyme and its c-met tyrosine kinase receptor, expressed on epithelial cells, participates in the regulation of cytotrophoblast differentiation and growth and may regulate the depth of invasion.[51]

Other factors involved in regulating trophoblast growth include IL-1, stem cell factor, macrophage colony stimulating factor (CSF-1), IGF, and T-helper (Th) cytokines. IL-1 and CSF-1 both stimulate trophoblast cell growth and function, whereas IGFBP-1 and the Th-1 cytokines IFN-γ and TNF may limit trophoblast growth.[52,53] These same cytokines/growth factors may also influence hCG[54] and progesterone[55] production from trophoblast cells.

Apoptotic factors are also involved in trophoblast growth. TNF and TGF-β are physiologic inducers of apoptosis, whereas apoptotic inhibitors include the extracellular matrix and growth factors.

Homeotic (HOXA) genes may also be involved in maternal–embryonic cross-talk. HOXA genes are regulatory genes encoding transcription factors essential to normal development. In the uterus, HOXA gene expression is normally regulated by gonadal steroids.[56] Gonadal steroid action in the uterus regulates HOXA-9, HOXA-10, and HOXA-11 expression, which may regulate stromal cell proliferation. HOXA-11 may also facilitate LIF expression. HOXA-10 and LIF within the uterus can affect prostaglandin receptor expression, facilitating decidualization.[56] IL-11 has recently been shown to be involved in decidualization, as genetically manipulated mice missing the IL-11 receptor were noted to have inadequate decidualization.[57]

SUMMARY

The human menstrual cycle evolved to prepare the uterus for blastocyst implantation, which is fundamentally under the control of gonadal steroids. Ovarian hormones induce marked morphological, physiological, and biochemical changes within reproductive tissues. These changes in turn induce alterations in the biosynthetic activity and release of a myriad of locally produced proteins into the microenvironment of the reproductive tract. These same factors may be further modified by proteins secreted by the developing embryo and accompanying cumulus cells in intimate contact with reproductive epithelium in a network signaling process known as maternal–embryonic cross-talk. Communication is not one-way, but rather a maternal–embryonic dialogue may occur as maternal proteins secreted into the microenvironment of the oviduct and uterus may facilitate fertilization and early embryo development and serve as homing beacons for blastocyst nidation. The communicating language facilitating this dialogue includes (1) cytokines, encompassing interleukins (1–18 at present), colony-stimulating factors, interferons, TNF, and chemokines; (2) growth factors such as FGF, KGF, EGF, LIF, IGFBPs, and the TGF superfamily including activin and inhibin; (3) angiogenic factors such as PAF, PDGF, VEGF, and angiopoietin; (4) apoptotic factors; (5) adhesion molecules and their modifiers; and (6) homeobox genes. These factors serve both paracrine and autocrine functions that may enhance and sustain fertilization, early cleavage stage embryo development, implantation events, and trophoblast growth and function, culminating in successful pregnancy. Dysregulation of these redundant, pluripotent, pleiotropic proteins leading to disrupted communication between a mother and her embryo may give rise to reproductive difficulty. This may occur either before or after fertilization or implantation and cause infertility or pregnancy loss.

Much remains to be learned concerning the nature, concentration, and interactions of the communicating signals comprising the maternal–embryonic cross-talk dialogue. Deciphering this language will undoubtedly lead to the development of new regulating agents with novel diagnostic, biological, and therapeutic potential for both facilitating and hindering normal reproductive function. The knowledge gained from such basic and translational research may also facilitate understanding the behavior of tumor cell metastasis, endometriosis, and, potentially, regenerative processes involved in angiogenesis, wound healing, and tissue repair.

REFERENCES

1. BERGH, P.A. & D. NARVOT. 1992. The impact of embryonic development and endometrium on the timing of implantation. Fertil. Steril. **58:** 537–542.
2. DEVOTO, L., M. VEGA, P. KOHEN, et al. 2000. Endocrine and paracrine–autocrine regulation of the human corpus luteum during mid-luteal phase. J. Reprod. Fertil. Suppl. **55:** 13–20.
3. JONES, T.H., & R.L. KENNEDY. 1993. Cytokines and hypothalamic–pituitary function. Cytokines **5:** 531.
4. HAIMOVICI, F. & J.A. HILL. 2000. In Cytokines in Human Reproduction. J.A. Hill, Eds.: 1–16. Wiley-Liss. New York.
5. CHEGINI, N. 1996. Oviductal-derived growth factors and cytokines. Implication in preimplantation. Semin. Reprod. **14:** 219–229.
6. BRABEC, C.M. & J.A. HILL. 2000. Cytokines/growth factors in the human fallopian tube. In Cytokines in Human Reproduction. J.A. Hill, Eds.: 221–237. Wiley-Liss. New York.
7. KAUMA, S.W. & D.W. MATT. 1995. Coculture cells that express leukemia inhibiting factor enhance mouse blastocyst development in vitro. J. Assist. Reprod. Genet. **12:** 153–156.
8. PARIA, B.C. & S.K. DEY. 1990. Preimplantation embryo development in vitro: cooperative interactions among embryos and the role of growth factors. Proc. Natl. Acad. Sci. USA **87:** 4756–4760.
9. ROBERTSON, S.A., R.F. SENMARK, L. GUILBERT, et al. 1994. The role of cytokines in cestation. Crit. Rev. Immunol. **14:** 239–292.
10. SCHULTZ, G.A. & S. HEYNER. 1993. Growth factors in preimplantation mammalian embryos. Oxford Rev. Reprod. **15:** 43–81.
11. BEST, C.L. & J.A. HILL. 2000. Cytokine in ovarian function. In Cytokines in Human Reproduction. J.A. Hill, Ed.: 43–77. Wiley-Liss. New York.
12. Adashi, E.Y. & P.C.K. Leung, Eds. 1993. The Ovary. Raven Press. New York. pp. 329–454.
13. SCHUST, D.J., D.J. ANDERSON & J.A. HILL. 1996. Progesterone-induced immunosuppression is not medicated through the progesterone receptor. Hum. Reprod. **11:** 980–985.
14. TABIBZADEH, S. 1991. Human endometrium: an active site of ctokine production and actin. Endocrniol. Rev. **12:** 272–290.
15. HILL, J.A. & D.J. ANDERSON. 1990. Evidence for the existence and significance of immune cells in male and female reproductive tissues. Immunol. Allerg. Clin. N. Am. **10:** 1–12.
16. CHEGINI, N. & R.S. WILLIAMS. 2000. Cytokines and growth factor networks in human endometrium from menstruation to embryo implantation. In Cytokine in Human Reproduction. J.A. Hill, Ed.: 93–132. Wiley-Liss. New York.
17. LOKE, Y.W. & A. KING. 2000. Immunological aspects of human implantation. J. Reprod. Fertil. Suppl. **55:** 88–90.
18. LOKE, Y.W. & A. KING. 2000. Decidual natural killer cell interaction with trophoblast: cytolysis or cytokine production? Biochem. Soc. Trans. **28:** 196–198.
19. CAROSELLA, E.D., N. ROUAS-FREISS, P. PAUL, et al. 1999. HLA-G: a tolerance molecule from the major histocompatibility complex. Immunol. Today **20:** 60–62.
20. LEBOUTEILLER, P. & A. BLASCHITZ. 1999. The functionality of ALA-G is emerging. Immunol. Rev. **167:** 233–244.
21. KAUMA, S.W. 2000. Cytokines in implantation. J. Reprod. Fertil. **55:** 31–40.
22. SIMON, C., G.N. PIQUETTE, A. FRANCES, et al. 1994. Embryonic implantation in mice is blocked by interleukin-1 receptor antagonist. Endocrinology **134:** 521–528.
23. ABBONDANZO, S.J., E.B. CULLINAN, K. MCINTYRE, et al. 1996. Reproduction in mice lacking a functional type 1 IL-1 receptor. Endocrinology **137:** 3598–3601.
24. PARIA, B.C., K.L. JONES, K.C. FLANDERS, et al. 1992. Localization and finding of transforming growth factor-B isoforms in mouse preimplantation embryos and is delayed and activated blastocysts. Rev. Biol. **151:** 91–104.

25. ADAMSON, E.D. 1993. Activities of growth factors in preimplantation embryos. J. Cell Biochem. **53:** 280.
26. CLARK, D.A. & R. COKER. 1998. Transforming growth factor-beta (TGF-beta). Int. J. Biochem. Cell Biol. **30:** 293–298.
27. CULINAN, E.B., S.S. ABDONDANZO, P.S. ANDERSON, et al. 1996. Leukemia inhibiting factor (LIF) and LIF receptor expression in human endometrium suggests a potential autocrine/paracrine function in regulating embryo implantation. PNAS USA. **93:** 3115–3120.
28. ROJIMA, K., H. KANZAKI, M. IWAI, et al. 1994. Expression of leukemia inhibiting factor in human endometrium and placenta. Hum. Reprod. **50:** 882–887.
29. DURGLISON, G.F., D.H. BARLOW & I.L. SARGENT. 1996. Leukemia inhibiting factor significantly enhances the blastocysts formation rates of human embryos cultured in serum-free medium. Hum. Reprod. **11:** 191–196.
30. JURISICOVA, A., A. BEN-CHETRIT, S.L. VASMUZA, et al. 1995. Recombinant human leukemia inhibiting factor does not enhance in vitro human blastocyst formation. Fertil. Steril. **64:** 999–1002.
31. BHATT, H., L.C. BRUNETT & C.C. STEWART. 1991. Uterine expression of leukemia inhibiting factor coincides with the onset of blastocyst implantation. PNAS USA **88:** 11401–11412.
32. STEWART, C.L., P. KASPAR, L.J. BRUNETT, et al. 1992. Blastocyst implantation depends on maternal expression of leukemia inhibitory factor. Nature **359:** 76–79.
33. NACHTIGALL, M.J. H.J. KLIMAN, et al. 1996. The effect of leukemia inhibitory factor on trophoblast differentiation: a potential role in human implantation. J. Clin. Endocrinol. Metab. **81:** 801–806.
34. BISCHOF, P., L. HAENGGELI & A. COMPANA. 1995. Effects of leukemia inhibitory factor on human cytotrophoblast differentiation along the invasive pathway. Am. J. Reprod. Immunol. **34:** 225–230.
35. GIPSON, I.K., S.B. HO, S.J. SPURS-MICHAUD, et al. 1997. Mucin genes expressed by human female reproductive tract epithelial. Biol. Reprod. **56:** 999–1011.
36. APLIN, J.D. 1999. MUC-1 glycosylation in endometrium: possible roles in the apical glycocalyx at implantation. **14:** 17–25.
37. APLIN, J.D., N.A. HEY & T.C. LI. 1996. MUC-1 as a cell surface at secretory component of endometrial epithelium: reduced levels in recurrent miscarriage. Am. J. Reprod. Immunol. **35:** 261–266.
38. NIKAS, G. 1999. Pinopodes as markers of endometrial receptivity in clinical practice. Hum. Reprod. **14:** 99–106.
39. BOWEN, J.A. & J.S. HUNT. 2000. The role of integrins in reproduction. Exp. Biol. Med. **223:** 331–343.
40. LESSEY, B.A., A.O. ILESANMI, M.A. LESSEY, et al. 1996. Luminal and glandular endometrial epithelium express integrins differentially throughout the menstrual cycle: implications for implantation, contraception, and infertility. Am. J. Reprod. Immunol. **35:** 195–204.
41. LESSEY, B.A. 1998. Endometrial integrins and the establishment of uterine receptivity. Hum. Reprod. **13**(Suppl. 3)**:** 247–258.
42. FUKUDA, M.N. & S. NOZAWA. 1999. Trophin, testin and bystin a complex mediating unique attachment between trophblastin and endometrial epithelial cells at their receptive opical cell membranes. Semin. Reprod. Endocrinol. **17:** 299–334.
43. SUZUKI, N., J. ZARA, T. SATO, et al. 1998. A cytoplasmia protein, bystin, interacts with trophinin, testin and cytokeratin and may be involved in trophinin-mediated cell and endometrial epithelial cells. PNAS USA **95:** 5027–5032.
44. ANDERSON, D.J., A.F. ABBOTT & R.M. JACK. 1993. The role of complement component C3b and its receptors in sperm–oocyte interaction. Proc. Natl. Acad. Sci. USA **90:** 10051–10055.
45. GUDEL, L., G. DENIZ, D. RUKAVINA, et al. 1996. Expression of functional molecules by human CD3-decidual granular leukocyte clones. Immunology **87:** 609–615,
46. ISAACSON, K.B., C. COUTIFARIS, C.R. GARCIA, et al. 1989. Production and secretion of complement component 3 by endometriotic tissue. J. Clin. Endocrinol. Metab. **69:** 1003–1009.

47. BISCHOF, P., A. MEISSER & A. COMPANA. 2000. Mechanisms of endometrial control of trophoblast invasion. J. Reprod. Fertil. Suppl. **55:** 65–71.
48. ALEXANDER, J.P., J.R. SAMPLES & T.S. ACOTT. 1998. Growth factor and cytokine modulation of trabecular meshwork matrix metalloproteinase and TIMP expression. Curr. Eye Res. **17:** 276–285.
49. DAMSKY, C.H., M.I. FITZGERALD & S.J. FISHER. 1992. Distribution patterns of extracellar matrix components and adhesion receptors are intricately modulated during first trimester cytotrophoblast differentiation along the invasive pathway, in vivo. J. Clin. Invest. **89:** 210–222.
50. RISAU, W. 1997. Mechanism of angiogenesis. Nature **386:** 671–674.
51. NASU, K., Y. ZHOU, M.T. MCMASTER, *et al.* 2000. Upregulation of human cytotrophoblast invasion by hepatocyte growth factor. J. Reprod. Fertil. Suppl. **55:** 73–80.
52. HUNT, J.S. 2000. Cytokine networks in the human placenta. *In* Cytokines in Human Reproduction. J.A. Hill, Ed.: 203–220. Wiley-Liss. New York.
53. HILL, J.A. 1995. T-helper 1-type immunity to trophoblast: evidence for a new immunological mechanism for recurrent abortion in women. Hum. Reprod. **10:** 114–120.
54. YANUSHPOLSKY, E.H., M. OZTURK, R.S. BERKOWITZ, *et al.* 1993. The effects of cytokines on human chorionic gonadotropin production by a trophoblast cell line. J. Reprod. Immunol. **25:** 235–247.
55. FEINBERG, B.B., D.J. ANDERSON, M.A. STELLAR, *et al.* 1994. Cytokine regulation of trophoblast steroidogenesis. J. Clin. Endocrinol. Metab. **78:** 586–591.
56. MA, L., M. YAO & R.I. MAAS. 1999. Genetic control of uterine receptivity during implantation. Sem. Reprod. Endocrinol. **17:** 205–206.
57. ROBB, L., R. LI, L. HARTLEY, *et al.* 1998. Infertility in female mice lacking the receptor for interleukin II is due to a defective uterine response to implantation. Nature Med. **4:** 303–308.

Fertility and Maternal Age

Strategies to Improve Pregnancy Outcome

LEWIS KREY, HUI LIU, JOHN ZHANG, AND JAMIE GRIFO

Program for In Vitro Fertilization, Reproductive Surgery, and Infertility,
Department of Obstetrics and Gynecology, New York University School of Medicine,
New York, New York 10016, USA

ABSTRACT: In humans, the live birth rate drops precipitously with increasing maternal age, and this decline is associated with increases in the incidence of oocyte and embryo aneuploidy. Preimplantation aneuploidy screening has improved pregnancy outcome by significantly lowering the miscarriage rate. Nevertheless, aneuploidy screening only identifies the affected embryos; it does not attempt to correct the underlying biologic problem. Anomalies in chromosome segregation can result from a dysfunctional first or second meiotic division in the egg or develop after fertilization during the first few mitoses of early embryonic development. In both instances, ooplasmic anomalies may account for the nuclear problem. Low cell levels of cytoplasmic proteins (e.g., cytoskeletal elements, enzymes, energy stores, cell cycle regulatory proteins) may lead to a dysfunctional division of chromosomes during egg maturation or following fertilization. Ooplasmic injection is a micromanipulation technique that has produced pregnancies in patients with a history of poor-quality, fragmented embryos. Germinal vesicle transfer is a research procedure used to investigate the ooplasmic–nuclear interplay regulating cell cycle, maturation, and fertilization. Both these techniques may prove to be effective in improving the quality of eggs from patients of advanced maternal age.

KEYWORDS: advanced maternal age; oocyte aneuploidy; embryo aneuploidy; preimplantation aneuploidy screening; ooplasmic injection; germinal vesicle transfer

INTRODUCTION AND BACKGROUND

In humans, the live birth rate drops precipitously with increasing maternal age (especially after 35 years of age), and this decline is accompanied by increases in the incidences of miscarriage and fetal and neonatal aneuploidy.[1] In 1998 the live birth rate associated with cycles utilizing assisted reproductive technology (ART) and fresh nondonor eggs or embryos for women ages 38–40 years of age fell by 50% when compared to those of women <35 years of age; moreover, the birth rate for women >40 years of age declined further by another 50% (see TABLE 1).[2]

Address for correspondence: Lewis Krey, Ph.D., Program for In Vitro Fertilization, Reproductive Surgery, and Infertility, NYU School of Medicine, 660 First Avenue, New York, NY 10016. Voice: 263-6418; fax: 263-0059.
    KREYIVF@yahoo.com

TABLE 1. Live birth rates for 1998 ART cycles using fresh, nondonor eggs or embryos

	Percentage of live births per ART cycle	
Age	No. prior live births	One or more previous live births
<35 years	31.0%	36.9%
35–37 years	25.1%	29.0%
38–40 years	17.0%	20.2%
>40 years	7.9%	9.0%

SOURCE: Data taken from Figure 16 of the 1998 Assisted Reproductive Technology Success Rates—National Summary and Fertility Clinic Reports.[1]

Examination of data from *in vitro* fertilization (IVF) cycles conducted at the Program for IVF, Reproductive Surgery, and Infertility at NYU School of Medicine reveals similar age-related trends. Looking at more than 3400 IVF cycles started between 1996 and 1999, there is clearly a progressive decline in the clinical pregnancy rate per cycle that first appears at 38 years of age (FIG. 1A). Similar declines were observed when the data was expressed as "per treatment start" or "per oocyte retrieval," indicating that poor responses to ovarian stimulation protocols were not a major issue. This fact is reinforced by looking at the average numbers of eggs retrieved and embryos transferred during these same IVF cycles (FIG. 1B). Although there was a very slight decline in egg number at retrieval, more than a sufficient number of eggs were retrieved, on average, to ensure the transfer of multiple embryos to the uterus. In fact, the mean number of embryos transferred per cycle actually increased with maternal age. Although there are a finite number of eggs in the human ovary and the number of eggs available for release drops progressively with age,[3] these data suggest that this phenomenon is not the primary cause of the decline in live birth rate.

If the fall in live birth rate is not related to the number of available eggs, then it must be the result of declining egg or embryo quality. Such a conclusion is confirmed by the data presented in FIGURE 1C, which shows the influence of maternal age on the implantation rate per transferred embryo. The decline in the ability of each embryo to implant is even more pronounced than that seen for the clinical pregnancy rate; moreover, it begins earlier—at a maternal age of 36 years. That this pattern reflects an embryo problem is indicated when one also examines the clinical pregnancy and implantation rates of oocyte donation cycles for women of 40+ years of age that are presented in the legends to FIGURES 1A and 1C. In these cycles the transferred embryos arose from oocytes donated by women 35 years of age or younger. Significantly, the clinical pregnancy and embryo implantation rates for these cycles matched those for <35-year-old women undergoing IVF. Such data indicate that maternal age–related uterine and male factor problems do not play a significant role.

The decline in embryo quality with increasing maternal age is most likely the result of an increase in the frequency of aneuploidy, which has been described to occur in the oocytes and embryos of older women.[4–11] Most embryonic aneuploidies are

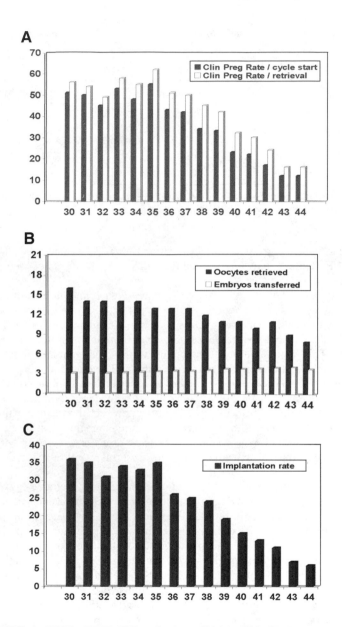

FIGURE 1. PIVF—NYU: IVF cycles from 1996 to 1999. (A) Clinical pregnancy rate per IVF cycle start (*open bar*) or per egg retrieval (*filled bar*) expressed as a function of maternal age at egg retrieval. Clinical pregnancy is defined as the presence of a gestational sac and fetal heartbeat activity. Data from 2500 IVF cycles were collected from 1996 through 1999 at the Program for IVF, Reproductive Surgery and Infertility at NYU School of Medicine. During these years the clinical pregnancy rates for oocyte donation cycles using eggs from young donors (<32 years of age) were 55% and 49% for recipients younger or older than 40 years of age, respectively. (B) Mean number of eggs collected and the mean number

thought to arise from a dysfunctional first meiotic division in the egg; this results in an inappropriate distribution of chromosomes between the egg and the first polar body.[7,10–12] Normally, this division is triggered by the periovulatory luteinizing hormone (LH) surge[13]; in an IVF cycle, it is triggered by a human chorionic gonadotropin (hCG) injection administered 36 hours before egg retrieval. Since an oocyte has few if any LH receptors, the LH surge or hCG injection appears to initiate meiosis indirectly by interacting with granulosa cells in the cumulus, cells that have LH receptors and that send projections through the zona pellucida to form gap junctions with the oolemma.[14,15] Before chromosome separation, ooplasmic factors initiate germinal vesicle membrane breakdown and chromosome condensation[13]; at the same time, construction of a meiotic spindle begins. The spindle can be visualized by tubulin immunocytochemistry, and structurally abnormal spindles have been reported to occur at an increased frequency in the eggs of older women.[16,17] These spindle irregularities are thought to be a primary cause of errors in chromosome segregation, although aberrations in other, as yet undefined, mechanisms in this hormonally activated process may also lead to a dysfunctional separation of chromosomes. Recent studies suggest that aneuploidy may also arise from a dysfunctional chromatid separation during the second meiotic division; in some eggs, separation errors during meiosis II may actually correct errors made during meiosis I.[9] In any event, any error in chromosome separation made in the egg is routinely passed on to the embryo, resulting in trisomic or monosomic embryos. Such a genetic heritage is not always indicated by fragmentation, slow development, or cell death during early embryonic life. Embryos from older women that are acceptable for elective transfer nonetheless show a fivefold increase in the incidence of aneuploidy.[8] Almost every aneuploidy compromises viability at some stage of embryonic or fetal development, resulting in a poor pattern of early embryonic development, a failure to progress to blastocyst, an inability to implant, or an early fetal loss.

In many embryos a postfertilization aneuploidy may arise during the first few mitoses of early embryonic development. Early cleavage stage embryos that contain multinucleated blastomeres have been described, as have embryos composed of a mosaic of blastomeres containing different but paired aneuploidies.[4,18–20] Although the impact of postfertilization aneuploidy on later embryo viability is not known, it may signal an early stage of cell death. Such a conclusion is suggested by the observation that the mosaic aneuploidies occur very frequently in embryos with extensive fragmentation, another sequela of cell death. In such affected embryos, low levels of cytoplasmic factors (e.g., mRNAs; enzymes; structural proteins such as tubulin-organizing centers, energy stores, and the mitochondria that generate them; and cell cycle–regulating proteins including putative checkpoint proteins in the MAD and BUB families[21–24]) may be the cause of inappropriate chromosome separation or failure for cytokinesis; they may also have an impact on embryo development, eventuating in a slow division rate or cell death and fragmentation.

---

of embryos transferred to the uterus in the IVF cycles depicted in (A). Transfers for oocyte donation cycles during this time were routinely two or three embryos. (**C**) Implantation rate (number of gestational sacs/number of embryos transferred) for the IVF cycles depicted in (A). The implantation rates for oocyte donation cycles were 34% and 30% for recipients younger and older than 40 years of age, respectively.

An increase in the incidence of aneuploidy not only decreases the pregnancy rate but also can have an adverse impact on pregnancy outcome. Spontaneous pregnancy losses due to fetal death during the first trimester are often the result of a nonviable aneuploidy. Similarly, elective termination of a pregnancy is invariably the response to the detection of aneuploidy by amniocentesis or chorionic villus sampling.

Other aspects of poor egg quality may also contribute to arrested embryo division, poor-quality embryos, or to embryos that fail to implant. Early embryonic development to at least the four-cell stage must also be directed by ooplasmic constituents, since the embryonic genome does not turn on immediately after fertilization.[13] Thus, abnormalities in level and/or distribution of metabolic stores, structural proteins, mitochondria, or transcription factors and other regulatory proteins may lead to aneuploidy as described above or to other cellular conditions that eventuate in a poor prognosis for the embryo. Hopefully, future research studies will focus on cytoplasmic analyses that characterize normal ooplasmic maturation in biochemical, morphologic, and molecular terms.

LABORATORY PROCEDURES TO IMPROVE PREGNANCY RATE AND PREGNANCY OUTCOME

Aneuploidies are present not only in poor-quality, fragmented embryos, but also in embryos of sufficient quality for elective transfer, which can show as much as a fivefold increase in chromosomal abnormalities when they arise from the eggs of older women.[8] During the past five years, preimplantation genetic diagnosis (PGD) of embryos for aneuploidy has become a popular procedure. According to the ESHRE PGD Consortium,[25] approximately 34% of all PGD cases in 1997–1998 were performed for aneuploidy screening. One can only expect this number to rise dramatically as more and more IVF programs are offering this screen. In this procedure one or two blastomeres are removed, irrespective of cell cycle stage, from a multicelled embryo before transfer and lysed. The nucleus is isolated and fixed; the numbers of specific chromosomes are determined by fluorescence *in situ* hybridization with nucleotide probes that bind to repeat DNA sequences on these chromosomes.[18] Currently, only a limited number of chromosomes are monitored in these PGD procedures. However, technologic advances in preimplantation genetic diagnosis should soon make it possible to count all chromosomes. In fact, the General Program Prize Paper at the Annual Meeting of the American Society for Reproductive Medicine in 2000 describes a novel technique based on whole-genome amplification and comparative genomic hybridization that "allows the copy number of every chromosome to be assessed in the majority of cells from a preimplantation embryo."[26]

PGD screening for aneuploidy has been reported to improve pregnancy outcome; significant decreases were noted in the spontaneous miscarriage rate and increases in live birth rate for transferred embryos.[27,28] Nevertheless, the overall pregnancy rate was not increased; many more cycles had no embryos to transfer because all available embryos for transfer were affected. Thus, although PGD clearly identifies the embryonic consequences of aneuploidy, it offers little hope for correcting the underlying biologic causes. More aggressive embryology procedures that focus on the egg appear to be necessary. Two such procedures have been described recently: cytoplasmic injection and germinal vesicle (GV) transfer.

Cytoplasmic injection is a micromanipulation procedure in which a small amount of ooplasm is withdrawn from a donor oocyte and injected into the patient's egg, often in conjunction with intracytoplasmic sperm injection. Presumably, this procedure is performed in an effort to boost the levels of key cell constituents in the patient's egg. A maximum of 15% of the cell volume is injected. Although not tested in the eggs of older women, this technique has been reported by several investigators to improve the pregnancy rates of patients with a history of fragmentation and poor embryo quality.[29–31] Because similar characteristics are often observed in the embryos of women of advanced maternal age, attempts to use this procedure for such patients might prove advantageous. Although cytoplasmic injection appears to result in the birth of healthy children, cells of these offspring can carry the mitochondrial DNA forms present in both the donor and recipient oocytes and the long-term biologic significance of this heteroplasmy is unknown.[32]

In nuclear transfer, the nucleus from one oocyte is transferred to another enucleated oocyte using micromanipulation and electrofusion techniques. Thus, virtually the entire cytoplasm is changed. Although we first utilized this procedure to exchange germinal vesicles (GV) between immature oocytes, we have subsequently expanded our range, performing metaphase II spindle and pronucleus transfer in different experiments.[33–37] Considering that nucleus transfer accomplishes a virtually complete exchange of ooplasm, the "reconstructed" oocytes are appropriate "cell models" to study the nuclear–cytoplasmic interrelationships underlying meiosis.

Over the past few years, we have focused our studies on mice. Initially, we reported that a transferred GV matured normally to metaphase II *in vitro* only when placed into an enucleated oocyte at the comparable stage of immaturity; such oocytes extruded a polar body and contained the appropriate diploid number of chromosomes.[33] Transfer of the GVs of cryopreserved oocytes have provided similar results.[36] Subsequent studies employed a sequential A23187-cyclohexamide treatment *in vitro* to stimulate mature oocytes to complete the second meiotic division normally and form a normal haploid pronucleus (PN); the reconstructed oocytes responded in similar fashion.[34] When exchanged with the female pronucleus from an *in vivo* fertilized zygote in a second transfer procedure, these PNs, even those that matured from a nucleus transferred at the GV stage, supported embryonic development to the blastocyst stage.[34] Further studies indicate that these embryos even support embryonic development to term, resulting in live births (Liu *et al.*, unpublished observations). We have also transferred the spindle at metaphase 2 between oocytes to examine for key events before and during an artificially induced second meiotic division.[35] This study indicates that the potential of an oocyte to support embryonic development to term depends on its maturation history, for example, site of maturation (*in vivo* vs. *in vitro*) and presence of cumulus cells at maturation.

In humans, oocytes "reconstructed" by GV transfer mature *in vitro* through the first stage of meiosis and can be fertilized by intracytoplasmic sperm injection. Embryo development following this union has been observed to progress at least to the 7- to 8-cell stage. That GV transfer may develop into a procedure to treat maternal age-related aneuploidy is suggested by the observations that, when a GV from an old patient's egg was transferred and matured in the ooplasm of a young patient, the metaphase II complement of chromosomes was normal in 80% of these "reconstructed" oocytes.[37] This data is still limited, however, and more extensive confirmatory studies are necessary before we can seriously consider GV transfer as a clinical procedure. Nonetheless, GV transfer must be cultivated, because it generates valuable research models that can be studied to characterize the cytoplasmic–nuclear interplay regulating cell cycle, maturation, and the postfertilization embryonic developmental potential of oocytes. With this information in hand, we may be able to design more precise and effective procedures to detect and correct the ooplasm-based problems that currently compromise fertility in women of advancing maternal age.

REFERENCES

1. HASSOLD, T. & D. CHIU. 1985. Maternal age-specific rates of numerical chromosome abnormalities with special reference to trisomy. Hum. Genet. **70:** 11–17.
2. CENTERS FOR DISEASE CONTROL AND PREVENTION. 2000. 1998 Assisted Reproductive Technology Success Rates. US Department of Health and Human Services. Atlanta, GA.
3. FADDY, M.J. & R.G. GOSDEN. 1995. A mathematical model of follicle dynamics in the human ovary. Hum. Reprod. **10:** 770–775.
4. MUNNE, S., *et al.* 1995. Embryo morphology, developmental rates and maternal age are correlated with chromosomal abnormalities. Fertil. Steril. **64:** 382–391.
5. VERLINSKY, Y. & A. KULIEV. 1996. A preimplantation diagnosis of common aneuploidies in fertile couples of advanced maternal age. Hum. Reprod. **11:** 2076–2077.
6. BENAVIDA, C.A., *et al.* 1996. Aneuploidy 16 in human embryos increases significantly with maternal age. Fertil. Steril. **66:** 248–255.
7. DAILEY, T., *et al.* 1996. Association between nondisjunction and maternal age in meiosis-II human oocytes. Am. J. Hum. Genet. **59:** 176–184.
8. PELLICER, A., *et al.* 1999. In vitro fertilization plus preimplantation genetic diagnosis in patients with recurrent miscarriage: an analysis of chromosome abnormalities in human preimplantation embryos. Fertil. Steril. **71:** 1033–1039.
9. VERLINSKY, Y., *et al.* 2000. High frequency of meiosis II aneuploidies in IVF patients of advanced maternal age (abstract). Fertil. Steril. **74(3s):** S33.
10. HASSOLD, T. & S. SHERMAN. 2000. Down syndrome: genetic recombination and the origin of the extra chromosome 21. Clin. Genet. **57:** 95–100.
11. MAY, K.M., *et al.* 1990. The parental origin of the extra X chromosome in 47, XXX females. Am. J. Hum. Genet. **46:** 754–761.
12. ANGELL, R., *et al.* 1994. First meiotic division abnormalities in human oocytes: mechanism of trisomy formation. Cytogenet. Cell. Genet. **65:** 194–202.
13. WASSARMAN, P.M. 1988. The mammalian ovum. *In* The Physiology of Reproduction. E. Knobil & J.D. Neill, Eds.: 69–102. Raven Press. New York.
14. BEERS, W.H. & N. DEKEL. 1981. Intracellular communication and the control of oocyte maturation. *In* Dynamics of Ovarian Function. N.B. Schwatz & M. Hunzicker-Dunn, Eds.: 95–108. Raven Press. New York.
15. LAWRENCE, T.S., *et al.* 1980. Binding of human chorionic gonadotropin by rat cumuli oophori and granulosa cells: a comparative study. Endocrinology **106:** 114–1122.
16. BATTAGLIA, D.E., *et al.* 1996. Influence of maternal age on meiotic spindle in oocytes from naturally cycling women. Hum. Reprod. **11:** 2217–2222.
17. PLACHOT, M. & N. CROZET. 1992. Fertilization abnormalities in human in vitro fertilization. Hum. Reprod. **7:** 89–94.
18. MUNNE, S. & U. WEIER,. 1996. Simultaneous enumeration of chromsomes 13,18,21,X and Y in interphase cells for preimplantation genetic diagnosis of aneuploidy. Cytogenet. Cell. Genet. **75:** 263–270.
19. DELHANTY, J.D.A., *et al.* 1997. Multicolour FISH detects frequent chromosomal mosaicism and chaotic division in normal preimplantation embryos from fertile patients. Hum. Genet. **99:** 755–760.
20. MUNNE, S., *et al.* Assessment of numeric abnormalities of X,Y, 18 and 16 chromosomes in preimplantation human embryos before transfer. Am. J. Obstet. Gynecol. **172:** 1191–1201.

21. KEEFE, D., *et al.* 1995. Mitochondrial deoxyribonucleic acid deletions in oocytes and reproductive aging in women. Fertil. Steril. **64:** 577–583.
22. VANBLERKOM, J., *et al.* 1998. Mitochondrial transfer between oocytes: potential applications of mitochondrial donation and the issue of heteroplasmy. Hum. Reprod. **13:** 2857–2868.
23. HANSIS, C., *et al.* 2001. Analysis of Oct-4 expression and ploidy in individual human blastomeres. Mol. Hum. Reprod. **7:** 155–161.
24. STEUERWALD, N., *et al.* 2001. Association between spindle assembly checkpoint expression and maternal age in human oocytes. Mol. Hum. Reprod. **7:** 49–55.
25. ESHRE PGD CONSORTIUM STEERING COMMITTEE. 1999. ESHRE Preimplantation Genetic Diagnosis (PGD) Consortium: preliminary assessment of data from January 1997 to September 1998. Hum. Reprod. **14:** 3138–3148.
26. WELLS, D. & J.D.A. DELHANTY. 2000. A novel methodology allows detection of every chromosome in single blastomeres from human preimplantation embryos and reveals aneuploidy, mosaicism and uniformly normal embryos (abstract). Fertil. Steril. **74(3s):** S1.
27. GIANAROLI, L., *et al.* 1999. Preimplantation diagnosis for aneuploidies in patients undergoing in vitro fertilization with a poor prognosis: identification of the categories for which it should be proposed. Fertil. Steril. **72:** 837–844.
28. MUNNE, S., *et al.* 1999. Positive outcome after preimplantation diagnosis of aneuploidy in human embryos. Hum. Reprod. **14:** 2191–2198.
29. COHEN, J., *et al.* 1997. Birth of infant after transfer of anucleate donor oocyte cytoplasm into recipient eggs. Lancet **350:** 186–187.
30. LAZENDORF, S., *et al.* 1999. Pregnancy following transfer of ooplasm from cryopreserved-thawed donor oocytes into recipient oocytes. Fertil. Steril. **71:** 575–577.
31. HUANG, C.C., *et al.* 1999. Birth after injection of sperm and the cytoplasm of tripronucleate zygotes into metaphase II oocytes in patients with repeated implantation failure after assisted fertilization procedures. Fertil. Steril. **71:** 702–706.
32. BRENNER, C.A., *et al.* 2000. Mitochondrial DNA heteroplasmy after human ooplasmic transplantation. Fertil. Steril. **74:** 573–578.
33. LIU, H., *et al.* 1999. Reconstruction of mouse oocytes by germinal vesicle transfer: maturity of host oocyte cytoplasm determines meiosis. Hum. Reprod. **14:** 2357–2361.
34. LIU, H., *et al.* 2000. In-vitro development of mouse zygotes following reconstruction by sequential transfer of germinal vesicles and haploid pronuclei. Hum. Reprod. **15:** 1997–2002.
35. LIU, H., *et al.* 2000. Evaluating the competency of the nucleus and ooplasm of in vitro matured, artificially activated oocytes. Fertil. Steril. **74(3s):** S65.
36. COMIGLIO, F., *et al.* 2000. Germinal vesicle transfer between fresh and cryopreserved immature mouse oocytes (Abstr.). Fertil. Steril. **74(3s):** S47.
37. ZHANG, J., *et al.*, 1999. In vitro maturation of human preovulatory oocytes reconstructed by germinal vesicle transfer. Fertil. Steril. **71:** 726–731.

Inhibin, Activin, and Follistatin in Human Fetal Pituitary and Gonadal Physiology

ZEEV BLUMENFELD AND MARINA RITTER

Reproductive Endocrinology, Department of Obstetrics and Gynecology, Rambam Medical Center and the B. Rappaport Faculty of Medicine, Technion, Israel Institute of Technology, Haifa, 31096, Israel

ABSTRACT: *Background*: Activin has been previously demonstrated to directly stimulate the synthesis of gonadotropin-releasing hormone (GnRH) receptors and to increase follicle-stimulating hormone (FSH) secretion in nonhuman pituitary cell cultures (PCCs). Currently, knowledge of the physiological role of these peptides in primates is still far from complete. Moreover, several results in macaque monkeys failed to support an unequivocal role for inhibin in FSH suppression. Whereas the bioactivity of inhibin and activin has been demonstrated in rat PCCs, no data exist on human pituitary response to these peptides either *in vivo* or *in vitro*. *Methods*: We studied the secretion of FSH and luteinizing hormone (LH) by dispersed human fetal pituitary cells from midtrimester abortions in response to recombinant human (rh-) activin-A, inhibin-A, and other secretagogues. After mechanical and enzymatic dispersion, the human fetal pituitary cells were cultured on an extracellular matrixlike-material-coated 24-well plate. After 3 days' incubation in serum-containing medium, the PCCs were washed and preincubated for 90 min in serum-free medium and incubated with activin-A, inhibin-A, TGF-β, follistatin, sex steroids, and GnRH, in quadruplicate. *Results*: Activin-A was a potent secretagogue for FSH secretion. GnRH (20 ng/ml) was more potent than rh-activin-A for LH secretion. Nevertheless, a significant increase in LH secretion into the medium was brought about by rh-activin-A. Inhibin decreased FSH and LH secretion, but the LH response to inhibin was less prominent than that of FSH. GnRH opposed the inhibitory effect of inhibin on LH secretion. In dynamic, short-term, repetitive exposure of fetal pituitary fragments to rh-activin-A (superfusion), we could not receive a similar increase in LH and FSH as in static incubations, as opposed to a short GnRH exposure. In addition to their endocrine, paracrine, and autocrine effects, and in addition to their role as possible markers, the TGF-β superfamily members may affect embryogenesis and possibly immunomodulation of the embryo and fetus. The role of activin and inhibin as intragonadal regulators is hypothesized. The pro-αC inhibin precursor may act as an FSH receptor antagonist. *Conclusions*: Human fetal PCCs express the previously reported physiologic responses to activin and inhibin generated in nonhuman experiments on gonadotropin secretion *in vitro* and may serve as a physiologic model for studying human gonadotrope responses to the TGF-β family of peptides.

KEYWORDS: inhibin; activin; follistatin; human fetal pituitary

Address for correspondence: Zeev Blumenfeld, Reproductive Endocrinology, Department of Obstetrics and Gynecology, Rambam Medical Center, The B. Rappaport Faculty of Medicine, Technion—Israel Institute of Technology, Haifa, 31096, Israel. Voice: 972-4-8542577; fax: 972-4-8542612.

bzeev@technix.technion.ac.il

INTRODUCTION

The history of inhibin, activin, and follistatin peptides is intermingled with the emergence of endocrinology as a specific scientific discipline and the concept that hormones produced in regulating organs can have an impact on distal target tissues.[1]

Regulation of gonadotropin secretion during the menstrual cycle involves a complex interplay between stimulation by gonadotropin-releasing hormone (GnRH) and feedback regulation by gonadal sex steroids (estradiol, progesterone) and peptides (inhibin) as well as pituitary factors (activin, follistatin). Although it was initially believed that two different hypothalamic factors regulated the secretion of luteinizing hormone (LH) and follicle-stimulating hormone (FSH), it is now generally accepted that GnRH is the stimulating factor for both gonadotropins and that any divergence in their secretion can be explained by differential sensitivity to the gonadal steroid milieu, alterations in GnRH pulse frequency, or the secretion of inhibin, activin, and/or follistatin.[2]

The existence of a nonsteroidal regulator of FSH secretion was first predicted almost 70 years ago, following the observation that a water-soluble extract of bovine testis prevented the development of so-called castration cells in the anterior pituitary gland.[3] Indeed, it was McCullagh who coined the name "inhibin" for the as-yet unidentified hormone. After this, there was little further progress until the 1970s when support for the inhibin hypothesis was offered by numerous studies showing that FSH could be selectively suppressed by various testicular fluids and extracts.[4-7] However, it was the novel observation that, in addition to the testis, follicular fluid containing large amounts of inhibinlike activity[8] facilitated more rapid progress. Bovine and porcine follicular fluids were readily available in large volumes,[9] and in 1985 inhibin was isolated and partially characterized, initially from a bovine source[10] and subsequently from porcine follicular fluid.[11] During the numerous extraction and purification steps developed to isolate inhibin, it became clear that another protein, similar to inhibin, existed. The protein was isolated and characterized the following year from porcine follicular fluid.[12] But, whereas inhibin suppressed FSH secretion, the new protein was found to stimulate it, and so was termed "activin." It soon became apparent that messenger ribonucleic acid (mRNA) for the inhibin and activin subunits was expressed in a variety of nongonadal sites,[13] suggesting that, in addition to regulating FSH secretion, these proteins possessed other functions.

Inhibins and activins are glycoproteins that belong to the transforming growth factor-β (TGF-β) superfamily. Inhibins are heterodimers consisting of disulfide-linked α (molecular mass, 18 kDa) and β (molecular mass, 14 kDa) subunits: inhibin A (α-β_A) and inhibin B (α-β_B) show considerable homology of amino acid sequence: The alpha subunits in the two different forms of inhibin are identical, whereas there is 70% homology between the β_A and β_B subunit amino acid sequences, and there is 30% homology between the sequences for the α and β subunits. Only the dimeric forms of inhibin are bioactive, although the α subunits circulate in excess as biologically inert monomers.[1,7] The activins are dimers of β subunits and act as functional antagonists of inhibin to increase FSH release by the pituitary. Other members of this family include Müllerian inhibiting substance, bone morphogenic proteins, and the amphibian protein VG1, which plays an important role during embryogenesis.[14,15]

Follistatin shows inhibin-like activities on FSH secretion *in vitro,* and activins stimulate the secretion of FSH. These proteins have been purified from the follicular fluid of various species, and their α, β_A, and β_B subunits' messenger RNA (mRNA) is expressed in the follicular granulosa cells of several species, including human, as well as in other tissues.[1,7,14–18] Although ligands that interact with the activin receptor show promise for the therapeutic regulation of the reproductive, hematopoietic, and central nervous systems, such applications have not yet been developed.[1,19–23]

Numerous publications and outstanding reviews have been published in the last decade on various aspects of activin and inhibin, including reception and action, binding proteins, malignancy, pregnancy and parturition, ovarian physiology, and possible markers in both female and male reproductive pathophysiology. It is beyond the scope of this manuscript to summarize the published data on all of these domains, each of them being an enormous chapter in itself. Instead, we will focus on our studies of inhibin/activin action in the human fetal pituitary and the intragonadal modulation of folliculogenesis. The ability of activin, inhibin, and follistatin to regulate gonadotropin biosynthesis and secretion has been established in a wide variety of *in vitro* and *in vivo* nonhuman experimental models.[24]

Injection of recombinant human (rh) inhibin into immature or ovariectomized animals has been shown to selectively suppress FSH-β mRNA and serum FSH levels, whereas rh-activin increased FSH-β gene expression. Conversely, infusion with antiserum against the inhibin α-subunit increased FSH secretion in rat and monkey.[24–26] Similar results have been detected with the use of *in vitro* systems in animal models. Treatment of static pituitary cell cultures with purified porcine inhibin or follistatin significantly decreases FSH β-subunit mRNA levels with parallel decreases in FSH secretion.[27]

In contrast, rh-activin stimulated FSH-β gene expression in rat primary pituitary cultures.[27] Weiss *et al.*[28] have shown, in a rat cell superfusion system, that activin increased and inhibin decreased FSH-β mRNA levels either alone or in combination with pulsatile GnRH. This activin effect was blunted by cotreatment with inhibin, consistent with a possible competition of activin and inhibin for identical receptors.[1,24,28]

Although a direct effect of activin and inhibin on gonadotropin secretion was previously reported, they were in nonhuman models.[1,2,19,20,29] Moreover, several results in macaque monkeys failed to support an unequivocal role for inhibin in suppression of FSH secretion.[21] Therefore, we attempted to explore the response of human fetal pituitary cells to rh-inhibin and rh-activin-A *in vitro.*

It has been demonstrated by us and others[30,31] that dispersed human fetal pituitary cells from between 14 and 25 weeks' gestation can accurately represent the endocrine activity of the adult human pituitary and may serve as an appropriate means to study the hypophysiotropic and neuroregulatory response of the human pituitary to various hypothalamic releasing factors (such as CRH, GH-RH) and other secretagogues.[30–33]

MATERIALS AND METHODS

Human fetal pituitaries from abortions that occurred between 15 and 22 weeks of gestation were removed by fetal craniotomy within 3 hours of fetal expulsion after pregnancy termination using intraamniotic insertion of prostaglandin F2α (PGF2α).

The experimental protocol was approved by the institutional and ministry of health committee for human experimentation (Helsinki II declaration). The time period from intraamniotic prostaglandin insertion until fetal expulsion ranged between 10 hours and 3 days. Each fetal pituitary was minced in M199 medium, and the fragments were transfered to a 15-ml conical tube and centrifuged at 300 × g for 1 minute, as previously described.[30] The buffer medium was aspirated, and 5 ml M199 containing 0.5% collagenase and 50 µg deoxyribonuclease (DNAase) were added. This was incubated for 1 hr at 37°C with agitation in a Dubnoff metabolic shaker, after which an additional 50 µg DNAase was added, and the tissue was mechanically dispersed in 5 ml M199 by trituration with a 5-ml pipette. Any remaining fibrous tissue fragments were allowed to settle and were then removed. The cell suspension was centrifuged at 150 × g for 5 min, and the cell pellet resuspended in M199 containing 10% fetal bovine serum (FBS), gentamycin 50 mg/ml, and 2 mM glutamine. Cells were plated at a density of 60–80 × 10^4 cells per well on an extracellular matrix–coated 24-well plate (Primaria, Falcon). After 3–4 days in culture, the cells were washed and preincubated with serum-free medium containing 0.1% BSA. After a 90-min preincubation, the cells were incubated with recombinant human (rh) activin-A, inhibin, transforming growth factor-β (TGF-β), and GnRH in quadruplicate wells. Experiments were performed in quadruplicate and repeated at least three times.

Recombinant human (rh) inhibin-A, activin-A, and follistatin were generously supplied by Dr. Teresa K. Woodruff (from Northwestern University, Evanston, IL) and later by the National Hormone and Pituitary Program (NIH NIDDK). Gonadotropin-releasing hormone (GnRH) was purchased from Serono (Relisorm L 100, Laboratoires Serono S.A., CH-1170 Aubonne, Switzerland), 17-β-estradiol (E_2), progesterone (P_4), testosterone (T), and TGF-β were purchased from Sigma (Sigma-Aldrich, Rehovot, Israel).

RESULTS AND DISCUSSION

After a 24-hr exposure to activin, responses in modulating gonadotropin secretion were observed. Mean ± SE ($n = 4$) FSH concentration increased significantly after incubation of dispersed human fetal pituitary cells (FIG. 1). The EC_{50} of rh activin-A for FSH secretion was around 10 ng/ml. Activin-A was a more potent secretagogue for FSH secretion than GnRH. However, GnRH at a concentration of 20 ng/ml was a more potent secretagogue than activin-A for LH secretion (TABLE 1). A significant increase in LH secretion into the medium was brought about by activin-A, at concentrations of 10 to 500 ng/ml.

Inhibin brought about a decrease in FSH and LH secretion into the medium by second-trimester human fetal pituitary cells (FIG. 2), an effect opposed by GnRH at levels of 20 ng/ml (TABLE 1). There was no significant difference in the qualitative results of gonadotropin secretion after either a 24- or 48-hr incubation.

Incubation of human fetal pituitary cells, at different gestational ages, with 17β-estradiol (1 ng/ml), progesterone (50 ng/ml), or testosterone (1 ng/ml) did not change either the basal gonadotropin secretion into the medium or the concentration after activin or inhibin coincubation (TABLE 1). However, pharmacologic levels of

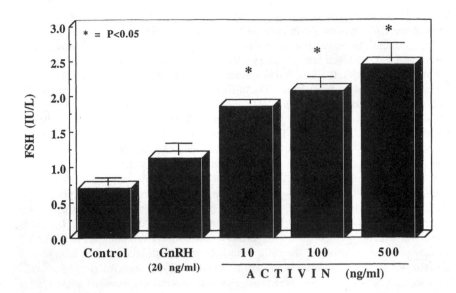

FIGURE 1. Increase in FSH secretion into the medium by 23-wk dispersed human fetal pituitary cells in response to activin and GnRH (mean ± SEM of quadruplicate wells).

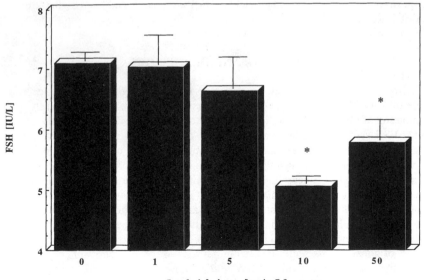

FIGURE 2. Decrease of FSH secretion by 18-wk dispersed human fetal pituitary cells in response to recombinant human inhibin-A (mean ± SEM, $n = 4$).

TABLE 1. Semiquantitative effects of various hypophysiotropic factors on gonadotropin secretion by second-trimester human fetal pituitary cells *in vitro*

	FSH	LH
Activin	↑↑↑	↑↑
Inhibin	↓↓↓	↓↓
GnRH	↑↑	↑↑↑
Activin + inhibin	−	−
Inhibin + GnRH	−	−/↑
Estradiol	−	−
Progesterone	−	−
Testosterone	−	−

SYMBOLS: ↑, ↑↑, ↑↑↑, Mild, moderate, significant secretory effect, respectively. ↓, ↓↓, ↓↓↓ Mild, moderate, significant inhibitory effect, respectively. − No significant effect.

E_2 inhibited the secretory action of activin. Follistatin modestly decreased both basal and GnRH-induced gonadotropin secretion.

Short-term (15 min), repetitive exposure of pituitary fragments to increasing concentrations of activin (0.1 to 500 ng/ml) at one-hour intervals did not bring about a significant increase in gonadotropin secretion, whereas 15 min of exposure to GnRH (20 ng/ml) at the end of the 8-hour experiment brought about a significant increase in both FSH and LH (FIG. 3 A,B).

Exposure of human fetal pituitary cells to activin or inhibin may affect the cells morphologically, in addition to modulating the secretory ability of FSH and LH, as suggested by our preliminary data in which exposure to rh-activin increased the secretory granules and affected ephithelial morphology of culture cells compared to control cells exposed to medium alone without secretagogue.

Inhibin/Activin Physiology

Whereas the α subunit of inhibin has been detected in granulosa cells, Sertoli cells, pituitary gonadotrophs, testicular interstitial cells, and prostatic epithelial cells, the β subunits have been found in many types of organs and tissues in addition to their classic description in the reproductive organs.[34] The β_A subunit of inhibin/activin has been detected in fibroblasts, endothelial cells, hepatocytes, vascular smooth muscle cells, macrophages, cuboidal epithelium, keratinocytes, osteoclasts, bone marrow monocytes, prostatic epithelium, neurons, chondrocytes, osteoblasts, Leydig cells, Sertoli cells, and granulosa cells.[34] The β_B subunit was found in pituitary gonadotrophs, Sertoli and Leydig cells, testicular interstitial cells, granulosa cells, and also in keratinocytes.[34]

More recently two additional β subunits have been found in animals but not in humans, β_C and β_D.[34] The β_C subunit has been described in the liver, ovary, testes, and in primary spermatocytes.[34] It is unknown yet whether these newer forms of β subunit possess any substantial and meaningful difference in tissue specificity, binding to carrier/binding proteins (such as follistatin and β_2 macroglobulin), plasma clearance, and, most importantly, function and activity or whether they are irrelevant to biological function.[34]

In most tissues and target organs, the functions of activin and inhibin are antagonistic. Whereas activin increases basal and GnRH-stimulated FSH secretion, inhibin decreases both. On the contrary, inhibin increases GRF-stimulated GH secretion, and activin suppresses this effect.

In the gonad, inhibin increases the effect of LH on theca cells to secrete androgens, whereas activin opposes this effect. Activin stimulates aromatase action, whereas inhibin decreases it. In the placenta, activin increases hCG-induced progesterone secretion, whereas inhibin suppresses this effect. Even the effects on bone marrow are antagonistic; activin stimulates erythropoiesis, whereas inhibin decreases it.[1,19-23]

Activin has been described as a paracrine hormone,[35] autocrine hormone,[36] possible endocrine hormone, growth and differentiation factor,[37] and later on even as a cytokine.[38] Molecules such as activin that break classical definitions of activity can be classified broadly as *multicrine,* that is, of multiple modes of activity.

Inhibin secretion differs between human and lower species. In the rat, LH causes a rapid decrease in inhibin concentration in the serum and in its mRNA levels.[1] The rat corpus luteum does not express inhibin subunit mRNA, whereas the primate corpus luteum is the principal source of luteal inhibin-A, demonstrated by: in situ hybridization, immunohistochemistry, ovarian vein, immunoreactive measurements, and by the increase in FSH levels following surgical luteectomy or hormonal ablation induced by GnRH-antagonist.[1] Whereas bovine follicular fluid (FF) is a rich source of dimeric inhibin, human FF has less than 2% of the activity of bovine FF.[1]

Activin/Inhibin in Folliculogenesis and Reproduction

Activin-A may function as an autocrine or paracrine regulator of follicular function in the human and primate ovary.[39-41] Activin binding sites were found in rat granulosa cells at a density of about 4000 binding sites per cell. Activin may decrease progesterone secretion, both basal and hCG-stimulated, aromatase activity in granulosa cells, both basal and FSH-stimulated, and androgen synthesis; and it may inhibit P_{450} cytochrome 17_α activity and mRNA, thus decreasing the function of the 17-α-hydroxylase/17,20 lyase steroidogenetic enzymes, resulting in a dose–response inhibition of estradiol secretion (FIG. 4).[39-41]

Activin suppressed the fetal zone and increased the ACTH-induced shift in the cortisol/dehydroepiandrosterone sulfate ratio.[39] Activin has been found to promote Graafian follicle growth, apoptosis, and ovulation and to block meiosis at metaphase I in the adult rat.[1,42-44]

The paracrine effect of inhibin on folliculogenesis was evaluated by injecting rh-inhibin-A directly into mature rat ovaries.[44] The diameter of the ovarian follicles increased in the rh-inhibin-A-treated group of rats compared to controls, suggesting a direct or indirect effect in folliculogenesis.[44] Inhibin may regulate follicular maturation, particularly in immature follicles, by stimulating theca cell androgen production, through the mechanism of the "two cell–two gonadotropin" theory.[1,40-45] It has been speculated[45] that inhibin-B, being secreted by the recently recruited cohort of follicles in response to FSH, may possibly limit the duration of the FSH rise, thus

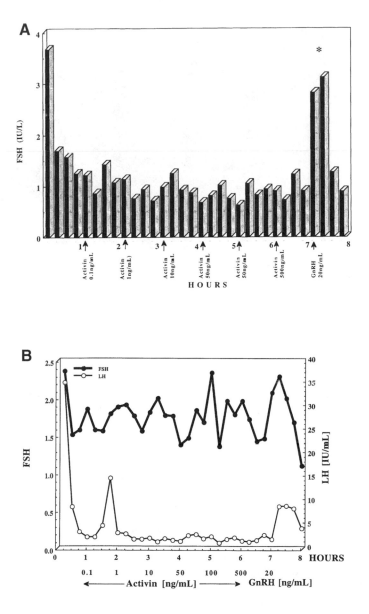

FIGURE 3. Short-term, repetitive exposure of 17-wk human fetal pituitary to increasing concentrations of hourly activin pulses (0.1 to 500 ng/ml) did not significantly affect gonadotropin secretion in perifusion-like experiments. At the end of the experiment, short-term (15-min) exposure to GnRH (20 ng/ml) brought about a significant increase in FSH **(A)** and LH **(B)** secretion into the medium.

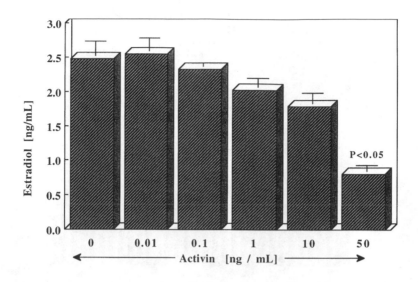

FIGURE 4. Decrease of 17-β-estradiol secretion by luteinized human granulosa cells retrieved by follicular aspiration for IVF in response to increasing concentrations of activin (mean ± SE, $n = 4$).

narrowing the "FSH window" of follicular recruitment through negative feedback at the pituitary level, a mechanism crucial for monofollicular development.[45]

More recently, Alak et al.[46] have monitored the breakdown of the germinal vesicle (GV), progression to metaphase II (M_{II}), and fertilization in vitro (IVF) of rhesus oocytes, recovered by oophorectomy, after 48 hours of culture with inhibin-A and/or activin-A. Activin-A alone (100 ng/ml) stimulated GV breakdown (GVBD), whereas both GVBD and M_{II} development was significantly enhanced by inhibin and activin coincubation.[46]

Follistatin abolished the stimulatory effect of activin and that of inhibin/activin coincubation. Exposure to inhibin and activin significantly increased the IVF of M_{II} oocytes from 25% to 68%,[46] suggesting that inhibin and activin are potent stimulators of primate oocyte maturation and possibly also fertilization.

In contrast to the reported antagonistic effects of inhibin and activin in different target organs and diverse gonadal and extragonadal cell types, it seems that, in the case of oocyte maturation and fertilization, inhibin and activin function synergistically with each other.[46] Also, the exogenous peptides may alter the dynamics of the receptors' mRNA expression in different compartments of the follicle (theca cell, granulosa cell, cumulus cell, or oocyte) with resulting alteration of the different cells and oocyte function and maturation.[46,47]

Usually, in vitro maturation is monitored by nuclear maturation alone since GVBD and polar body extrusion are easily observed.[46] However, a study by Alak et al.[46] suggests a beneficial effect on cytoplasmic maturation as well, since activin and/or inhibin elevated the fertilization of mature (M_{II}) oocytes to 50–68% versus 17–32%, as previously reported for the macaque's unstimulated oocytes. Indeed, in a previous study, in humans, Cha *et al.*[48] achieved a fertilization rate of 32–81% of human unstimulated oocytes after incubation with follicular fluid known to contain inhibin and activin, and, following *in vitro* maturation and fertilization, one successful pregnancy was generated. More recently, it was also shown that activin-A has accelerated meiotic maturation of human oocytes and has modulated granulosa cell steroidogenesis *in-vitro.*[49]

In human ovaries, immunohistochemical and *in situ* hybridization studies have revealed that the expression patterns of the α, β_A, and β_B inhibin subunits and follistatin are modulated during folliculogenesis,[50] suggesting that a dynamic but tightly regulated pattern of inhibin, activin, and follistatin biosynthesis occurs during follicular maturation.[51–53]

The α subunit of inhibin is produced in vast excess over the amount necessary to produce dimeric inhibin.[54] This results in various forms of monomeric α subunit in follicular fluid and serum, including the full-length precursor protein and a form containing a short segment of the pro-region disulfide linked to the mature α subunit, creating a 26-kDa peptide known as pro-αC.[55,56] Although the physiologic significance of free α subunit is not known, these proteins may inhibit FSH binding to its receptor,[57] influence follicle development,[58] or inhibit postcleavage development of bovine embryos derived from cumulus–oocyte complexes matured and fertilized *in vitro.*[59] Taken together, these results suggest that free α subunit, dimeric inhibins, activin, and/or follistatin may influence human follicle and oocyte development.

To test this hypothesis, the mRNA for the inhibin–activin–follistatin system and hormone concentrations were recently examined in granulosa cells and follicular fluids retrieved by follicular aspiration from patients undergoing IVF.[54] The results of this study indicate that some α-subunit mRNA biosynthesis is associated with normal oocyte and follicle maturation but that excessive α subunit is associated with lower quality embryos. In addition, levels of both follistatin and progesterone were higher in follicles with more mature oocytes.[54] None of the analyzed hormones were associated with oocyte or embryo quality.[54]

Of note, granulosa-cell inhibin α-subunit mRNA levels were associated with several aspects of oocyte maturation and competence. Significantly higher inhibin α-subunit mRNA levels were associated with more mature, higher grade, and successfully fertilized oocytes, suggesting that inhibin α-subunit protein, either alone or as dimeric inhibin, is produced in follicles that contain mature, healthy oocytes. However, inhibin α-subunit mRNA levels were significantly higher in poorer quality embryos that were not developing properly. This later observation suggests that too much inhibin α subunit can detrimentally affect the developmental competence of oocytes, as manifested by poorer quality embryos.[54]

If indeed the α-inhibin precursor, pro-αC protein, is an FSH-receptor binding competitor that antagonizes FSH's bioactivity, follicles with high pro-αC levels would be resistant to FSH, which provides a new perspective on the pathogenesis of the idiopathic premature ovarian failure (POF) and the so-called "gonadotropin-resistant ovary" syndrome in young women.[57,60] Alternatively, follicles with more dimeric inhibin (α-β), which do not possess the FSH-receptor binding competitor activity of the α subunit, might be more sensitive to FSH and therefore proceed to dominance and ovulation. On the basis of these assumptions and hypotheses, one may view the complex process of folliculogenesis as a balanced interplay between activin, inhibin, and their subunits (FIG. 5).

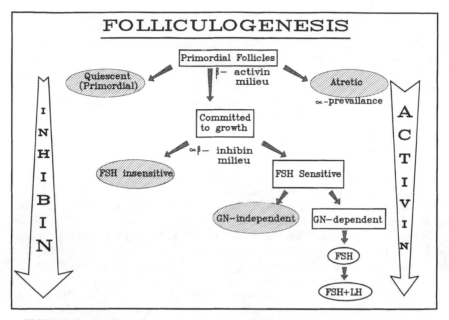

FIGURE 5. Suggested interaction between inhibin/activin and their subunits in the process of folliculogenesis.

Activin may have a crucial role in promoting the receptivity of the undifferentiated granulosa cells to FSH. Therefore, at the beginning of the folliculogenetic process, the primordial, uncommitted follicles need a β-activin milieu in order to proceed to the stage of primary follicles committed to growth and differentiation (FIG. 5). Those small follicles exposed to an excess of α subunit will become atretic, whereas those that will acquire the ability to differentiate and grow will be gradually exposed to the increasing influence of α-β inhibin dimer and in parallel a gradual decrease in the β-β activin dimer influence.[35] The increasing concentrations of inhibin will, in an endocrine mechanism, suppress the pituitary FSH release, enabling the selection of one dominant follicle that would have acquired the ability to grow and develop continuously in spite of lower FSH concentrations. Concomitantly, increased inhibin would restrict the growth of the nondominant follicles (FIGS. 5, 6).[1,35] The increased need for androstenedione, produced by the theca cells, as a substrate for estradiol production by the granulosa cells according to the "two cells–two gonadotropins" theory, is met by the increasing inhibin concentrations. The action of activin to increase FSH receptors and granulosa cell responsiveness to FSH at the early stage of folliculogenesis in an autocrine or paracrine manner is significantly diminished or even shut off at the selection and dominance periods of the mid- and late-follicular phase, thus preventing additional follicles from reaching the dominant stage (FIGS. 5, 6). Moreover, increased activin concentrations in the mid- or latefollicular phase may induce follicular atresia.[35]

The possible detrimental effect of the pro-αC protein/α-inhibin precursor is relevant to several areas of future study, including the area focusing on whether the con-

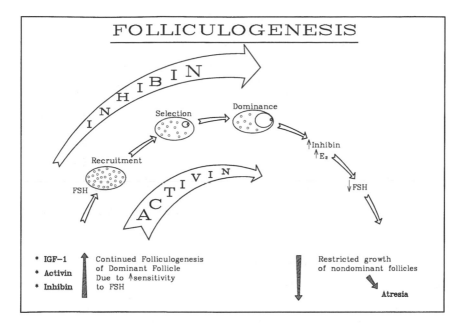

FIGURE 6. Increasing inhibin influence concomitantly with decreasing activin effect acting in concert to affect monofollicular ovulation.

centrations of α-inhibin precursors/pro-αC are really increased in young women with unexplained POF. If indeed increased α-inhibin precursors are involved in the pathophysiologic process of POF, a possible mechanism is suggested for the reported beneficial effect of the GnRH-agonist/glucocorticosteroids/hMG cotreatment in POF.[60] The GnRH agonist, by decreasing FSH levels, could suppress inhibin subunit production by granulosa cells, facilitating temporary release from α-inhibin precursor-mediated competitive binding at the FSH receptor. The concurrent administration of exogenous FSH or hMG may thus induce folliculogenesis and, in some cases, even ovulation and conception.[60] Of course, this speculative explanation awaits future scientific substantiation. Thus, levels of the pro-αC/α-inhibin precursor may be of prognostic value in examining the efficacy of hormone treatments in patients with POF.[60]

The precise physiologic role of inhibin α subunit and, in particular, the forms of inhibin α-subunit protein that may influence oocyte and follicle maturation merits further investigation.

ACKNOWLEDGMENTS

The help of Dr. Teresa K. Woodruff, Dr. Marina Ritter, Dr. Er'ela Livne, Mrs. Batia Navar, Architect Ruth Blumenfeld, and the pathology and gynecology departments is acknowledged with thanks. This work was supported by the Binational U.S.–Israel Grant #181-173.

REFERENCES

1. WOODRUFF, T.K. & J.P. MATHER. 1995. Inhibin, activin and the female reproductive axis. Annu. Rev. Physiol. **57:** 219–244.
2. HAYES, F.J., J.E. HALL & W.F. CROWLEY, JR. 1998. Inhibin secretion in men and women during the menstrual cycle. In Treatment of Infertility: The New Frontiers. Marco Filicori & Carlo Flamigni, Eds.: 85–96. Communications Media for Education, Inc. Princeton Junction, NJ.
3. MCCULLAGH, D. 1932. Dual endocrine activity of the testis. Science **76:** 19–20.
4. FRANCHIMONT, P., D. MILLET, E. VENDRELLY, et al. 1972. Relationship between spermatogenesis and serum gonadotrophin levels in azoospermia and oligospermia. J. Clin. Endocrinol. Metab. **34:** 1003–1008.
5. SETCHELL, B.P. & F. JACKS. 1974. Inhibin-like activity in rete testis fluid. Endocrinology **62:** 675–676.
6. KEOGH, E.J., V.L.W.K. LEE, G.C. RENNIE, et al. 1976. Selective suppression of FSH by testicular extracts. Endocrinology **98:** 997–1004.
7. WALLACE, E.M. & D.L. HEALY. 1996. Inhibins and activins: roles in clinical practice. Br. J. Obstet. Gynaecol. **103:** 945–956.
8. DE JONG, F.H. & R.M. SHARPE. 1976. Evidence for inhibin-like activity in bovine follicular fluid. Nature **263:** 71–72.
9. BURGER, H.G. 1992. The story of inhibin—the Melbourne version. Endocrinology **131:** 1585–1586.
10. ROBERTSON, D.M., L.M. FOULDS, L. LEVERSHA, et al. 1985. Isolation of inhibin from bovine follicular fluid. Biochem. Biophys. Res. Commun. **126:** 220–226.
11. LING, N., S-Y. YING, N. UENO, et al. 1985. Isolation and partial characterization of a Mr 32,000 protein with inhibin activity from porcine follicular fluid. Proc. Natl. Acad. Sci. USA **82:** 7217–7221.
12. VALE, W., J. RIVIER, J. VAUGHAN, et al. 1986. Purification and characterization of an FSH-releasing protein from porcine ovarian follicular fluid. Nature **321:** 776–779.
13. MEUNIER, H.C., C. RIVIER, R.M. EVANS & W. VALE. 1988. Gonadal and extragonadal expression of inhibin α, β_A and β_B subunits in various tissues predicts diverse functions. Proc. Natl. Acad. Sci. USA **85:** 247–251.
14. MESSINIS, I.E. 2000. Ovarian regulation of gonadotropin secretion. Ann. N.Y. Acad. Sci. **900:** 10–15.
15. LOCKWOOD, G.M., S. MUTUKRISHNA & W.L. LEDGER. 1998. Inhibins and activins in human ovulation, conception and pregnancy. Hum. Reprod. Update **4:** 284–295.
16. WOODRUFF, T.K., J.B. D'AGOSTINO, N.B. SCHWARTZ & K.E. MAYO. 1988. Dynamic changes in inhibin/activin subunit mRNA in rat ovarian follicles during the reproductive cycle. Science **239:** 1296–1299.
17. SCHWALL, R.H., A.J. MASON, J.N. WILCOX, et al. 1990. Localization of inhibin/activin subunit mRNA within the primate ovary. Mol. Endocrinol. **4:** 75–79.
18. YAMOTO, M., S. MINAMI, R. NAKANO & M. KOBAYASHI. 1992. Immunohistochemical localization of inhibin/activin subunits in human ovarian follicles during the menstrual cycle. J. Clin. Endocrinol. Metab. **74:** 989–993.
19. VALE, W.W., A. HSUEH, C. RIVIER & L. YU. 1990. The inhibin/activin family of growth factors. In Peptide Growth Factors and Their Receptors. Handbook of Experimental Pharmacology. 95/II. M.A. Sporn & A.B. Roberts, Eds.: 211–248. Springer-Verlag. Heidelberg.
20. VALE, W., C. RIVIER, A. HSUEH, et al. 1988. Chemical and biological characterization of the inhibin family of proteins. Recent Prog. Horm. Res. **44:** 1–34.
21. FRASER, H.M., S.F. LUNN, K.B. SMITH & P.T.K. SAUNDERS. 1993. Synthesis, control and endocrine function of inhibin during the primate menstrual cycle. In GnRH, GnRH Analogs, Gonadotropins and Gonadal Peptides. P. Bouchard, A. Caraty, H.J.T. Coelingh-Bennink & S.N. Pavlou, Eds.: 545–557. Parthenon Publ. Group. London.
22. BURGER, H.G. 1993. Clinical utility of inhibin measurements. J. Clin. Endocrinol. Metab. **76:** 1391–1396.

23. MASON, A.S., V.S. HAYFLICK, N. LING, et al. 1985. Complementary DNA sequences of ovarian follicular fluid inhibin show precursor structure and homology with transforming growth factor-beta. Nature **318:** 659–663.
24. HALVORSON, L.M. & W.W. CHIN. 1999. Gonadotropic hormones: biosynthesis, secretion, receptors, and action. In Reproductive Endocrinology. 4th ed. S.S.C. Yen, R.B. Jaffe & R.L. Barbieri, Eds.: 94–97. W.B. Saunders. Philadelphia.
25. DALKIN, A.C., C.D. KNIGHT, M.A. SHUPNIK, et al. 1993. Ovariectomy and inhibin immunoneutralization acutely increase follicle-stimulating hormone-β messenger ribonucleic acid concentrations: evidence for a nontranscriptional mechanism. Endocrinology **132:** 1297–1304.
26. MEDHAMURTHY, R., M.D. CULLER, V.L. GAY, et al. 1991. Evidence that inhibin plays a major role in the regulation of follicle-stimulating hormone secretion in the fully adult male rhesus monkey (Macaca mulatta). Endocrinology **129:** 389–395.
27. CARROL, R.S., A.Z. CORRIGAN, S.D. GHARIB, et al. 1989. Inhibin, activin, and follistatin: regulation of follicle-stimulating hormone messenger ribonucleic acid levels. Mol. Endocrinol. **3:** 1969–1976.
28. WEISS, J., W.F. CROWLEY, L.M. HALVORSON & J.L. JAMESON. 1993. Perifusion of rat pituitary cells with gonadotropin-releasing hormone, activin, and inhibin reveals distinct effects on gonadotropin gene expression and secretion. Endocrinology **132:** 2307–2311.
29. WOODRUFF, T.K., R. LYON, S.E. HANSEN & J.P. MATHER. 1993. ^{125}I-recombinant human activin A accumulates in the ovary of the immature female rat following intravenous injection. In GnRH, GnRH Analogs, Gonadotropins and Gonadal Peptides. P. Bouchard, A. Caraty, H.J.T. Coelingh-Bennink, S.N. Pavlou, Eds.: 529–534. Parthenon. London.
30. BLUMENFELD, Z. & R.B. JAFFE. 1986. Hypophysiotropic and neuroregulatory modulation of ACTH secretion by human fetal pituitary. J. Clin. Invest. **78:** 288–294.
31. BLUMENFELD, Z., R.W. KUHN & R.B. JAFFE. 1986. Corticotropin-releasing factor can stimulate gonadotropin secretion by human fetal pituitaries in superfusion. Am. J. Obstet. Gynecol. **154:** 606–612.
32. JAFFE, R.B., J.J. MULCHAHEY, A.M. DiBLASIO, et al. 1988. Peptide regulation of pituitary and target tissue function and growth in the primate fetus. Proceedings of the Laurenthian Hormone Conference. Recent Prog. Horm. Res. **44:** 431–449.
33. BLUMENFELD, Z., P. TAPANAINEN, S. KAPLAN, et al. 1989. Partial loss of responsiveness of human fetal pituitary cells to hGHRH after chorionic exposure. Acta Endocrinol. **121:** 721–726.
34. MATHER, J.P., A. MOORE & R.H. LI. 1997. Activins, inhibins and follistatin: further thoughts on a growing family of regulators. Proc. Soc. Exp. Biol. Med. **215:** 209–222.
35. MATHER, J.P., T.K. WOODRUFF & L. KRUMMEN. 1992. Paracrine regulation of reproductive function by inhibin and activin. Proc. Soc. Exp. Biol. Med. **201:** 1–15.
36. SUZUKI, A., T. MAGAI, S. NISHIMATSU, et al. 1994. Autoinduction of activin genes in early Xenopus embryos. Biochem. J. **298:** 275–280.
37. DePAOLO, L, T. BICSAK, G. ERICKSON, et al. 1991. Follistatin and activin: potential intrinsic regulatory system within diverse tissues. Proc. Soc. Exp. Biol. Med. **198:** 500–512.
38. FANN, M.F. & P. PATTERSON. 1994. Neuropoietic cytokines and activin A differentially regulate the phenotype of cultured sympathetic neurons. Proc. Natl. Acad. Sci. USA **91:** 43–47.
39. SPENCER, S.J., J. RABINOVICI, S. MESIANO, et al. 1992. Activin and inhibin in the human adrenal gland. Regulation and differential effects in fetal and adult cells. J. Clin. Invest. **90:** 142–149.
40. YEN, S.S.C. 1999. The human menstrual cycle: neuroendocrine regulation. In Reproductive Endocrinology. 4th ed. S.S.C. Yen, R.B. Jaffe & R.L. Barbieri, Eds.: 191–217. W.B. Saunders. Philadelphia.
41. YEH, J. & E.Y. ADASHI. 1999. The ovarian life cycle. In Reproductive Endocrinology. 4th ed. S.S.C. Yen, R.B. Jaffe & R.L. Barbieri, Eds.: 173–174. W.B. Saunders. Philadelphia.

42. DePaolo, L., T. Bicsak, G. Erickson, *et al.* 1991. Follistatin and activin: a potential intrinsic regulatory system within diverse tissues. Proc. Soc. Exp. Biol. Med. **198:** 500–512.
43. Woodruff, T.K. 1998. Regulation of cellular and system function by activin. Biochem. Pharmacol. **55:** 953–963.
44. Woodruff, T.K., R.J. Lyon, S.E. Hansen, *et al.* 1990. Inhibin and activin locally regulate rat ovarian folliculogenesis. Endocrinology **127:** 3196–3205.
45. Fauser, B.C. & A.M. van Heusden. 1997. Manipulation of human ovarian function: physiological concepts and clinical consequences. Endocr. Rev. **18:** 71–106.
46. Alak, B.H., G.D. Smith, T.K. Woodruff, *et al.* 1996. Enhancement of primate oocyte maturation and fertilizatin in vitro by inhibin A and activin A. Fertil. Steril. **66:** 646–651.
47. Cameron, V., E. Nishimura, L. Mathews, *et al.* 1994. Hybridization histochemical localization of activin receptor subtypes in rat brain, pituitary, ovary, and testis. Endocrinology **134:** 799–808.
48. Cha, K.Y., J.J. Koo, D.H. Choi, *et al.* 1991. Pregnancy after in vitro fertilization of human follicular oocytes collected from non-stimulated cycles, their culture in vitro and their transfer in a donor oocyte program. Fertil. Steril. **55:** 109–113.
49. Alak, B.M., S. Coskun, C.I. Friedman, *et al.* 1998. Activin A stimulates meiotic maturation of human oocytes and modulates granulosa cell steroidogenesis in vitro. Fertil. Steril. **70:** 1126–1130.
50. Roberts, V.J., S. Barth, A. El-Roeiy & S.S. Yen. 1993. Expression of inhibin/activin subunits and follistatin messenger ribonucleic acids and proteins in ovarian follicles and the corpus luteum during the human menstrual cycle. J. Clin. Endocrinol. Metab. **77:** 1402–1410.
51. Yamoto, M., S. Minami, R. Nakano & M. Kobayashi. 1992. Immunohistochemical localization of inhibin/activin subunits in human ovarian follicles during the menstrual cycle. J. Clin. Endocrinol. Metab. **74:** 989–993.
52. Sadatsuki, M., O. Tsutsumi, R. Yamada, *et al.* 1993. Local regulatory effects of activin A and follistatin on meiotic maturation of rat oocytes. Biochem. Biophys. Res. Commun. **196:** 388–395.
53. Silva, C.C. & P.G. Knight. 1998. Modulatory actions of activin A and follistatin on the developmental competence of in vitro matured bovine oocytes. Biol. Reprod. **58:** 558–565.
54. Fujiwara, T., G. Lambert-Messerlian, Y. Sidis, *et al.* 2000. Analysis of follicular fluid hormone concentrations and granulosa cell mRNA levels of the inhibin–activin–follistatin system: relation to oocyte and embryo characteristics. Fertil. Steril. **74:** 348–355.
55. Robertson, D.M., M. Giacometti, L.M. Foulds, *et al.* 1989. Isolation of inhibin alpha subunit precursor proteins from bovine follicular fluid. Endocrinology **125:** 2141–2149.
56. Schneyer, A.L., A.J. Mason, L.E. Burton, *et al.* 1990. Immunoreactive inhibin alpha subunit in human serum: implications for RIA. J. Clin. Endocrinol. Metab. **70:** 1208–1212.
57. Schneyer, A.L., P.M. Sluss, R.W. Whitcomb, *et al.* 1991. Precursors of alpha-inhibin modulate FSH receptor binding and biological activity. Endocrinology **129:** 1987–1999.
58. Dhar, A., L.A. Salamonsen, B.W. Doughton, *et al.* 1998. Effect of immunization against the amino-teminal peptide (alpha N) of the alpha 43-subunit of inhibin on follicular atresia and expression of tissue inhibitor of matrix metalloproteinase (TIMP-1) in ovarian follicles of sheep. J. Reprod. Fertil. **114:** 147–155.
59. Silva, C.C., N. Groome & P.G. Knight. 1999. Demonstration of a suppressive effect of inhibin α subunit on the developmental competence of in vitro matured bovine oocytes. J. Reprod. Fertil. **115:** 381–388.
60. Blumenfeld, Z., S. Halachmi, B.A. Peretz, *et al.* 1993. Premature ovarian failure—the prognostic application of autoimmunity conception after ovulation induction. Fertil. Steril. **59:** 750–755.

Gonadotropin-Releasing Hormone Antagonists

Implications for Oocyte Quality and Uterine Receptivity

KEITH GORDON

Reproductive Medicine, Organon Inc., West Orange, New Jersey 07052, USA

ABSTRACT: Until recently, gonadotropin-releasing hormone (GnRH) agonists were the only choice available to physicians for prevention of premature luteinizing hormone (LH) surges in women undergoing controlled ovarian stimulation. The recent FDA approval of GnRH antagonists for this indication gives clinicians some new options. Results of clinical trials to date suggest that, with GnRH antagonists, much shorter treatment regimens with fewer injections and possibly less gonadotropin can achieve good clinical results. In most of the trials performed to date, however, the GnRH antagonist regimens have been associated with a slightly lower pregnancy and implantation rate than the established GnRH agonist protocols. This remains the biggest hurdle to their more general acceptance. Herein, the possible contributing factors are discussed, and the proposal made that differences in serum estradiol patterns preceding oocyte retrieval are the most likely contributing factor.

KEYWORDS: GnRH antagonist; controlled ovarian (hyper)stimulation; *in vitro* fertilization/embryo transfer; uterine receptivity

Although *in vitro* fertilization (IVF) was first successfully performed with an oocyte retrieved from a natural cycle,[1] the vast majority of IVF/ICSI cycles now employ controlled ovarian (hyper)stimulation (COH). In simple terms, the purpose of COH is to maximize the number of fertilizable oocytes obtainable at the time of oocyte retrieval. Initially, COH was achieved via the administration of exogenous gonadotropins, either alone or in combination with clomiphene citrate. Despite close monitoring of follicular growth (via ultrasound and serum estradiol determinations), 10–25% of cycles were canceled due to premature luteinizing hormone (LH) surges. During the early to middle 1980s, with new knowledge of how the pattern of gonadotropin-releasing hormone (GnRH) release regulated the secretion of LH and follicle-stimulating hormone (FSH), clinicians started to employ GnRH agonists to achieve a state of hormonally selective temporary hypophysectomy, thereby negating any chance of a premature LH surge occurring.

Address for correspondence: Keith Gordon, Ph.D., Associate Director, Reproductive Medicine, Organon Inc., 375 Mt. Pleasant Ave., West Orange, NJ 07052. Voice: 973-325-5403; fax: 973-325-4699.

k.gordon@organoninc.com

Thus, although not specifically developed for the indication, GnRH agonists became part of the standard therapy for preventing premature LH surges during COH. By using these GnRH agonists, clinicians have benefited in terms of fewer cancellations, more flexible scheduling of patients, more oocytes, and ultimately higher pregnancy rates.[2] However, these gains are associated with certain costs. Stimulations require more injections, use more gonadotropin, and are consequently more costly.

According to Akira Arimura (one of the members of A. V. Schally's team that first elucidated the structure of LH-releasing hormone [LHRH]), the structure of LHRH (GnRH) was finally confirmed at 09:00 on Sunday April 25th, 1971.[3] Within one year, synthetic analogues of GnRH (both agonists and antagonists) were being developed[4,5] and tested for their ability to stimulate (agonists) or inhibit (antagonists) the secretion of LH and FSH. Relatively few modifications were needed to produce potent GnRH agonists, and these compounds quickly passed through the various stages of drug development, appearing on the U.S. market in the early 1980s. In contrast, the early GnRH antagonists were plagued with relative lack of potency and an unexpected side effect. When administered to lab animals, they caused marked histamine release that could potentially lead to an anaphylactic reaction.[6]

It has taken many years to optimize their design, but clinically useful GnRH antagonists are now available. Their arrival has been met with mixed emotions. Many clinicians have embraced these new compounds as a much needed and more logical choice for the temporary inhibition of pituitary function during COH.[7-9] Others are more cautious.[10,11] Numerous trials have now been performed comparing classical GnRH agonist protocols with the newer GnRH antagonist protocols.[12-14] These trials and other noncomparative trials[15,16] have revealed numerous advantages of the stimulation regimens incorporating GnRH antagonists versus those employing GnRH agonists. Advantages include much shorter total treatment duration, fewer injections, the need for less gonadotropin, and also possible options if the patient is at risk of ovarian hyperstimulation syndrome (OHSS).[17] However, some disadvantages have also been identified. There appears to be a learning curve associated with the introduction of these new compounds into treatment regimens; scheduling of patients is more challenging, and there is a perception that the achieved pregnancy rates are lower with the antagonist protocols than with the established agonist protocols.

Factors that could contribute to lower pregnancy rates include the number of follicles stimulated and the resultant number of oocytes retrieved, the fertilization rate, the numbers of embryos obtained, embryo quality, developmental competency, and implantation rates. In the studies performed to date, slightly fewer follicles are obtained in the antagonist cycles than in the agonist cycles. Consequently, fewer oocytes are obtained. Fertilization rates appear identical but, not surprisingly, the total number of embryos obtained is slightly lower. Trials performed to date have standardized the number of embryos to be transferred in the antagonist and agonist regimens, yet the implantation and pregnancy rates have been lower for the antagonist regimen.

In a recent double-blind dose-finding study[15] performed in 333 women, six different doses of the GnRH antagonist ganirelix, ranging between 0.0625 and 2 mg, were tested. In this study, women undergoing ovarian stimulation with recombinant FSH were treated with a fixed daily dose of 150 IU for 5 days before initiating

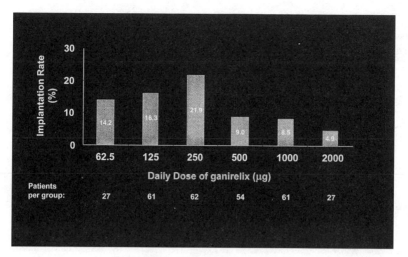

FIGURE 1. Mean implantation rate.

ganirelix therapy. The study revealed that a daily dose of 250 μg of ganirelix prevented premature LH surges and gave the best clinical outcome, with ongoing-pregnancy rates (at 12–16 weeks after transfer) of 34% per attempt and 37% per transfer. Nevertheless, the results also showed that high doses of GnRH antagonist (0.5, 1, or 2 mg once daily) were associated with relatively low implantation rates (FIG. 1). No obvious explanation could be provided for these lower rates, but the authors suggested that it did not appear to be the result of lower levels of serum estradiol on the day of hCG or due to differences in the numbers of oocytes retrieved. Excess embryos from this study were frozen. A follow-up study attempted to replace these cryopreserved embryos into the women who did not become pregnant from replacement of fresh embryos (TABLE 1).[18] The data from this study suggested that high doses of ganirelix do not adversely affect the potential of embryos to establish clinical pregnancies in freeze–thaw cycles.

Recently, these issues have been synthesized into a provocative debate article that concluded that implantation was the likely bottleneck.[11] The author of that article proposed that a direct effect of the GnRH antagonists at the endometrial level may be responsible for the outcomes. I would like to reexamine this issue and offer a slightly different hypothesis.

TABLE 1. Outcome after replacement of thawed embryos

	Original after replacement of thawed embryos						
	0.0625	0.125	0.25	0.5	1.0	2.0	Overall
No. of cycles	7	8	8	7	17	11	58
Ongoing-pregnancy rate	0	37.5	14.3	14.3	36.4	25.0	23.9

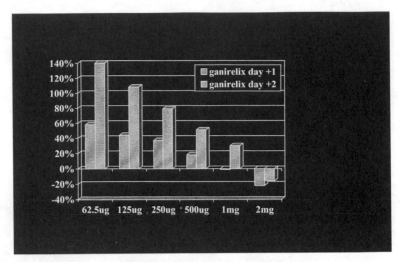

FIGURE 2. Change in estradiol.

As part of an ongoing effort to investigate this issue, we reevaluated the pattern of estradiol before administration of hCG in women who participated in the dose-finding study. In FIGURE 2, the mean percent change in serum estradiol levels relative to the value drawn immediately before ganirelix administration is shown for days +1 and +2 for all doses. As can clearly be seen, with increasing doses of ganirelix there is a progressive decline in the estradiol rises seen on the first and second day after initiation of ganirelix therapy. This actually becomes negative in the highest dose (2 mg) group, in which serum estradiol levels fell on the day after initiation of ganirelix therapy.

In FIGURE 3, these results are expressed slightly differently. For each ganirelix dose group, the bars depict the percentage of women for whom serum estradiol levels declined, rose by 0–25%, or rose by more than 25%. Again we see a reciprocal relationship. The higher the dose of ganirelix, the greater the percentage of women who experienced a decline in serum estradiol levels 24 hours after the first injection of ganirelix. Conversely, the lower the dose of ganirelix, the greater the percentage of women whose serum estradiol levels rose by more than 25%. Thus, it appears that with higher doses of ganirelix, the progressive daily increases in serum estradiol that usually accompany COH were not seen.

In the ganirelix efficacy and safety trials conducted so far, treatment is initiated with recombinant FSH (Puregon®, NV Organon, Oss, The Netherlands/Follistim®, Organon Inc., West Orange, NJ) on day 2 or 3 of the menstrual cycle by a once-daily s.c. injection. After 5 days of recombinant FSH treatment, ganirelix treatment was started by daily s.c. administration of 250 μg and was continued up to and including the day of hCG administration. The daily dose of recombinant FSH was fixed for the first five treatment days. From day 6 onwards, the dose of FSH could be adjusted depending on the ovarian response, as monitored via ultrasound and/or serum estradiol levels. Serum estradiol levels on the day of the first monitoring visit (day 6) were

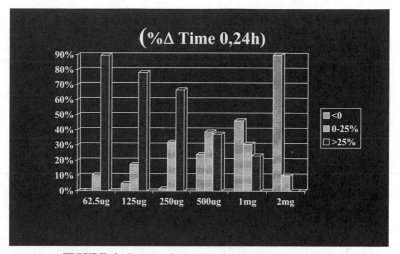

FIGURE 3. Impact of ganirelix dose on serum estradiol.

considerably higher than those usually seen in downregulated protocols and may have prompted a clinical decision to decrease the exogenous FSH dose. When ganirelix is initiated, however, dose-dependent decreases in pituitary FSH and LH levels occur, which may be viewed as an iatrogenic "step-down." In certain women, the decrease in pituitary gonadotropin secretion induced by ganirelix (coupled with a significant decrease in the amount of exogenous gonadotropin administered) may have had adverse clinical consequences due to the excessive total decline in circulating gonadotropins.

It has also been noted[15] that the ongoing-pregnancy rates for ganirelix patients treated at study sites that had previous experience with the ganirelix regimen were better (and no different from agonist patients at those sites) than for patients treated at sites without prior antagonist experience. Taken together, I think, these observations point towards differences in patient management and resultant serum estradiol patterns preceding oocyte retrieval as the most likely contributing factor, rather than direct effects of the GnRH antagonist at the endometrial level.

REFERENCES

1. STEPTOE, P.C. & R.G. EDWARDS. 1978. Birth after the reimplantation of a human embryo. Lancet **12(2):** 366.
2. HUGHES, E.G., *et al.* 1992. The routine use of gonadotropin-releasing hormone agonists prior to in vitro fertilization and gamete intrafallopian transfer: a meta analysis of randomized controlled trials. Fertil. Steril. **58(5):** 888–896.
3. ARIMURA, A. 1991. The backstage story of the discovery of LHRH. Endocrinology **129(4):** 1687–1689.
4. SCHALLY, A.V. & A.J. KASTIN. 1971. Stimulation and inhibition of fertility through hypothalamic agents. Drug Ther. **1(11):** 29–32.
5. VALE, W., *et al.* 1972. Synthetic polypeptide antagonists of the hypothalamic luteinizing hormone releasing factor. Science **176:** 933–934.

6. SCHMIDT, F., *et al.* 1984. [Ac-D-Nal(2)^1,4F-D-Phe^2,D-Trp^3,D-Arg^6]-LHRH, a potent antagonist of LHRH, produces transient edema and behavioral changes in rats. Contraception **29:** 283–289.
7. BOUCHARD, P. & B.C.J.M. FAUSER. 2000. Gonadotropin-releasing hormone antagonists: new tools vs. old habits. Fertil. Steril. **73(1):** 18–20.
8. FAUSER, B.C.J.M., *et al.* 1999. Minimal ovarian stimulation for IVF: appraisal of potential benefits and drawbacks. Hum. Reprod. **14(11):** 2681–2686.
9. FELDERBAUM, R. & K. DIEDRICH. 1999. Ovarian stimulation for in-vitro fertilization/intracytoplasmic sperm injection with gonadotrophins and gonadotrophin-releasing hormone analogues: agonists and antagonists. Hum. Reprod. **14(Suppl. 1):** 207–221.
10. CRAFT, I., *et al.* 1999. Will GnRH antagonists provide new hope for patients considered "difficult responders" to GnRH agonist protocols? Hum. Reprod. **14(12):** 2959–2962.
11. HERNANDEZ, E.R. 2000. Embryo implantation: the Rubicon for GnRH antagonists. Hum. Reprod. **15(6):** 1211–1216.
12. OLIVENNES, F., *et al.* 2000. Prospective, randomized, controlled study of in vitro fertilization–embryo transfer with a single dose of a luteinizing hormone-releasing hormone (LH-RH) antagonist (cetrorelix) or a depot formula of an LH-RH agonist (triptorelin). Fertil. Steril. **73(2):** 314–320.
13. ALBANO, C., *et al.* 2000. Ovarian stimulation with HMG: results of a prospective randomized phase III European study comparing the luteinizing hormone-releasing hormone (LHRH)-antagonist cetrorelix and the LHRH-agonist buserelin. Hum. Reprod. **15(3):** 526–531.
14. BORM, G. & B. MANNAERTS FOR THE EUROPEAN ORGALUTRAN® STUDY GROUP. 2000. Treatment with the gonadotrophin-releasing hormone antagonist ganirelix in women undergoing ovarian stimulation with recombinant follicle stimulating hormone is effective, safe and convenient: results of a controlled, randomized, multicentre trial. Hum. Reprod. **15(7):** 1490–1498.
15. THE GANIRELIX DOSE-FINDING STUDY GROUP. 1998. A double-blind, randomized, dose-finding study to assess the efficacy of the gonadotrophin-releasing hormone antagonist ganirelix (Org 37462) to prevent premature luteinizing hormone surges in women undergoing ovarian stimulation with recombinant follicle stimulating hormone (Puregon®). Hum. Reprod. **13(11):** 3023–3031.
16. FELBERBAUM, R.E., *et al.* 2000. Ovarian stimulation for assisted reproduction with HMG and concomitant midcycle administration of the GnRH antagonist cetrorelix according to the multiple dose protocol: a prospective uncontrolled phase III study. Hum. Reprod. **15(5):** 1015–1020.
17. OLIVENNES, F., *et al.* 1996. Triggering of ovulation by a gonadotropin releasing hormone (GnRH) agonist in patients pretreated with a GnRH antagonist. Fertil. Steril. **66(1):** 151–153.
18. KOL, S., *et al.* 1999. High doses of gonadotrophin-releasing hormone antagonist in in-vitro fertilization cycles do not adversely affect the outcome of subsequent freeze–thaw cycles. Hum. Reprod. **14(9):** 2242–2244.

Ovulation Induction Disrupts Luteal Phase Function

ASIMINA TAVANIOTOU,[a] JOHAN SMITZ,[a] CLAIRE BOURGAIN,[b] AND
PAUL DEVROEY[a]

[a]Centre for Reproductive Medicine and [b]Department of Pathology, Dutch-Speaking Free
University of Brussels, 1090 Brussels, Belgium

ABSTRACT: Abnormalities in the luteal phase have been detected in virtually all
the stimulation protocols used in *in vitro* fertilization, on both the hormonal
and endometrial levels. Supraphysiological follicular or luteal sex steroid serum concentrations, altered estradiol:progesterone (E_2/P) ratio, and disturbed
luteinizing hormone pituitary secretion leading to corpus luteum insufficiency
or a direct drug effect have been postulated as the main etiologic factors.
Luteinizing hormone supports corpus luteum function, and low LH levels have
been described after human menopausal gonadotropin treatment, after gonadotropin-releasing hormone (GnRH)-agonist treatment, or after GnRH-antagonist treatment. These low luteal LH levels may lead to an insufficient corpus
luteum function and consequently to a shortened luteal phase or to the low
luteal progesterone concentrations frequently described after ovulation induction. A direct effect of the GnRH agonist or GnRH antagonist on human corpus
luteum or on human endometrium and thus on endometrial receptivity cannot
be excluded, as GnRH receptors have been described in both compartments.
Endometrial histology has revealed a wide range of abnormalities during the
various stimulation protocols. In GnRH-agonist cycles, mid-luteal biopsies
have revealed increased glandulo-stromal dyssynchrony and delay in endometrial development, strong positivity of endometrial glands for progesterone receptors, decreased $\alpha_v\beta_3$-integrin subunit expression, and earlier appearance of
surface epithelium pinopodes. These factors suggest a shift forwards of the implantation window. Progesterone supplementation improves endometrial histology, and its necessity has been well established, at least in cycles using GnRH
agonists.

KEYWORDS: luteal phase function; GnRH-agonist treatment; GnRH-antagonist
treatment; corpus luteum; endometrium

INTRODUCTION

Abnormalities in the luteal phase have been shown in virtually all the stimulation
protocols used in ovarian stimulation, on the hormonal, as well as on the endometrial
level.[1,2,3] All three aspects of a defective luteal phase, that is, a shortened luteal
phase and/or low mid-luteal serum progesterone concentrations and/or abnormal endometrial histology, have been regularly observed in *in vitro* fertilization cycles.
Luteal-phase supplementation with human chorionic gonadotropin (hCG) or progesterone increases pregnancy rates, and its necessity has been well established, at least

Address for correspondence: Asimina Tavaniotou, AZ-VUB, Centre for Reproductive Medicine, Laarbeeklaan 101,1090 Brussels, Belgium. Voice: 0032-2-4776501; fax: 0032-2- 4776549.
mtavaniotou@hotmail.com

in gonadotropin-releasing hormone (GnRH)-agonist cycles.[4] Currently, the most frequently used protocols for *in vitro* fertilization are those that associate a gonadotropin-releasing hormone agonist with gonadotropins. Recently, the GnRH antagonists that prevent the luteinizing hormone surge have been introduced in ovarian stimulation cycles. As both protocols have been associated with a defective luteal phase despite their different modes of action, the aim of this article is to provide a review of the hormonal and histological correlates of the luteal phase after GnRH-agonist or GnRH-antagonist treatment.

HORMONAL CORRELATES OF THE LUTEAL PHASE IN GnRH CYCLES

The lifespan and steroidogenic capacity of the human corpus luteum is dependent on continuous tonic luteinizing hormone (LH) secretion.[5] Feedback mechanisms from ovarian steroids and GnRH pulses regulate LH secretion during the luteal phase, but a number of autocrine and paracrine factors within the ovary might also play a role in controlling corpus luteum function.

Low luteal LH levels have been described after human menopausal gonadotropin treatment[6] and after GnRH-agonist treatment[2,7] or after GnRH-antagonist treatment.[8,9] These low, almost undetectable, luteal LH levels may not be able to support corpus luteum. As a result, a shortened luteal phase and low mid-luteal progesterone concentrations have been described in cycles stimulated with the association either of a GnRH agonist or a GnRH antagonist.[2,8]

Luteal LH Secretion in GnRH-Agonist Cycles

Because pituitary LH secretion is dependent on GnRH stimulus and feedback mechanisms from ovarian steroids, any alteration may be deleterious. In cycles using GnRH agonists for ovarian stimulation, a significant drop in mid-luteal progesterone concentrations was observed, consistent with corpus luteum insufficiency.[10] Long-term GnRH-agonist administration has been associated with a profound desensitization of the pituitary cells. In fact, studies on pituitary gonadotropin secretory capacity after GnRH-agonist treatment have indicated that this remains impaired for at least 14 days after the discontinuation of the GnRH-agonist and for the whole length of the luteal phase.[2,11] In a recent randomized trial, it was also demonstrated that, despite the early cessation of the GnRH agonist in the follicular phase, luteal-phase characteristics were abnormal.[7]

Luteal LH Secretion in GnRH-Antagonist Cycles

GnRH-antagonist treatment has been shown to be effective in blocking the LH surge. GnRH antagonists bind competitively to pituitary GnRH receptors and cause an immediate inhibition of gonadotropin release. In contrast to GnRH agonists, it was suggested that treatment with GnRH antagonists may not adversely affect luteal LH secretion, since the pituitary maintains its responsiveness to the endogenous GnRH stimulus.[12] A normal luteal phase, in terms of duration and serum progesterone concentrations, was observed in natural cycles in which an antagonist was administered to prevent the LH surge.[13] However, data on the luteal phase from unsupplemented cycles after antagonist administration are limited as a result of the small number of patients involved and are rather controversial. Four out of six patients had either a shortened luteal phase or low progesterone concentrations in cycles stimulated with HMG and the GnRH antagonist Cetrorelix and receiving no luteal-phase supplementation.[3] This finding has not been confirmed in another recent trial.[9] However, with[8] or without[9] luteal-phase supplementation, luteal LH levels were low, indicating that another mechanism might be involved.

Luteal-Phase Defect in Ovarian Stimulation: Role of Ovarian Steroids

In the pre-agonist era, the alteration of the estradiol:progesterone (E_2/P) ratio was considered a main cause of luteal-phase inadequacy, possibly through the luteolytic action of E_2.[14] Recent studies support this hypothesis: Different estrogen receptors have been detected in the corpus luteum, and estradiol may play a role in luteolysis and corpus luteum apoptosis.[15,16] Supraphysiological estrogen and progesterone serum concentrations, routinely attained after ovarian stimulation, may also interfere with the pituitary's luteinizing hormone secretion by disturbing the feedback control mechanisms and may result in a reduction of the LH serum levels.[17]

Direct Effect of GnRH on Human Corpus Luteum

GnRH receptors[18] and GnRH receptor mRNA[19] were found to be expressed in human granulosa-luteal cells. In *in vitro* studies, it was demonstrated that the administration of GnRH agonists may directly affect the steroidogenic capacity of the human corpus luteum, particularly progesterone secretion.[20] Additionally, luteinized-granulosa aromatase activity was found to be reduced after GnRH antagonist treatment, in contrast to GnRH agonist treatment.[21] Data from the literature are rather controversial, however, and there are concerns about the effect that GnRH analogue treatment may exert on ovarian steroidogenesis and subsequent progesterone production from the corpus luteum.[18,22]

ENDOMETRIAL CORRELATES OF THE LUTEAL PHASE IN GnRH AGONIST OR ANTAGONIST CYCLES

In clinical practice, endometrial assessment is usually carried out by dating the endometrium according to the criteria of Noyes *et al.*[23] Different timing of the biopsies, different stimulation protocols, different routes or dosages of progesterone supplementation, and differences in the interpretation of biopsy specimens may explain the different findings in endometrial biopsy studies. The adverse effect that ovulation induction might exert on endometrial receptivity has been demonstrated in a study in which implantation rates were significantly lower in oocyte donors than in the matched recipients for age and embryo quality.[24] Endometrial receptivity is defined as a temporally unique sequence of factors that make the endometrium receptive to embryonic implantation. Implantation of the human embryo may occur only during a regulated "implantation window" on days 6–10 postovulation or from day 20 to day 24 of a normalized 28-day cycle.[25]

Studies performed in GnRH-agonist cycles have investigated endometrial histology in terms of dating or the presence of endometrial steroid receptors. Not many studies, however, have evaluated the impact that ovarian stimulation exerts on potential functional markers of uterine receptivity and, to the best of our knowledge, there are no studies on endometrial histology after GnRH-antagonist treatment.

Etiology of Abnormal Endometrial Histology

Altered endometrial development in ovarian stimulation cycles may be due to supraphysiological steroid serum concentrations and altered E_2/P ratio in the early luteal phase. A high E_2/P ratio has been connected with failures of conception probably due to altered endometrial receptivity, because progesterone levels may not be high enough to balance the high estrogen levels.[26] However, corpus luteum insufficiency and impaired progesterone secretion may also result in an abnormal endometrial histology. A direct effect of the drugs on the endometrium cannot be excluded. Except for the well-known antiestrogenic effect of clomiphene citrate on the endometrium, GnRH analogues may also directly affect endometrial receptivity. Endometrial cells express GnRH receptor mRNA,[27] and there are also assumptions that GnRH-antagonist treatment may adversely affect endometrial receptivity in a dose-dependent manner.[28]

Endometrial Histology

Classically, the endometrium is characterized as "out of phase," following the Noyes criteria, if its histology does not correspond within two days with the expected day of the natural cycle. Synchronization between embryo and endometrium is important: No pregnancies were observed if the endometrium was more than three days ahead of what would normally be expected.[29] Early luteal-phase biopsies have shown advanced or in-phase endometrial maturation.[29,30] On day hCG + 7, the endometrium was more advanced in the stimulated cycles by 1.8 days than in HRT control recipients.[31] However, midluteal biopsies showed a significant maturation delay in half of the endometria from nonsupplemented cycles, which was corrected only after luteal-phase supplementation with hCG or progesterone[32] (TABLE 1). Endometrial biopsies from nonsupplemented cycles revealed distinct ultrastructural abnormalities, consistent with low progesterone bioavailability, that is, absence of nucleolar channel systems and giant mitochondria, even when the light microscopy was in phase.[32]

A second common finding from endometrial biopsies in stimulated cycles is the asynchronous maturation between the endometrial glands and stroma, with the stroma being more than two days in advance of the endometrial glands. Both in early and mid-luteal biopsies, a high percentage of glandular-stroma asynchrony has been detected.[33–35] In mid-luteal biopsies, dissociated maturation was more pronounced in cycles supplemented with hCG or with progesterone IM than vaginal progesterone.[32] Supraphysiological steroid serum concentrations or altered steroid serum ratios[34] may be an etiologic factor. It has been indicated that progesterone concentrations five times higher than physiological values in combination with normal estrogen concentrations might not affect endometrial glandular maturation in artificial cycles, but may affect the stroma.[36]

TABLE 1. Summary of studies with endometrial biopsies in GnRH/HMG or recFSH cycles, where no luteal-phase supplementation was given

Author	Number	Protocol	Timing	Finding
Macrow, 1994[34]	11	GnRH/HMG	OPU + 4	Glands 11/11 in-phase Stroma 5/11 advanced
	11	Natural	Ovul + 4	Glands 11/11 in-phase Stroma 2/11 advanced
Bourgain, 1994[32]	10	GnRH/HMG	OPU+6–10	6/10 delayed
Kolb, 1997[31]	7	GnRH/HMG	hCG + 7	1.8 days advanced than
	20	HRT	P for 7 days	recipients
Lass, 1998[44]	33	GnRH/FSH	OPU	15/33 advanced 3/33 delayed
Meyer, 1999[36]	9	GnRH/HMG	hCG + 8	3/9 in-phase
	20	Natural	LH + 8	12/20 in phase

ABBREVIATIONS: OPU: the day of oocyte retrieval; hCG: the day of injection of the ovulatory hCG; P: progesterone.

Endometrial Steroid Receptors

Ovarian steroid hormones exert their effect on the endometrium after they have bound to their specific nuclear receptors in endometrial glands and stroma. The expression of endometrial steroid receptors varies during the menstrual cycle in humans. In the follicular and early luteal phase of the normal menstrual cycle, both endometrial estrogen receptors (ERs) and progesterone receptors (PRs) are found in the endometrial glands and stroma.[37,38] In the mid-luteal phase, and under the action of progesterone, there is an initial disappearance of ERs from the glandular cells, followed by a subsequent disappearance of the PRs from the same cells (FIG. 1). This variability of the steroid receptors indicates that they may play a role in mediating the endometrial response to steroids from the corpus luteum around the time of implantation.[37,38]

There is evidence that ovulation induction may affect the level of steroid receptors present within endometrial epithelial or stromal cells, although there are conflicting results among the different studies.[32,39,40] The presence of nuclear glandular and stromal PRs and ERs was found to be significantly reduced in the early luteal phase of stimulated cycles compared to natural (control) cycles,[30] although the endometrial biopsies were in phase. In mid-luteal biopsies, after GnRH/HMG stimulation, the presence of glandular progesterone receptors was significantly higher in nonsupplemented than in supplemented cycles, suggesting a low exposure to progesterone.[32] This high glandular PR positivity corresponded to cycles with maturation delay or dissociated maturation.[32] No differences in PR expression were found between natural and stimulated cycles. However, the presence of a protein (ubiquitin) that modifies PR was affected in the stimulated cycles.[40] The decline of glandular PRs and ERs occurs during the implantation window. Because an earlier decline in epithelial ERs and PRs was observed in stimulated cycles compared to natural cycles, it has been suggested that a shift forward of the implantation window might take place in stimulated cycles.[41]

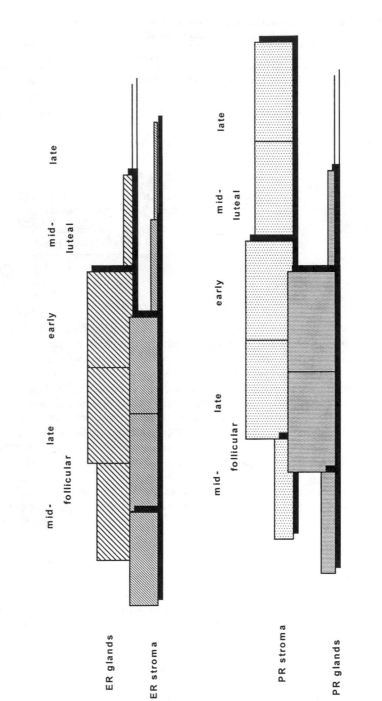

FIGURE 1. Variation of endometrial estrogen and progesterone receptors during the menstrual cycle.

Potential Functional Markers of Uterine Receptivity

A. Cell Adhesion Molecules

Integrins are cell adhesion molecules involved in cell–cell and cell–matrix interactions and contributing to cell migration and signal transduction. It has been suggested that the coexpression of three integrins—α_1, α_4, and $\alpha_v\beta_3$—might frame the putative implantation window.[42] The lack of $\alpha_v\beta_3$ in women with minimal or mild endometriosis, luteal-phase deficiency, and hydrosalpinx is consistent with a role that this molecule might play in the implantation process.[42] However, lower midluteal $\alpha_v\beta_3$ integrin was found in a stimulated cycle than in natural cycles, indicating a probable adverse effect from ovarian stimulation.[35]

B. Pinopodes

Pinopodes appear on the apical surface of luminal epithelium around the 20th day of the menstrual cycle, and it has been suggested that pinopode formation might be a functional marker of uterine receptivity.[43] Advanced endometrial histological features, in terms of dating[31] or in terms of earlier reduction in ERs and PRs, are correlated with the earlier appearance of pinopodes in stimulated cycles, further supporting the concept of a probable shift forward in the implantation window in these cycles.[41]

CONCLUSION

Ovarian stimulation with GnRH agonists is associated with luteal-phase defects in terms of endocrinological and histological features. Endometrial dating, steroid receptors, and functional markers appear to be altered, indicating altered endometrial receptivity and impaired embryo–endometrial synchronization. Treatment with GnRH antagonist may also adversely effect the luteal phase, either because of low LH secretion or because of a direct effect on the endometrium. Although the need for luteal phase supplementation is well established in GnRH-agonist cycles, data from the literature are rather scarce regarding the GnRH-antagonist cycles, and further studies are needed to investigate the effect that GnRH analogues exert on the luteal phase.

REFERENCES

1. EDWARDS, R.G., P.C. STEPTOE & J.M. PURDY. 1980. Establishing full-term pregnancies using cleaving embryos grown in vitro. Br. J. Obstet. Gynaecol. **87:** 737–756.
2. SMITZ, J., P. DEVROEY, et al. 1988. The luteal phase and early pregnancy after combined GnRH-agonist/HMG treatment for superovulation in IVF or GIFT. Hum. Reprod. **3:** 585–590.
3. ALBANO, C., G. GRIMBIZIS, et al. 1998. The luteal phase of nonsupplemented cycles after ovarian superovulation with human menopausal gonadotropin and the gonadotropin-releasing hormone antagonist Cetrorelix. Fertil. Steril. **70:** 357–359.
4. SOLIMAN, S., S. DAYA, et al. 1994. The role of luteal phase support in infertility treatment: a meta-analysis of randomized trials. Fertil. Steril. **61:** 1068–1076.
5. JONES, G.S. 1991. Luteal phase defect: a review of pathophysiology. Curr. Opin. Obstet. Gynecol. **3:** 641–668.

6. MESSINIS, I.E. & A.A. TEMPLETON. 1987. Disparate effects of endogenous and exogenous oestradiol on luteal phase function in women. J. Reprod. Fertil. **79:** 549–554.
7. BECKERS, N.G, J.S. LAVEN, *et al.* 2000. Follicular and luteal phase characteristics following early cessation of gonadotrophin-releasing hormone agonist during ovarian stimulation for in vitro fertilization. Hum. Reprod. **15:** 43–49.
8. ALBANO, C., J. SMITZ, *et al.* 1999. Luteal phase and clinical outcome after human menopausal gonadotrophin/gonadotrophin releasing hormone antagonist treatment for ovarian stimulation in in-vitro fertilization/intracytoplasmic sperm injection cycles. Hum. Reprod. **14:** 1426–1430.
9. DE JONG, D., N.S. MACKLON & B.C.J.M. FAUSER. 2000. A pilot study involving minimal ovarian stimulation for in-vitro fertilization: extending the "follicle-stimulating hormone window" combined with the gonadotropin releasing hormone antagonist cetrorelix. Fertil. Steril. **73:** 1051–1054.
10. SMITZ, J., P. DEVROEY, *et al.* 1987. Management of failed cycles in an IVF/GIFT programme with the combination of a GnRH analogue and HMG. Hum. Reprod. **2:** 309–314.
11. SMITZ, J., P. ERARD, *et al.* 1992. Pituitary gonadotrophin secretory capacity during the luteal phase in superovulation using GnRH agonists and HMG in a desensitization or flare-up protocol. Hum. Reprod. **7:** 1225–1229.
12. FELBERBAUM, R.E., T. REISSMANN, *et al.* 1995. Preserved pituitary response under ovarian stimulation with HMG and GnRH antagonists (Cetrorelix) in women with tubal infertility. Eur. J. Obstet. Gynecol. Reprod. Biol. **61:** 151–155.
13. DITKOFF, E.S., D. CASSIDENTI, *et al.* 1991. The gonadotropin-releasing hormone antagonist (Nal-Glu) acutely blocks the luteinizing hormone surge but allows for resumption of folliculogenesis in normal women. Am. J. Obstet. Gynecol. **165:** 1811–1817.
14. GORE, B.Z., *et al.* 1973. Estrogen-induced human luteolysis. J. Clin. Endocrinol. Metab. **36:** 615–617.
15. MISAO, R., Y. NAKANISHI, *et al.* 1999. Expression of oestrogen receptor α and β mRNA in corpus luteum of human subjects. Mol. Hum. Reprod. **5:** 17–21.
16. KHAN-DAWOOD, F.S., J. YANG & M.Y. DAWOOD. 1996. Expression of gap junction protein connexin-43 in the human and baboon (*Papio anubis*) corpus luteum. J. Clin. Endocrinol. Metab. **81:** 835–842.
17. GIBSON, M., *et al.* 1991. Short-term modulation of gonadotropin secretion by progesterone during the luteal phase. Fertil. Steril. **55:** 522–528.
18. BRUS, L., *et al.* 1997. Specific gonadotrophin-releasing hormone analogue binding predominantly in human luteinized follicular aspirates and not in human preovulatory follicles. Hum. Reprod. **12:** 769–773.
19. PENG, C., N.C. FAN, *et al.* 1994. Expression and regulation of gonadotropin-releasing hormone (GnRH) and GnRH receptor messenger ribonucleic acids in human granulosa-luteal cells. Endocrinology. **135:** 1740–1746.
20. PELLICER, A. & F. MIRO. 1990. Steroidogenesis in vitro of human granulosa-luteal cells pre-treated in vivo with gonadotropin-releasing hormone analogs. Fertil. Steril. **54:** 590–596.
21. MINARETZIS, D., *et al.* 1995. Gonadotropin-releasing hormone antagonist versus agonist administration in women undergoing controlled ovarian hyperstimulation: cycle performance and in vitro steroidogenesis of granulosa-lutein cells. Am. J. Obstet. Gynecol. **172:** 1518–1525.
22. DODSON, W., *et al.* 1988. Leuprolide acetate: serum and follicular fluid concentrations and effects on human fertilization, embryo growth and granulosa-lutein cell progesterone accumulation in vitro. Fertil. Steril. **50:** 612–617.
23. NOYES, R.W., A.T. HERTIG & J. ROCK. 1950. Dating the endometrial biopsy. Fertil. Steril. **1:** 3–25.
24. CHECK, J.H., K. NOWROOZI, *et al.* 1992. Comparison of pregnancy rates following in vitro fertilization-embryo transfer between the donors and the recipients in a donor oocyte program. J. Assist. Reprod. Genet. **9:** 248–250.
25. BERGH, P.A. & D. NAVOT. 1992. The impact of embryonic development and endometrial maturity on the timing of implantation. Fertil. Steril. **58:** 537–542.

26. GIDLEY-BAIRD, A.A., *et al.* 1986. Failure of implantation in human in vitro fertilization and embryo transfer patients: the effects of altered progesterone/estrogen ratios in humans and mice. Fertil. Steril. **45:** 69–74.
27. IMAI, A., T. OHNO, *et al.* 1994. Presence of gonadotropin releasing hormone receptor and its messenger ribonucleic acid in endometrial carcinoma and endometrium. Gynecol. Oncol. **55:** 144–148.
28. KOL, S., *et al.* 1999. High doses of gonadotrophin-releasing hormone antagonist in *in vitro* fertilization cycles do not adversely affect the outcome of subsequent freeze–thaw cycles. Hum. Reprod. **14:** 2242–2244.
29. UBALDI, F., C. BOURGAIN, H. TOURNAYE, *et al.* 1997. Endometrial evaluation by aspiration biopsy on the day of oocyte retrieval in the embryo transfer cycles in patients with serum progesterone rise during the follicular phase. Fertil. Steril. **67:** 521–526.
30. HADI, F.H., E. CHANTLER, E. ANDERSON, *et al.* 1994. Ovulation induction and endometrial steroid receptors. Hum. Reprod. **9:** 2405–2410.
31. KOLB, B.A. & R.J. PAULSON. 1997. The luteal phase of cycles utilizing controlled ovarian hyperstimulation and the possible impact of this hyperstimulation on embryo implantation. Am. J. Obstet. Gynecol. **176:** 1262–1269.
32. BOURGAIN, C., J. SMITZ, *et al.* 1994. Human endometrial maturation is markedly improved after luteal supplementation of gonadotrophin-releasing hormone analogue/human menopausal gonadotrophin stimulated cycles. Hum. Reprod. **9:** 32–40.
33. SEIF, M.W., J.M. PEARSON, *et al.* 1992. Endometrium in in-vitro fertilization cycles: morphological and functional differentiation in the implantation phase. Hum. Reprod. **7:** 6–11.
34. MACROW, P.J., *et al.* 1994. Endometrial structure after superovulation: a prospective controlled study. Fertil. Steril. **61:** 696–699.
35. MEYER, W.R. 1999. Effect of exogenous gonadotropins on endometrial maturation in oocyte donors. Fertil. Steril. **71:** 109–114.
36. LI, T.C., S.S. RAMESEWAK, E.A. LENTON, *et al.* 1992. Endometrial responses in artificial cycles: a prospective randomized study comparing three different progesterone dosages. Br. J. Obstet. Gynaecol. **99:** 319–324.
37. LESSEY, B.A., A.P. KILLAM, *et al.* 1988. Immunohistochemichal analysis of human uterine estrogen and progesterone receptors throughout the menstrual cycle. J. Clin. Endocrinol. Metab. **67:** 334–340.
38. GARCIA, E., P. BOUCHARD, *et al.* 1988. Use of immunocytochemistry of progesterone and estrogen receptors for endometrial dating. J. Clin. Endocrinol. Metab. **67:** 80–87.
39. BALASCH, J., *et al.* 1991. Hormonal and histological evaluation of the luteal phase after combined GnRH-agonist/gonadotrophin treatment for superovulation and luteal phase support in *in vitro* fertilization. Hum. Reprod. **6:** 914–917.
40. BEBINGTON, C., *et al.* 2000. The progesterone receptor and ubiquitin are differentially regulated within the endometrial glands of the natural and stimulated cycle. Mol. Hum. Reprod. **6:** 264–268.
41. DEVELIOGLOU, O.H., J-G. HSIU, *et al.* 1999. Endometrial estrogen and progesterone receptor and pinopode expression in stimulated cycles of oocyte donors. Fertil. Steril. **71:** 1040–1047.
42. LESSEY, B.A. 1998. Endometrial integrins and the establishment of uterine receptivity. Hum. Reprod. **13(Suppl. 3):** 247–261.
43. NIKAS, G. 1999. Pinopodes as markers of endometrial receptivity in clinical practice. Hum. Reprod. **14(Suppl. 2):** 99–106.
44. LASS, A., *et al.* 1998. Histological evaluation of endometrium on the day of oocyte retrieval after gonadotrophin-releasing hormone agonist/follicle stimulating hormone ovulation induction for in vitro fertilization. Hum. Reprod. **13:** 3203–3205.

Perifollicular Vascularity and Its Relationship with Oocyte Maturity and IVF Outcome

ANDREA BORINI,[a] ANDREA MACCOLINI,[a] ALESSANDRA TALLARINI,[a] MARIA ANTONIETTA BONU,[a] RAFFAELLA SCIAJNO,[a] AND CARLO FLAMIGNI[b]

[a]Tecnobios, Center for Reproductive Health, 40125 Bologna, Italy

[b]First Clinic of Obstetrics and Gynaecology, Department of Obstetric and Gynaecology, University of Bologna, Bologna, Italy

ABSTRACT: New markers of embryo ability to implant are pursued continuously. Understanding whether an oocyte is really "mature," that is, ready to be fertilized, would be of great help in choosing an embryo that will implant. It is usual to pay attention to the phase of meiosis, considering the extrusion of the polar body (metaphase II) to be the only sign of the maturity of the oocytes. Nevertheless, understanding more about how the cytoplasm contributes to an oocyte's competency also shows promise as a method of predicting which embryos will implant. Some studies about perifollicular vascularity have demonstrated that embryos originating from oocytes developed in well-vascularized follicles have a higher implantation rate than those originating from oocytes developed in follicles with poor vascularization. Here, we report our results from a preliminary study in which embryos were transferred according to the degree of vascularization of the follicle. Women who received embryos originating from oocytes developed in well-vascularized follicles had a statistically higher pregnancy rate than women who received embryos deriving from oocytes grown in more poorly vascularized follicles (34% vs. 13.7%).

KEYWORDS: perifollicular vascularity; oocyte maturity; implantation rate; power Doppler imaging

BACKGROUND

Despite advances in assisted reproduction over the last decade, the number of embryos that implant is still low. Many factors have been claimed to be prognostic of outcome. These factors include advanced maternal age. Biochemical markers such as level of follicle-stimulating hormone (FSH) in the early follicular phase and inhibin concentration are able to detect reduced ovarian reserve associated with reduced ovarian responsiveness to stimulation and reduced pregnancy rate. Transvaginal ultrasound during assisted conception therapy has significantly enhanced the accuracy of folliculogenesis monitoring. Usually, mean follicular diameters >18 mm are considered a criterion of preovulatory status, but we know that during spontaneous cycles ovulation can occur with a leading follicle ranging from

Address for correspondence: Andrea Borini, M.D., Director Tecnobios, Center for Reproductive Health, Via Dante 15, 40125 Bologna, Italy. Voice: +39 051 2867511; fax: +39 051 2867512. borini@tecnobios.it

15 to 29 mm. Ovulation in the mammalian ovary involves changes in the blood flow to the follicle. *In vivo* studies in the rat with acute ligation of one of the two arteries supplying the ovary are suggestive of the role of a continuous high or increased blood flow to the follicle at ovulation.[1] Chui *et al.* have demonstrated changes in overall ovarian vascularity in both natural and stimulated cycles using color Doppler imaging.[2] Campbell *et al.* have shown that there is a significant increase in perifollicular blood flow in the periovulatory follicle, although this is not related to a decrease in vascular resistance.[3] Power Doppler imaging is a new modality, which unlike conventional color Doppler, maps the amplitude of the frequency shift to produce a color image. As a result, power Doppler is more effective than the conventional color Doppler and enables flows with lower volumes and velocities to be displayed.

A developmentally significant association between the chromosomal normality of the human oocyte and the level of intrafollicular oxygen was proposed by Gaulden.[4] He suggested that hypoxic intrafollicular conditions that result from the failure of an appropriate microvasculature to develop around the growing or preovulatory follicle could be a proximate cause of the maternal age-related increase in the incidence of trisomic conditions. The effect of hypoxia on the oocyte could include reduced levels of metabolism and lower intracellular pH, which in turn could influence the organization and the stability of the meiotic metaphase spindle. Van Blerkom *et al.* found that developmentally significant defects in chromosome number, spindle organization, and cytoplasmic structure occurred in oocytes derived from follicles with dissolved oxygen contents of $\leq 1\%$ at a significantly higher frequency than in oocytes from follicles with dissolved oxygen content $\geq 3\%$.[5] Furthermore, they observed a significant reduction in the ability of fertilized eggs from follicles with relatively low oxygen contents to develop to the six- to eight-cell stage *in vitro*.

Several studies using perifollicular blood flow measurement demonstrated that each fully grown follicle has a unique blood flow characteristic and perifollicular capillary bed development.[2,5,6] Therefore, color-pulsed Doppler ultrasonography can detect differences between follicles that by conventional ultrasound appear to be equivalent.

Results from studies in which follicles were divided according to the degree of vascularization show that a significant fraction of fully grown follicles are poorly vascularized. Some have no detectable perifollicular blood flow, whereas for others perifollicular circulation appears to be limited to one region of the follicle. At the same time, other follicles from the same ovary appear well vascularized. In recent studies,[2,5] pregnancy rates of 60% and >50%, respectively, were reported when the embryos transferred derived from well-vascularized follicles; no pregnancies occurred when all of the transferred embryos originated from poorly vascularized follicles. Van Blerkom[7,8] described significant differences in the occurrence of spindle defects and the frequency of aneuploidy if oocytes were derived from well (<5%) or poorly (>35%) vascularized follicles. Bhal *et al.* stated that these results support the concept that embryo developmental potential is largely determined by intrafollicular influences that can be detected by analysis of perifollicular vascularity.[9]

Bhal *et al.* studied vascular perfusion using a grading system based on the percentage of follicular circumference (grade 1 <25%, grade 2 <50%, grade 3 <75% and grade 4 >75%) that depicted an echo signal. A total of 1285 follicles were studied, of which 64% were of high (3 or 4) and 36% were low (1 or 2) grade vascularity.

TABLE 1. Pregnancy rates from two groups of transferred embryos

	Group A	Group B
Transfers	41	34
Pregnancies (%)	14 (34)*	4 (13.7)*
Singletons	10	4
Twins	4	0
Abortions (%)	1 (7)	0

*$p < 0.05$

Mean follicular diameter, oocyte retrieval rate, number of mature oocytes recovered, and fertilization rates were all significantly higher ($p < 0.05$) and triploidy rate significantly lower ($p < 0.05$) from the cohort of follicles with high-grade vascularity. No correlation between embryo morphology and vascularity grade was found. The pregnancy rate for cycles where the embryos transferred were derived from follicles with uniformly high-grade (3 or 4 only) vascularity was significantly higher than for those cycles where the embryos transferred were derived from mixed (1 to 4) or low (1 or 2 only) grade follicles (34% versus 18%; $p < 0.05$).

OUR EXPERIENCE

Women up to 38 years of age were included in this study. The stimulation protocol was as previously described.[10] On the day of oocyte retrieval, each woman underwent a transvaginal Doppler ultrasound scan. The vascularity of each follicle was subjectively graded. Seventy-five patients undergoing assisted reproduction treatments in our center agreed to using Power Doppler imaging. The grading system was based on the percentage of vascularization of the follicle circumference according to Chui et al.[2]

Patients were divided into two subgroups: (A) 41 patients receiving embryos originating from oocytes derived from follicles graded 3 or 4 and (B) 34 patients receiving embryos originating from oocytes derived from follicles graded 1 or 2. A maximum of two embryos was replaced with the aim of avoiding a high rate of twin and triplet pregnancies.

Our results are summarized in TABLE 1. We found a statistically higher pregnancy rate in group A, for which the embryos transferred originated from oocytes grown in follicles with high grades of vascularization.

CONCLUSIONS

Our data show the same results already described in the literature; they are a further suggestion that perifollicular vascularization may play a role in the developmental competence of the oocyte after fertilization. The possibility of studying the degree of vascularization with Power Doppler ultrasonography makes the procedure relatively easy to perform. If the data are confirmed with increased test cases, it appears reasonable that in the future embryos originating from oocytes developed in well-vascularized follicles will be the first priority for transfer.

REFERENCES

1. ZACKIRISSON, U., *et al.* 1996. Ovulation rate in the rat is decreased by acute ligation of the ovarian artery or the ovarian branch of the uterine artery (abstract). Biol. Reprod. **54:** 68.
2. CHUI, D.K.C., *et al.* 1997. Follicular vascularity—the predictive value of transvaginal power Doppler ultrasonography in an in-vitro fertilization programme: a preliminary study. Hum. Reprod. **12:** 191–196.
3. CAMPBELL, S., *et al.* 1993. Transvaginal color blood flow imaging of the periovulatory follicle. Fertil. Steril. **60:** 433–438.
4. GAULDEN, M. 1992. The enigma of Down syndrome and other trisomic conditions. Mutat. Res. **269:** 69–88.
5. VAN BLERKOM, J., *et al.* 1997. The developmental potential of human oocyte is related to the dissolved oxygen content of follicular fluid: association with vascular endothelial growth factor levels and perifollicular blood flow characteristics. Hum. Reprod. **12:** 1047–1055.
6. NURGUND, G., *et al.* 1996. Association between ultrasound indices of follicular blood flow, oocyte recovery and preimplantation embryo quality. Hum. Reprod. **11:** 109–113.
7. VAN BLERKOM, J. 1997. Can the developmental competence of early human embryos be predicted effectively in the clinical IVF laboratory? Hum. Reprod. **12:** 1610–1614.
8. VAN BLERKOM, J. 1998 Epigenetic influences on oocyte developmental competence: perifollicular vascularity and intrafollicular oxygen. J. Assist. Reprod. Genet. **15:** 226–234.
9. BHAL, P.S., *et al.* 1999. The use of transvaginal power Doppler ultrasonography to evaluate the relationship between perifollicular vascularity and outcome in in-vitro fertilization treatment cycles. Hum. Reprod. **14:** 939–945.
10. BORINI, A., *et al.* 1996. Oocyte donation programme: results obtained with intracytoplasmic sperm injection in cases of severe male factor infertility or previous failed fertilization. Hum. Reprod. **11:** 548–550.

Role of Steroid Hormone–Regulated Genes in Implantation

INDRANI C. BAGCHI, QUANXI LI, AND YONG PIL CHEON

The Population Council, 1230 York Avenue, New York, New York 10021, USA

ABSTRACT: The endometrium acquires the ability to implant the developing embryo within a specific time window, termed the "receptive phase." During this period, the endometrium undergoes pronounced structural and functional changes induced by the ovarian steroids, estrogen and progesterone, which prepare it to be receptive to invasion by the embryo. These steroid-induced molecules, when identified, may serve as useful markers of uterine receptivity. In this article, we provide a brief description of one such molecule that has emerged as candidate marker of steroid hormone action in rats and humans during implantation.

KEYWORDS: endometrium; ovarian steroids; estrogen; progesterone; uterine receptivity; calcitonin

INTRODUCTION

Initiation of implantation leading to the establishment of pregnancy results from the culmination of a series of complex interactions between the developing embryo and the uterus.[1–4] Although the details of implantation vary in different species, the basic features of the blastocyst attachment and penetration of the uterine surface epithelium are common to many mammals. It is generally believed that the embryo–uterine interactions leading to implantation can only succeed when embryonic development is synchronized with the preparation of the uterus to the receptive state. Typically, this means that the embryos have reached the blastocyst stage and that the endometrium has undergone certain hormone-dependent changes during a specific time window in the preimplantation phase that prepare it to be receptive to the developing blastocyst.

UTERINE RECEPTIVITY

The concept of an "implantation window" or "receptive endometrium" was initially established in rodents. In the rat, the fertilized embryo reaches the uterus on

Current address for correspondence: Indrani C. Bagchi, Department of Veterinary Biosciences, University of Illinois at Urbana/Champaign, 2001 S. Lincoln, Urbana, IL 61802. Voice: 217-333-7986; fax: 217-244-1652.

ibagchi@uiuc.edu

day 4 of pregnancy, and implantation occurs in the afternoon of day 5.[5–7] Studies by Psychoyos demonstrated that rat uterus can accept the blastocyst to implant only for a brief period of time on day 5 of gestation, known as the receptive phase.[5–7] The uterus enters a nonreceptive phase on the following day (day 6), when it is refractory to implantation. In humans, the ovum is fertilized in the fallopian tube, arrives in the uterine cavity around day 17 (day 14 is taken as day of ovulation of a 28-day cycle), and remains there as a free-floating embryo until about day 19; implantation then occurs between day 19 to 22.[8–12] The precise timing and molecular basis of the receptive window in the human remain undefined.

STEROID HORMONES REGULATE EMBRYO IMPLANTATION

The specific modifications leading to acquisition of the receptive state of the uterus are regulated by a timely interplay of the maternal steroid hormones, estrogen and progesterone.[5,6] It is known that the completion of a hormonal sequence of progesterone and estrogen action in rats is achieved by day 4 of gestation, resulting in the creation of a receptive uterine state that allows implantation on day 5.[1] In the rat the level of progesterone is low during the estrous cycle, increases markedly after fertilization, and remains high until the end of gestation.[13,14] The circulating level of estrogen is high in nonpregnant animals at estrus stage. After fertilization, the level of estrogen declines and remains low throughout gestation, except for a transitory rise in estrogen level that occurs on day 4 of pregnancy.[15] This transitory rise in estrogen, termed nidatory estrogen, is essential for embryo implantation in rodents. Steroid hormones also regulate uterine receptivity in the human. In the first half of the menstrual cycle during the proliferative phase, the level of estrogen is high. Following ovulation in the later half of the cycle, progesterone is the dominant hormone.[16] The endometrium undergoes pronounced morphological and physiological alteration in response to these hormones. Estrogen initiates hypertrophy and hyperplasia of endometrial epithelia. Progesterone transforms this prepared endometrium into a secretory tissue and creates an environment within the uterine milieu that is conducive to embryo attachment.[1–4,16] Although previous research has established that estrogen and progesterone regulate the events leading to implantation, relatively little is known of the molecular mechanisms through which these hormones promote uterine receptivity. Steroid hormones act through their intracellular receptors, which are ligand-inducible gene regulatory factors.[17–19] It is therefore likely that steroids trigger the expression of a unique set of genes during the early stages of pregnancy and that these eventually lead to synthesis of new proteins that prepare the uterus to accept the invading blastocyst. To investigate the molecular basis of the hormonal regulation of uterine receptivity and implantation, we sought to identify the genes whose expression in the uterus temporally coincides with the steroid hormone surge at the preimplantation phase of pregnancy. By employing differential gene expression screening techniques, we isolated a number of putative implantation stage-specific genes.[20,21] One of these genes has been identified by DNA sequence analysis as that for calcitonin.

EXPRESSION OF CALCITONIN IN THE RECEPTIVE
ENDOMETRIUM DURING IMPLANTATION

Calcitonin, a 32 amino acid peptide hormone, has long been known to be synthesized and secreted primarily by the parafollicular C cells of the thyroid gland.[22–25] Its most well-characterized physiological role is to regulate calcium levels in bone and kidney cells. In response to hypercalcemia, the C cells release calcitonin rapidly, which in turn lowers blood calcium by inhibiting osteoclast activity and thereby reducing bone resorption and remodeling.[22–25] The hormone is also present, although in miniscule amounts, in tissues such as lung, liver, intestine, pituitary, and the central nervous system (CNS).[26,27] The precise site of synthesis and function of calcitonin in these tissues remains unknown. Its wide distribution throughout the body, including the CNS, and its presence in animals that have no bony skeleton suggest that calcitonin may possess other properties in addition to its action in bones.[28] The common denominator in the various physiological actions of calcitonin could well be the modulation of calcium flux across the membranes of a number of different types of cells, and thus of the intracellular–extracellular distribution of calcium in various systems.

Our studies revealed the uterus as a novel site of calcitonin synthesis. The level of uterine calcitonin mRNA in cycling rats is low (less than 1% of the mRNA present in the thyroid gland) but rises dramatically (to about 10–20% of that synthesized by the thyroid gland) during the preimplantation phase of gestation.[29,30] The expression of the calcitonin gene increases by day 2 (post fertilization) of gestation and reaches

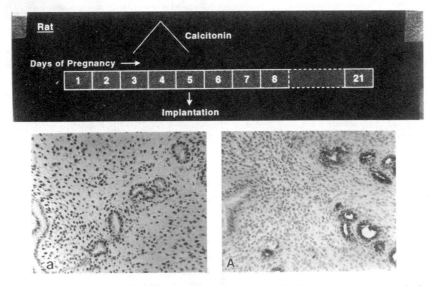

FIGURE 1. *Upper panel*: The profile of expression of calcitonin in rat uterus during early pregnancy. *Lower panel*: Immunocytochemistry was performed employing polyclonal rabbit anti-rat calcitonin using sections from day 4 pregnant rat uterus. **Panel a**: Control sections of day 4 pregnant uterus incubated with preimmune serum. **Panel A**: Immunostaining of calcitonin in uterine sections from day 4 pregnant animals.

a peak on day 4, the day before implantation. On day 5, the day implantation occurs, the expression of the gene starts to decline; and by day 6, when implantation is completed, the calcitonin level falls to below detection limits.[30] The transient burst of calcitonin expression at the time of implantation is restricted to the glandular epithelial cells of the endometrium (FIG. 1). In immunocytochemical experiments as well as in *in situ* hybridization analysis, no significant calcitonin mRNA or protein signal has been detected in the stromal cells or in the myometrium.[31] We also detected significant amounts of calcitonin in the luminal secretions collected on days 4–5 of gestation, indicating that this hormone is secreted from its glandular site of synthesis immediately preceding implantation.[31] Collectively, these observations lead us to propose that calcitonin is a measurable marker that forecasts the receptive state of rat endometrium during blastocyst implantation.

Our recent studies in the human also suggest that calcitonin is an excellent candidate marker of uterine receptivity during implantation. We observed that calcitonin mRNA and protein is expressed in the glandular epithelial cells of the human endometrium during the postovulatory mid-secretory phase (days 17–25) of the menstrual cycle with maximal expression occurring between days 19 and 21.[32] Very little calcitonin expression was detected in the endometrium, either in the preovulatory proliferative (days 5–14) or in the late secretory (days 26–28) phase. The timing and location of its synthesis in the glands prompt us to speculate that, as in the rat, calcitonin is secreted into the uterine lumen at the time of implantation in the human, and its principal function may be to regulate blastocyst implantation in a paracrine manner (FIG. 2).

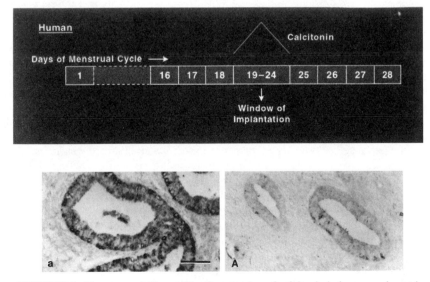

FIGURE 2. *Upper panel*: The profile of expression of calcitonin in human endometrium during the menstrual cycle. *Lower panel*: Immunohistochemistry was performed with endometrial sections in the mid-secretory phase (day 20) employing a polyclonal rabbit anti-human calcitonin antibody. **Panel a**: Immunostaining of calcitonin in endometrial sections at day 20 of the menstrual cycle. **Panel A**: Control endometrial sections at day 20 of the menstrual cycle incubated with preimmune serum.

PROGESTERONE AND ESTROGEN REGULATE CALCITONIN
EXPRESSION IN THE UTERUS DURING IMPLANTATION

Calcitonin expression in the uterus is regulated by progesterone. Treatment of ovariectomized rats with progesterone leads to a 20-fold increase in the synthesis of calcitonin.[29] In pregnant rats, the rise in calcitonin expression on day 2 of gestation coincides with the surge in circulating progesterone level following fertilization. Previous studies indicated that serum progesterone concentration increases at least threefold on day 2 of pregnancy.[13,14] The level of progesterone rises further on day 4 and remains high until term.[14] The fact that progesterone is indeed an inducer of calcitonin gene expression in the uterus during pregnancy is confirmed by experiments employing the antiprogestin drug RU486.[29,32] In rodents and humans, treatment with RU486 during early pregnancy disrupts progestational action and terminates pregnancy.[33,34] Treatment of pregnant rats during the preimplantation stage (day 3) with a single dose of RU486 abolishes calcitonin expression within 24 hours.[29] Similarly, administration of RU486 in women drastically reduces calcitonin expression in the endometrium.[32] It is believed that RU486 exerts its inhibitory effects by impairing the gene regulatory activity of the progesterone receptor.[35,36] It is, therefore, likely that progesterone influences calcitonin gene transcription. Consistent with this prediction, it was observed that cotransfection of progesterone receptor and a reporter gene linked to a 1.3-kb fragment of calcitonin promoter into human endometrial Ishikawa cells led to a significant progesterone-dependent enhancement of reporter gene expression.[31] These results indicate that the regulatory effects of progesterone is indeed exerted at the level of transcription of the calcitonin gene.

Estrogen has no significant effect on calcitonin gene expression when administered alone to ovariectomized rats. In ovariectomized animals, it has been shown that administration of estrogen together with progesterone inhibits progesterone-mediated calcitonin gene induction.[29] Such antagonistic interactions between estrogen and progesterone pathways have been documented previously in breast and uterine cells.[37,38] It has been proposed that these phenomena reflect transcriptional cross-talk occurring between estrogen and progesterone receptors coexpressed in the same target tissue.[37,38] During pregnancy in the rat, the circulating levels of estrogen do not change on day 2 after fertilization, increase sharply on the evening of day 4, decline again by day 5 of pregnancy, and remain low throughout gestation until term.[15] It is interesting to note that the transient surge of estrogen on the evening of day 4 of pregnancy is coincident with the decline in calcitonin expression. To understand how the interplay of progesterone and estrogen through their respective nuclear receptors may regulate calcitonin promoter function, the expression of calcitonin in a delayed implantation model was analyzed. It is observed that in the absence of estrogen, progesterone alone stimulates calcitonin mRNA synthesis.[31] Continued administration of this hormone maintains calcitonin expression in the glands, while the embryo remains free-floating but viable.[31] Administration of estrogen, which triggers implantation, also reduces the progesterone-mediated enhancement of calcitonin expression.[31] These events, therefore, mimic the physiological pattern of calcitonin expression during early pregnancy. These results suggest that a complex interplay of the two ovarian hormones, progesterone and estrogen, in the uterine milieu is critical for optimal calcitonin gene expression.

CALCITONIN PLAYS A CRITICAL ROLE DURING IMPLANTATION

One way of investigating the biological role of calcitonin during implantation is by analyzing a calcitonin-deficient mutant mouse model system. Surprisingly, however, calcitonin production is not induced in the mouse uterus at the time of implantation. Therefore, to understand the role of calcitonin in rat uterus, an alternative approach was undertaken whereby calcitonin gene expression was blocked by using antisense ODNs targeted against calcitonin mRNA. Administration of antisense oligodeoxynucleotides (ODNs), targeted specifically against calcitonin mRNAs, into the lumen of the preimplantation-phase uterus resulted in a dramatic reduction in the number of implanted embryos.[39] Similar treatment with the corresponding sense ODNs exhibited no effect on implantation. The antisense ODN intervention also markedly suppressed the steady-state level of the calcitonin mRNA and protein in the uterus, without affecting the expression of nontarget genes.[39] These results strongly suggest that a transient expression of calcitonin in the preimplantation rat uterus is crucial for blastocyst implantation.

REGULATION OF CELLULAR FUNCTION BY CALCITONIN AND ITS RECEPTOR

The emergence of calcitonin as a candidate marker of uterine receptivity in both rat and human makes it important to study the mechanism of signal transduction by this hormone during embryo–uterine interactions. Intracellular signaling by calcitonin is initiated upon binding of this peptide hormone to its specific receptor on the target cell.[40] Previous studies have shown that binding of calcitonin to its receptor on the target cell leads to a rise in intracellular calcium and cAMP, which in turn regulate cellular functions.[41–43] To analyze the signaling pathway of calcitonin in the endometrium, we investigated the ability of calcitonin to regulate cellular functions in the Ishikawa endometrial cell line, which harbors abundant calcitonin receptors. Our studies showed that binding of calcitonin to its cell surface receptor elicits a transient rise in intracellular calcium level (Q. Li and I. Bagchi, unpublished observation). An alteration in intracellular calcium is known to control adhesiveness of epithelial cells by changing the expression or triggering redistribution of critical cell adhesion molecules or junctional complexes. E-cadherin is a cell surface glycoprotein that mediates calcium-dependent cell–cell adhesion and is critical in the establishment and maintenance of adherent junctions in epithelial cells.[44,45] We observed that calcitonin-dependent elevation of intracellular calcium in Ishikawa cells leads to the disappearance of E-cadherin from cell–cell contact sites. Our studies further revealed that calcitonin treatment of Ishikawa cells results in downregulation of E-cadherin mRNA. We next investigated whether the expression of calcitonin in rat uterine tissue during implantation influences expression of E-cadherin mRNA. In pregnant rats, uterine epithelial cells expressed a high level of E-cadherin mRNA during the first three days of gestation, while the calcitonin level remained low. Concomitant with a transient rise in calcitonin level during days 4–5 of pregnancy, there was a marked decline in the level of E-cadherin mRNA on these days. Consistent with this observation, administration of exogenous calcitonin to animals on day 2 of pregnancy triggered a premature downregulation of E-cadherin mRNA level. On the basis of these *in vitro* and *in vivo* studies, we favor the hypothesis that elevation of calcitonin in endometrial cells leads to downregulation of E-cadherin, which in turn results in relaxation of adherent junctions between epithelial cells, facilitating implantation of the blastocyst.

CALCITONIN: A POTENTIAL MARKER OF UTERINE RECEPTIVITY

The peptide hormone calcitonin is currently being evaluated as a potential marker of the fertile human endometrium. An ideal marker of uterine receptivity should fulfill a number of important criteria. It should be present in the endometrium, preferably in the surface epithelium near the site of implantation. It is also possible that a marker or effector of the receptive endometrium might be synthesized in the glandular epithelium and secreted at or near the implantation sites at the appropriate time. It should appear within the window of implantation or precede it by a certain amount of time and disappear with the termination of the receptive phase. The marker should be present in the nonconception cycle independent of embryo-derived signals. Most importantly, an appropriate marker should also have a unique biological function during the implantation process.

In light of the implantation stage-specific expression of uterine calcitonin in species as diverse as rat and human, this hormone displays the potential to serve as a dependable marker of the endometrium that is receptive for blastocyst implantation. Studies using antisense ODNs have shown that calcitonin is critical for implantation. Studies have also shown that a possible function of this hormone is to downregulate E-cadherin in order to relax the adherent junctions between the epithelial cells to facilitate the invasion of the embryo during implantation. More importantly, the fact that calcitonin is synthesized in the endometrial glands allows us to speculate that it might be secreted into the human uterine lumen. This scenario, if validated by future experiments, may permit the development of sensitive methods (such as radioimmunoassay) for detection of this hormone in uterine secretions or other body fluids of the human. This will give calcitonin a clear advantage over other potential markers of uterine receptivity that are not secretory proteins. From a clinical point of view, this finding will have important implications for *in vitro* fertilization/embryo transfer (IVF/ET) procedures. Despite the recent progress in reproductive techniques, the majority of IVF attempts end in failure, as endometrial receptivity remains one of the rate-limiting factors in the establishment of a successful pregnancy in this setting. The timely transfer of embryos fertilized *in vitro* to the recipient uterus for successful implantation in IVF depends on the ability to evaluate whether and when the endometrium is receptive and able to support the implantation. There is, therefore, an urgent need in this field for measurable markers indicative of the receptive state of human endometrium. The identification of a marker, such as calcitonin, may assist in the diagnosis of female infertility due to failure of implantation and facilitate management of clinical therapy for affected women.

ACKNOWLEDGMENTS

The research summarized in this article was supported by research grants HD-34527, HD-39291, and HD-34760 (National Cooperative Program on Markers of Uterine Receptivity for Blastocyst Implantation) from NIH. We thank Dr. M. K. Bagchi for his valuable comments and criticisms of the work.

REFERENCES

1. PSYCHOYOS, A. 1973. Endocrine control of egg implantation. *In* Handbook of Physiology. R.O. Greep & E.G. Astwood, Eds.: 187–215. American Physiological Society. Washington, DC.
2. YOSHINAGA, K. 1988. Uterine receptivity for blastocyst implantation. Ann. N.Y. Acad. Sci. **541:** 424–431.
3. PARR, M.B. & E.L. PARR. 1989. The implantation reaction. *In* Biology of the Uterus. R.M. Wynn & W.P. Jollie, Eds.: 233–277. Plenum Press. New York.
4. WEITLAUF, H.M. 1994. Biology of implantation. *In* The Physiology of Reproduction. E. Knobil & J.D. Neill, Eds.: 391–440. Raven Press. New York.
5. PSYCHOYOS, A. 1973. Hormonal control of ovoimplantation. Vitam. Horm. **31:** 205–255.
6. PSYCHOYOS, A. 1976. Hormonal control of uterine receptivity for nidation. J. Reprod. Fertil. Suppl. **25:** 17–28.
7. PSYCHOYOS, A. 1986. Uterine receptivity for nidation. Ann. N.Y. Acad. Sci. **476:** 36–42.
8. HERTIG, A.T., J. ROCK & E.C. ADAMS. 1956. A description of 34 human ova within the first 17 days of development. Am. J. Anat. **98:** 435–493.
9. FORMIGLI, L., G. FORMIGLI & C. ROCCIO. 1987. Donation of fertilized uterine ova to infertile women. Fertil. Steril. **47:** 62–65.
10. ROGERS, P.A.W. & C.R. MURPHY. 1989. Uterine receptivity for implantation: human studies. *In* Blastocyst Implantation. K. Yoshinaga, Ed.: 231–238. Serono Symposia. Norwell, MA.
11. NAVOT, D.M., T.L. ANDERSON, K. DROESCH, *et al.* 1989. Hormonal manipulation of endometrial maturation. J. Clin. Endocrinol. Metab. **68:** 801–807.
12. NAVOT, D.M., R.T. SCOTT, K. DROESCH, *et al.* 1991. The window of embryo transfer and the efficiency of human conception in vitro. Fertil. Steril. **55:** 114–117.
13. KALRA, S.P. & P.S. KALRA. 1974. Temporal interrelationships among circulating levels of estradiol, progesterone and LH during the rat estrous cycle: effects of exogenous progesterone. Endocrinology **95:** 1711–1718.
14. WIEST, W.G. 1970. Progesterone and 20α–Hydroxypregn-4-en-3-one in plasma, ovaries and uteri during pregnancy in the rat. Endocrinology **87:** 43–48.
15. YOSHINAGA, K., R.A. HAWKINS & J.F. STOCKER. 1969. Estrogen secretion by the rat ovary in vivo during the estrous cycle and pregnancy. Endocrinology **85:** 103–112.
16. STRAUSS, J.F. & E. GURPIDE. 1991. The endometrium: regulation and dysfunction. *In* Reproductive Endocrinology. S.S.C. Yen & R.B. Jaffe, Eds.: 309–356. W.B. Saunders. Philadelphia.
17. EVANS, R.M. 1988. The steroid and thyroid hormone receptor superfamily. Science **240:** 889–895.
18. BEATO, M. 1989. Gene regulation by steroid hormones. Cell **56:** 335–344.
19. TSAI, M.J. & B.W. O'MALLEY. 1994. Molecular mechanisms of action of steroid/thyroid receptor superfamily members. Annu. Rev. Biochem. **63:** 451–486.
20. WANG, Z. & D.D. BROWN. 1991. A gene expression screen. Proc. Natl. Acad. Sci. USA **88:** 11505–11509.
21. LIANG, P. & A.B. PARDEE. 1992. Differential display of eukaryotic messenger RNA by means of polymerase chain reaction. Science **257:** 967–971.
22. FRIEDMAN, J. & L.G. RAISZ. 1965. Thyrocalcitonin: inhibitor of bone resorption in tissue culture. Science **150:** 1465–1467.

23. FOSTER, G.V. 1968. Calcitonin (thyrocalcitonin). N. Engl. J. Med. **279:** 349–360.
24. AUSTIN, L.A. & H. HEATH. 1981. Calcitonin. N. Engl. J. Med. **304:** 269–278.
25. WIMALAWANSA, S.J. 1990. Calcitonin: molecular biology, physiology, pathophysiology and its therapeutic uses. *In* Advances in Bone Regulatory Factors: Morphology, Biochemistry, Physiology and Pharmacology. A.A.B. Pecile, Ed.: 121–160. Plenum Press. England.
26. BECKER, K.L., R. SNIDER, C.F. MOORE, *et al.* 1979. Calcitonin in extrathyroidal tissues of man. Acta Endocrinol. (Copenhagen) **92:** 746–751.
27. FISCHER, J.A., P.H. TOBLER, M. KAUFMANN, *et al.* 1981. Calcitonin: regional distribution of the hormone and its binding sites in the human brain and pituitary. Proc. Natl. Acad. Sci. USA **78:** 7801–7805.
28. COPP, D.H. 1982. Modern view of the physiological role of calcitonin in vertebrates. *In* The Effects of Calcitonin in Man: Proceedings of the First International Workshop in Florence, Italy. C. Gennari & G. Segre, Eds.: 3–12.
29. DING, Y.Q., L.J. ZHU, M.K. BAGCHI & I.C. BAGCHI. 1994. Progesterone stimulates calcitonin gene expression in the uterus during implantation. Endocrinology **135:** 2265–2274.
30. DING, Y.Q., M.K. BAGCHI, C.W. BARDIN & I.C. BAGCHI. 1995. Calcitonin gene expression in the rat uterus during pregnancy. Rec. Progr. Horm. Res. **50:** 373–378.
31. ZHU, L.J., K.C. BOVE, M. POLIHRONIS, *et al.* 1998. Calcitonin is a progesterone-regulated marker which forecasts the receptive state of endometrium during implantation. Endocrinology **139:** 3923–3934.
32. KUMAR, S., L.Z. ZHU, M. POLIHRONIS, *et al.* 1998 Calcitonin is a progesterone-regulated marker of uterine receptivity for implantation in the human. J. Clin. Endocrinol. Metab. **83:** 4443–4450.
33. PHILIBERT, D., M. MOGUILEWSKY, I. MARY, *et al.* 1985. Pharmacological profile of RU 486 in animals. *In* The Antiprogestin Steroid RU 486 and Human Fertility Control. Plenum Press. New York.
34. SITRUK-WARE, R., L. BILLAUD, I. MOWSZOWICA, *et al.* 1985. The use of RU 486 as an abortifacient in early pregnancy. *In* The Antiprogestin Steroid RU 486 and Human Fertility Control. E.E. Baulieu & S.J. Segal, Eds.: 243–248. Plenum Press. New York.
35. BAULIEU, E.E. 1989. Contragestion and other clinical applications of RU 486, an antiprogesterone at the receptor. Science **245:** 1351–1357.
36. BAULIEU, E.E. 1991. The antisteroid RU 486: its cellular and molecular mode of action. Trends Endocrinol. Metab. **2:** 233–239.
37. KIRKLAND, J.L., L. MURTHY & G.M. STANCEL. 1992. Progesterone inhibits the estrogen-induced expression of c-fos messenger ribonucleic acid in the uterus. Endocrinology **130:** 3223–3230.
38. KRAUS, W.L. & X. KATZENELLENBOGEN. 1993. Regulation of progesterone receptor gene expression and growth in the rat uterus: modulation of estrogen action by progesterone and sex steroid hormone antagonists. Endocrinology **132:** 2371–2379.
39. ZHU, L.J., M.K. BAGCHI & I.C. BAGCHI. 1998. Attenuation of calcitonin gene expression in pregnant rat uterus leads to a block in embryonic implantation. Endocrinology **139:** 330–339.
40. MARX, S.J., C.J. WOODWARD & G.D. AURBACH. 1972. Calcitonin receptors of kidney and bone. Science **178:** 999–1001.
41. CHABRE, O., B.R. CONKIN, H.Y. LIN, *et al.* 1992. A recombinant calcitonin receptor independtly stimulates $3',5'$-cyclic adenosine monophosphate and Ca^{2+}/inositol phosphate signaling pathways. Mol. Endocrinol. **6:** 551.
42. FORCE, T., I.V. BONVENTRE, M.R. FLANNERY, *et al.* 1992. A cloned porcine renal calcitonin receptor couples to adenyl cyclase and phospholipase C. Am. J. Physiol. **262:** F1110–F1115.
43. HEERSCHE, J.N.M., R. MARCUS & G.D. AURBACH. 1974. Calcitonin and the formation of $3',5'$-AMP in bone and kidney. Endocrinology **94:** 251.
44. POTTER, E., C. BERGWITZ & G. BRABANT. 1999. The cadherin–catenin system: implications for growth and differentiation of endocrine tissues. Endocr. Rev. **20:** 207–239.
45. GUMBINAR, B.M. 2000. Regulation of cadherin adhesive activity. J. Cell. Biol. **148:** 399–404.

Decidual Cell-Expressed Tissue Factor Maintains Hemostasis in Human Endometrium

CHARLES J. LOCKWOOD, GRACIELA KRIKUN, AND FREDERICK SCHATZ

Department of Obstetrics and Gynecology, New York University School of Medicine, New York, New York 10016, USA

ABSTRACT: We showed that decidualized stromal cells of luteal phase and pregnant human endometrium express tissue factor (TF), the primary initiator of hemostasis, thereby suggesting a mechanism by which perivascular decidual cells can mitigate the risk of hemorrhage during endovascular trophoblast invasion. Progestins enhanced TF mRNA and protein levels in monolayers of human endometrial stromal cells (HESCs), with estradiol (E_2) + progestin, further enhancing TF levels despite a lack of response to E_2 alone. This differential ovarian steroid response has been found for several decidualization markers. Further studies with cultured HESCs established that elevated TF levels are mediated by the progesterone receptor and are maintained for weeks in response to E_2 plus progestin, thus simulating the chronic upregulation of TF levels observed in decidualized HESCs *in vivo*. Recent studies revealed that elevated TF expression during *in vitro* decidualization of HESCs involved both the EGFR and progesterone receptor. Thus, enhancement of TF mRNA and protein levels in the HESCs required co-incubation with a progestin (MPA) and an EGFR agonist such as EGF or TGF-α. In correspondence with co-elevation of EGFR and TF in decidualized HESCs in sections of luteal phase and pregnant endometrium, EGFR levels proved to be progestin-enhanced in the cultured HESCs. We established that progestin-enhanced TF expression in HESCs was trancriptionally regulated, then evaluated the relative roles of SP and EGR-1 sites on the TF promoter in regulating this expression. Transient transfections with a series of promoter constructs containing overlapping SP and EGR-1 sites and with constructs in which the EGR-1 and SP sites were systematically inactivated by site-directed mutagenesis established the dominance of SP sites in both basal and progestin-enhanced TF transcriptional activity. Additional experiments involving transient transfections with SP1overexpressing vectors and with a specific blocker of if Sp1 binding to its corresponding GC box specified the importance of the Sp1 transcription factor. These results were further validated by immunostaining, which revealed that the ratio of Sp1 to Sp3 increased during progestin-regulated decidualization of HESCs *in vitro* and *in vivo*. The absence of canonical estrogen and progesterone response elements from either the TF or Sp1 gene promoters suggests that the EGFR may help to mediate progestin-enhanced TF expression during decidualization of HESCs.

KEYWORDS: tissue factor; human endometrium; hemostasis; human endometrial stromal cells

Address for correspondence: Charles J. Lockwood, M.D., Professor and Chairman, Department of Obstetrics and Gynecology, New York University School of Medicine, 550 First Avenue, New York, NY 10016. Voice: 212-263-8579; fax: 212-263-5742.

schatf01@popmail.med.nyu.edu

INTRODUCTION

Decidual Cells Are Positioned to Modulate Endometrial Hemostasis during Human Implantation

Progesterone stimulates the estrogen-primed human endometrium to undergo decidualization, the process of growth and differentiation that transforms precursor stromal cells into decidual cells. Decidualization begins around blood vessels of the midluteal-phase endometrium. Under the continued influence of estradiol (E_2) and progesterone, the decidualization reaction spreads throughout the late luteal phase and gestation.[1] Implantation is initiated by attachment of the blastocyst to the uterine luminal epithelium. Subsequently, syncytiotrophoblasts invade the underlying endometrial stromal compartment. They breach capillaries and venules that are enmeshed in stromal cells at various stages of decidualization to establish the primordial utero-placental circulation. Extravillous cytotrophoblasts then penetrate the uterine spiral arteries and initiate morphological changes that increase intervillous blood flow.[2] These processes provide the developing embryo with essential oxygen and nutrients before placentation.[3] They risk decidual hemorrhage, however, which can lead to spontaneous abortion, placental abruption, and preterm birth.[4-6] In species with a hemochorial placenta, the degree of trophoblast invasiveness is positively corrrelated with the extent of decidualization with human trophoblasts and human endometrium, respectively, displaying the most invasiviness and most extensive decidualization.[7] Moreover, the association of ectopic pregnancy with hemorrhage is highest in species lacking a true decidua. Their localiziation at perivascular sites postions decidual cells to promote local hemostasis, thus counteracting the threat of hemorrhage during endovascular trophoblast invasion and subsequent remodeling of endometrial blood vessels.

Decidual Cell-Expressed Tissue Factor Modulates Endometrial Hemostasis

Previous work in our laboratory demonstrated that decidualized stromal cells in sections of luteal-phase and gestational endometium displayed enhanced immunohistochemical staining for tissue factor (TF),[8,9] a cell membrane–bound glycoprotein (46 kDa) and a member of the class 2 cytokine receptor family. TF is composed of a hydrophilic extracellular domain, a membrane-spanning hydrophobic domain, and a cytoplasmic tail.[10-12] Upon exposure to blood, perivascular cell-bound TF binds to factor VII. Cleavage of factor VII to VIIa by thrombin, factor IXa, or Xa increases its activity 100-fold, thereby accelerating the hemostatic process. The TF–factor VIIa complex can directly or indirectly activate factor X and thence generate thrombin.[13-15]

Studies in embryonic lethal TF knock-out mice confirmed that the expression of TF by decidualized endometrial stromal cells is crucial in maintaining decidual hemostasis. These mice die *in utero* from hemorrhage and development of fragile vessels.[16] Rescue of the TF-knockout embryos by incorporation of the human TF minigene expressed at approximately 1% of wild-type levels resulted in live-born pups. However, almost half of the pregnancies in which both mother and fetus were homozygotic, low TF expressors were associated with multiple intrauterine hemorrhages and intraplacental "blood pools" in the labyrinth, leading to fatal hemorrhage. About 20% of these mice also suffered fatal postpartum hemorrhage, irrespective of embryonic genotype.[17,18]

TF is expressed by mesenchymal and epithelial cells of several tissues including placental villous stromal cells.[19,20] Under physiological conditions, TF is not expressed by cells in contact with the circulation such as endothelial and trophoblast cells. However, expression of TF by perivascular decidual cells is positioned to create a hemostatic "envelope" that prevents hemorrhage during endovascular trophoblast invasion and subsequent remodeling of the vasculature.

TF Expression Is Enhanced during in Vitro Decidualization of Human Endometrial Stromal Cells

The relationship between TF expression and decidualization was evaluated in monolayers of stromal cells isolated from specimens of cycling human endometrium. Progestins affect the expression of several *in vivo* decidualization markers in these cultures. These include prolactin,[21] insulin-like growth factor binding protein-1,[22,23] the ECM proteins fibronectin and laminin,[24,25] and plasminogen activator (PA) inhibitor type-1 (PAI-1),[26] which are elevated. By contrast, the proteases uPA, tPA,[26] stromelysin-1,[27,28] and interstitial collagenase[29] are inhibited. The human endometrial stromal cell (HESC) monolayers are refractory to E_2 alone. However, E_2 augments these effects when added with progestins. These changes simulate the differential effects elicited by ovarian steroids *in vivo*, whereby E_2 primes the endometrium for the decidualizing effects of progestins by enhancing progesterone receptor levels.[30,31] These results therefore validate HESCs as a relevant decidualization model.

In cultured cells derived from diverse tissues, cytokines, growth factors, and serum transiently enhance TF mRNA and protein levels (1–4 hours).[32–37] However, we observed that TF expression in HESC monolayers in response to the progestin medroxyprogesterone acetate (MPA) was upregulated for several days.[8] Moreover, co-incubation with E_2 plus MPA extended the induction period to at least three weeks,[38] thereby mimicking the chronic induction of TF expression observed in decidualized stromal cells of late luteal phase and pregnant endometrium.[8,9] That this process is mediated by the progesterone receptor was confirmed by observations that the glucocorticoid dexamethasone did not affect TF expression, whether added alone or with E_2, and that both RU486 and the the purer antiprogesterone onapristone blocked progestin-induced TF mRNA and protein levels in cultured HESCs.[39]

RESULTS

To elucidate mechanisms underlying the novel chronic upregulation of TF expression during decidualization, cultured HESCs were used to investigate (1) the role of progestin–growth factor interactions in the regulation of TF and (2) the molecular level of this regulation.

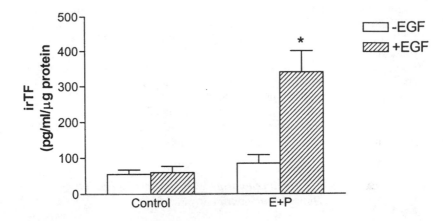

FIGURE 1. Effects of EGF and steroids on immunoreactive (ir) TF levels. HESCs were incubated for 4 days in basal medium plus 10% stripped calf serum[8] containing either vehicle control or 10^{-8} mol/l E_2 (E) + 10^{-7} mol/l MPA (P), and then exposed to the corresponding control or E + P with or without 50 ng/ml EGF in a defined medium[38] for 36 hours. Cell-associated TF measured by ELISA and normalized to cell protein in 10 separate experiments. * control (±EGF) versus E + P + EGF ($p < 0.0001$). (From Lockwood et al.[44] Reprinted with permission.)

Progestin–Growth Factor Interactions Regulate TF Expression in Cultured HESCs

The published sequence of the TF gene promoter lacks estrogen and progesterone response elements, suggesting that autocrine and/or paracrine factors mediate steroid effects on TF expression. In HESC monolayers, progestin–epidermal growth factor (EGF) interactions regulate growth, prolactin, and extracellular matrix protein expression.[40] The cellular effects of EGF are initiated by binding to the cell surface-sequestered EGF receptor (EGFR), which is a structural homologue of the c-ErbB oncogene protein product.[41] Ligand binding induces the EGFR to homodimerize or to form heterodimers with other EGF/ErbB receptor family members. Consequently, complex intracellular gene-activating phosphorylation pathways are triggered.[42,43]

Paracrine and/or Steroid Effects on HESC-Expressed TF

FIGURE 1 displays the separate and interactive effects of EGF and E_2 plus MPA on TF expression in confluent HESCs. Incubating the cultures with EGF together with E_2 plus MPA elicited a statistically significant sevenfold increase in immunoreactive TF levels. By contrast, neither EGF alone, nor the steroids added without EGF, affected TF levels. Consistent with the differential response to E_2 and progestins revealed by our previous studies,[38] TF levels were enhanced when EGF was added with MPA, but not with E_2. Northern blot analysis indicated that elevation of TF mRNA levels also required co-incubation with progestin and EGF. Moreover, transforming growth factor–α (TGF-α), which binds to and activates the EGFR with affinity similar to EGF,[42] replaced EGF in upregulating TF expression. Unlike the EGFR agonists, nei-

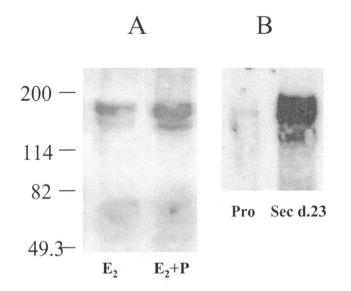

FIGURE 2. EGFR levels in cultured HESCs, and endometrial biopsies. (A) Conflu-ent cultures were maintained in basal medium plus 10% stripped calf serum[44] with either 10^{-8} mol/l E_2 or 10^{-8} mol/l $E_2 + 10^{-7}$ mol/l MPA (P) for 4 days. The medium was removed; and the cells were washed with HBSS, harvested, and analyzed by Western blotting for the presence of EGFR. Densitometric comparisons in cultures derived from three specimens in-dicated an increase of 253% ± 94 (mean ± SEM) in HESCs from three specimens treated with E_2 plus MPA versus E_2. (From Lockwood *et al.*[44] Reprinted with permission.) **(B)** Western blotting for the EGFR in extracts from proliferative phase (Pro), day 23 secretory phase (d23), and 9-week gestational endometrium.

ther transforming growth factor–β (TGF-β, nor interleukin-1 β (IL-1β) affected TF expression in the cultured HESCs whether added alone or with E_2 plus MPA. The lack of binding of these agents to the EGFR further emphasizes the involvement of the EGFR in elevating TF levels during progestin-regulated decidualization.[44]

Progestin Effects on HESC-Expressed EGFRs

Recently, we observed an association between an increase in immunohistochem-ical (IHC) EGFR levels in the stromal cells of specimens of cycling and gestational endometrium and progestin-enhanced decidualization.[45] To study direct progestin effects on stromal cell–expressed EGFR, confluent HESCs were incubated in paral-lel with E_2 or with E_2 + MPA, and Western blot analysis was carried out to detect the presence of the EGFR. FIGURE 2A demonstrates that the HESCs contain a doublet at 170 kDa that corresponds to the EGFR. Moreover, its magnitude increased two- to threefold in incubations with E_2 plus MPA compared with E_2 alone. The results shown in FIGURE 2B are consistent with previous reports that EGFR levels are much higher in endometrial extracts from the secretory than from the proliferative phase.[46,47]

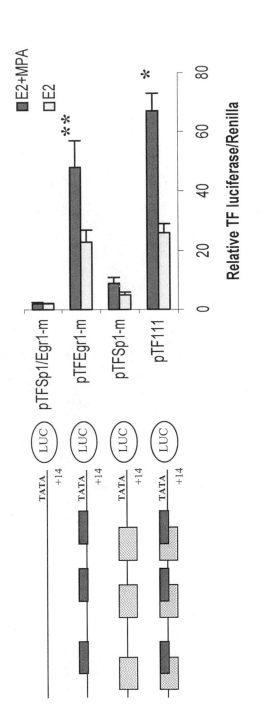

FIGURE 3. Transfection of mutant TF promoters. Cultured HESCs were treated with E_2 or E_2 +MPA. Transfections were carried out with the minimal TF promoter −111 to +14 bp (pTF111) and with promoters mutated in the three Sp1 (pTFSp1-m), the three Egr-1 (pTFEgr1-m), or all six Sp1 and Egr-1 (pTFSp1/Egr1-m). A schematic of these is shown on the left. Levels of luciferase activity were corrected for transfection efficiency ($n = 9$, triplicates from three separate experiments). *$p < 0.0001$, comparing E_2 vs. E_2 + MPA for pTF111 and **$p < 0.002$ comparing E_2 vs. E_2 + MPA for pTFEgr1-m. (From Krikun et al.[50] Reprinted with permission.)

Molecular Level of Regulation of TF Expression in HESCs

The transient upregulation of TF expression that characterizes several cell types is reportedly under transcriptional control.[32–37] Therefore, we questioned whether a similar mechanism mediated the uniquely prolonged enhancement of TF expression elicited by progestins in the cultured HESCs. Message stability studies revealed that MPA did not affect turnover of TF mRNA, thus ruling out progestin-mediated inhibition of TF mRNA degradation.[48] The alternative possibility that MPA increased transcription of TF mRNA was evaluated by transiently transfecting HESC monolayers with TF promoter constructs. In these experiments, cultures were incubated in parallel with E_2 and with E_2 plus MPA in a serum-containing medium. The former was used as a control condition to simulate estrogen priming of the stromal cells for the decidualizing effects of the progestin. Moreover, since serum contains several EGFR agonists, the EGFR is presumed to be maximally stimulated during the transient transfections.

In several cell types, control of TF expression involves several regulatory sites on the TF gene promoter including AP-1, Egr-1, and those for the SP family.[49] Transient transfections of HESCs were carried out with a series of truncated TF promoter constructs. FIGURE 3 indicates that both basal (E_2) and progestin (E_2 + MPA) mediated upregulatory effects are retained following transfection with a luciferase-linked "minimal wild-type promoter" construct (pTF 111), which contains three overlapping Sp1 and Egr-1 sites.[50] FIGURE 3 also extends this basic finding by examining the effects of site-directed mutagenesis of the Sp1 and Egr-1 sites on progestin-enhanced TF transcription. Thus, promoter activity observed with pTF Egr1-m, in which all three Egr-1 sites were mutated, is similar to that of the the wild-type pTF 111 promoter in response to both E_2 and to E_2 + MPA. By contrast, promoter activity is significantly reduced during incubation with either E_2 or E_2 + MPA after transfection with promoter constructs in which the three Sp1 sites are mutated, either alone (pTF Sp1-m) or together with the three Egr-1 sites (pTF Sp1/Egr1-m).

In view of the involvement of Sp1 in regulating TF expression suggested by FIGURE 3, confluent HESCs were incubated with medium containing vehicle control, E_2, or E_2 + MPA with and without 10 nM mithramycin, an inhibitor of Sp1 binding to its corresponding GC box. FIGURE 4 reveals that mithramycin abrogated the progestin induction of TF mRNA levels, which further supports the role of Sp1 in enhanced TF expression by HESCs. Moreover, co-transfection with vectors overexpressing Sp1 mRNA enhances TF promoter activity, while overexpression of its antagonist, Sp3, had no effect alone and inhibited the action of Sp1 overexpression.[50] That the ratio of Sp1 to Sp3 is important in progestin-enhanced TF expression was further indicated by immunostaining for the presence of these transcription factors. These results showed that the ratio of Sp1 to Sp3 was increased during progestin-regulated decidualization *in vitro*, as well as in decidualized stromal cells *in vivo*.[50]

DISCUSSION

Previous studies from our laboratory suggested that decidual cell-expressed TF, the primary initiator of hemostasis, could prevent hemorrhage during endovascular

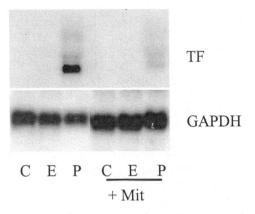

FIGURE 4. Effect of mithramycin on progestin induction of TF mRNA expression.
Control (C), E_2 (E), or E_2+MPA (P) treated HESCs were incubated with and without 10 nM mithramycin (Mit). Northern blots were performed for TF, and loading efficiencies were assessed with glyceraldehyde 3-phosphate dehydrogenase (GAPDH). (From Krikun et al.[50] Reprinted with permission.)

invasion by implanting syncytiotrophoblasts. Thus, TF protein and mRNA levels, as determined by immunohistochemical staining and *in situ* hybridization,[8,51] respectively, were elevated in decidualized stromal cells in sections of luteal phase and gestational endometium. TF expression was also augmented during progestin-initated decidualization of stromal cell monolayers (HESCs) derived from specimens of cycling endometrium. Progestins alter the expression of several *in vivo* decidualization markers in the cultured HESCs. Because of its stability in culture, we have used MPA in these experiments. Although the HESCs are refractory to E_2 alone, the responses to MPA are enhanced when the cultures are incubated with MPA and E_2. Thus, this well-characterized decidualization model mimics the differential actions of ovarian steroids *in vivo*, in which E_2 enhances progesterone receptor levels,[30,31] thereby priming the endometrium for the decidualizing effects of progestins. Accordingly, TF mRNA and protein levels are elevated by progestins, but not by E_2, whereas TF expression was further elevated by incubating the HESCs with progestins plus E_2.[8,38]

The characteristically transient (order of hours) upregulation of TF expression elicited by cytokines, growth factors, and serum in various cell types[32–37] contrasts with the several-day augmentation of TF expression elicited by MPA in HESCs. This period was increased to weeks by incubating the HESCs with E_2 plus MPA.[38] The latter simulates both the elevated circulating levels of E_2 and progesterone and the chronic increase of TF expression observed in decidualized stromal cells of the secretory-phase and pregnant endometrium.[8,9] Subsequent studies in which steroid specificity and the effects of antiprogestins were evaluated[39] implicated the progesterone receptor in the uniquely prolonged enhancement of TF expression in the HESCs elicited by progestins.

The reported involvement of EGF–progestin interactions in controlling the expression of decidualization-related endpoints in the HESC monolayers[40] prompted evaluation of the separate and interactive effects of EGF and progestin on TF expression in these cells. Initial results established the co-involvement of both the EGFR and progsterone receptor in mediating this TF upregulation. Thus, enhancement of TF mRNA and protein levels required incubation of the HESCs with a progestin (MPA) together with an EGFR agonist such as EGF or TGF-α. Moreover, neither TGF-β nor IL-1β could substitute for an EGFR agonist despite the general effectivness of growth factors and cytokines in enhancing TF expression in an array of cell types. Additional *in vitro* observations taken together with *in vivo* results indicated that enhancement of TF expression in HESCs was linked to a decidualization-related increase in EGFR expression. Thus, EGFR levels, as determined by Western blotting, were found to be progestin-enhanced in the cultured HESCs.[44] Finally, IHC measurements indicated that the EGFR and TF are coordinately upregulated in stromal cells undergoing decidualization in luteal-phase and pregnant endometrium.[8,45]

Our initial studies determined that progestin enhancement of TF expression in HESCs involves trancriptional control. Subsequently, several lines of evidence stressed the regulatory role played by the Sp family of transcription factors in the uniquely prolonged enhancement of TF expression during decidualization of HESCs. First, transfection of HESCs with a series of truncated TF promoter constructs showed that basal and progestin-elevated TF promoter activity was retained by a construct containing overlapping SP and EGR-1 sites. Second, mutation of the SP sites virtually eliminated basal and progestin-enhanced transcriptional activity, whereas these were unaffected by mutation of the EGR-1 sites. Third, a specific inhibitor of Sp1 binding to its corresponding GC box inhibited progestin induction of TF mRNA levels. Fourth, co-transfection with overexpressing Sp1 mRNA vectors enhanced TF promoter activity, whereas overexpression of its anatgonist, Sp3, was ineffective alone and inhibited the effects of overexpressed Sp1.[50] Finally, immunostaining for the presence of the Sp family of transcription factors indicated an increase in the ratio of Sp1 to Sp3 during progestin-regulated decidualization *in vitro* and *in vivo*.[50]

In summary, our recent studies reveal that progestin-elicited decidualization of HESCs involves enhancement of EGFR levels as well as a shift in the ratio of the Sp family of transcription factors (Sp1 and Sp3) in favor of Sp1. The absence of canonical estrogen and progesterone response elements from either the TF or Sp1 gene promoters suggests the importance of carrying out experiments in the presence of varying concentrations of EGFR agonists.

ACKNOWLEDGMENTS

This work was supported in part by grants from the National Institutes of Health, 5RO1 HL33937-06 (CJL), and from the NIH General Clinical Research Center, M01 RR00096.

REFERENCES

1. BELL, S.C. 1990. Decidualization and relevance to menstruation. *In* Contraception and Mechanisms of Endometrial Bleeding. C. D'Arcangues, I.S. Fraser, J.R. Newton & V. Odlind, Eds.: 188. Cambridge University Press. Cambridge, U.K.

2. DE WOLF, F., C. WOLF-PEETERS & I. BROSENS. 1973. Ultrastructure of the spiral arteries in the human placental bed at the end of normal pregnancy. Am. J. Obstet. Gynecol. **117:** 833–848.
3. MOORE, K.L. 1988. The Developing Human, 4th ed. W.B. Saunders. Philadelphia, PA.
4. EDMONDS, D.K., K.S. LINDSAY, J.F. MILLER, et al. 1982. Early embryonic mortality in women. Fertil. Steril. **38:** 447–453.
5. McCORMICK, M.C. 1985. The contribution of low birth weight to infant mortality and childhood morbidity. N. Engl. J. Med. **312:** 82–90.
6. STROBINO, B. & J. PANTEL-SILVERMAN. 1989. Gestational vaginal bleeding and pregnancy outcome. Am. J. Epidemiol. **129:** 806–815.
7. RAMSEY, E.M., M.L. HOUSTON & J.W. HARRIS. 1976. Interactions of the trophoblast and maternal tissues in three closely related primate species. Am. J. Obstet. Gynecol. **124:** 647–652.
8. LOCKWOOD, C.J., Y. NEMERSON, S. GULLER, et al. 1993. Progestational regulation of human endometrial stromal cell tissue factor expression during decidualization. J. Clin. Endocrinol. Metab. **76:** 231–236.
9. LOCKWOOD, C.J., G. KRIKUN, C. PAPP, et al. 1994. The role of progestationally regulated stromal cell tissue factor and type-1 plasminogen activator inhibitor (PAI-1) in endometrial hemostasis and menstruation. Ann. N.Y. Acad. Sci. **734:** 57–79.
10. NEMERSON, Y. 1988. Tissue factor and hemostasis. Blood **71:** 1–8.
11. GUHA, A., R. BACH, W. KONIGSBERG & Y. NEMERSON. 1986. Affinity purification of human tissue factor: interaction of factor VII and tissue factor in detergent micelles. Proc. Natl. Acad. Sci. USA **83:** 299–302.
12. BACH, R.R. 1988. Initiation of coagulation by tissue factor. C.R.C. Crit. Rev. Biochem. **23:** 339–368.
13. HAGEN, F.S., C.L. GRAY, P. O'HARA, et al. 1986. Characterization of a cDNA coding for human factor VII. Proc. Natl. Acad. Sci. USA **83:** 2412.
14. ZUR, M., R.D. RADCLIFFE, J. OBERDICK & Y. NEMERSON. 1982. The dual role of factor VII in blood coagulation. J. Biol. Chem. **257:** 5623–5631.
15. CARMELIET, P. & D. COLLEN. 1998. Tissue factor. Int. J. Biochem. Cell Biol. **30:** 661–667.
16. CARMELIET, P., N. MACKMAN, L. MOONS, et al. 1996. Role of tissue factor in embryonic blood vessel development. Nature **383:** 73–75.
17. PARRY, G.C., J.H. ERLICH, P. CARMELIET, et al. 1998. Low levels of tissue factor are compatible with development and hemostasis in mice. J. Clin. Invest. **101:** 560–569.
18. ERLICH, J.H., G.C. PARRY, C. FEARNS, et al. 1999. Tissue factor is required for uterine hemostasis and maintenance of the placental labyrinth during gestation. Proc. Natl. Acad. Sci. USA **96:** 8138–8143.
19. DRAKE, T.A., J.H. MORRISSEY & T.S. EDGINGTON. 1989. Selective cellular expression of tissue factor in human tissues. Am. J. Pathol. **134:** 1087–1112.
20. FAULK, W.P., C.A. LABARRERE & S.D. CARSON. 1990. Tissue factor: identification and characterization of cell types in human placentae. Blood **76:** 86–96.
21. HUANG, J.R., L. TSENG, P. BISCHOF & O.A. JANNE. 1987. Regulation of prolactin production by progestin, estrogen, and relaxin in human endometrial stromal cells. Endocrinology **121:** 2011–2017.
22. GIUDICE, L.C., D.A. MILKOWSKI, G. LAMSON, et al. 1991. Insulin-like growth factor binding proteins in human endometrium: steroid-dependent messenger ribonucleic acid expression and protein synthesis. J. Clin. Endocrinol. Metab. **72:** 779–787.
23. BELL, S.C., J.A. JACKSON, J. ASHMORE, et al. 1991. Regulation of insulin-like growth factor-binding protein-1 synthesis and secretion by progestin and relaxin in long term cultures of human endometrial stromal cells. J. Clin. Endocrinol. Metab. **72:** 1014–1024.
24. IRWIN, J.C., D. KIRK, R.J.B. KING, et al. 1989. Hormonal regulation of human endometrial stromal cells in culture: an in vitro model for decidualization. Fertil. Steril. **52:** 761–768.
25. ZHU, H.H., J.R. HUANG, J. MAZELA, et al. 1992. Progestin stimulates the biosynthesis of fibronectin and accumulation of fibronectin mRNA in human endometrial stromal cells. Hum. Reprod. **7:** 141–146.

26. SCHATZ, F., C. PAPP, S. AIGNER, *et al.* 1995. Plasminogen activator activity during decidualization of human endometrial stromal cells is regulated by plasminogen activator inhibitor 1. J. Clin. Endocrinol. Metab. **80:** 2504–2510.
27. SCHATZ, F., C. PAPP, E. TOTH-PAL & C.J. LOCKWOOD. 1994. Ovarian steroid-modulated stromelysin-1 expression in human endometrial stromal and decidual cells. J. Clin. Endocrinol. Metab. **78:** 1467–1472.
28. OSTEEN, K.G., W.H. RODGERS, M. GAIRE, *et al.* 1994. Stromal–epithelial interaction mediates steroidal regulation of metalloproteinase expression in human endometrium. Proc. Natl. Acad. Sci. USA **91:** 10129–10133.
29. LOCKWOOD, C.J., G. KRIKUN, V. HAUSKNECHT, *et al.* 1998. Matrix metalloproteinase and matrix metalloproteinase inhibitor expression in endometrial stromal cells during progestin-initiated decidualization and menstruation-related progestin withdrawal. Endocrinology **139:** 4607–4613.
30. LUBBERT, H., K. POLLOW, A. ROMMLER & J. HAMMERSTEIN. 1982. Estradiol and progesterone receptor concentrations and 17β-hydroxysteroid-dehydrogenase activity in estrogen–progestin-stimulated endometrium of women with gonadal dysgenesis. J. Steroid Biochem. **17:** 143–148.
31. ECKERT, R.L. & B.S. KATZENELLENBOGEN. 1981. Human endometrial cells in primary tissue culture: modulation of the progesterone receptor level by natural and synthetic estrogens *in vitro*. J. Clin. Endocrinol. Metab. **52:** 699–708.
32. CUI, M.Z., G.C.N. PARRY, P. OETH, *et al.* 1996. Transcriptional regulation of the tissue factor gene in human epithelial cells is mediated by SP1 and EGR-1. J. Biol. Chem. **271:** 2731–2739.
33. DONOVAN-PELUSO, M., L.D. GEORGE & A.C. HASSET. 1994. Lipopolysaccharide induction of tissue factor expression in THP-1 monocytic cells, protein–DNA interactions with the promoter. J. Biol. Chem. **269:** 1361–1369.
34. FELTS, S.J., E.S. STOFLET, C.T. EGGERS & M.J. GETZ. 1995. Tissue factor gene transcription in serum-stimulated fibroblasts is mediated by recruitment of c-fos into specific AP-1 DNA-binding complexes. Biochemistry **34:** 12355–12362.
35. GALDAL, K.S., T. LYBERG, S.A. EVENSEN, *et al.* 1985. Thrombin induces thromboplastin synthesis in cultured vascular endothelial cells. Thromb. Haemost. **54:** 373–376.
36. BARTHA, K., C. BRISSON, G. ARCHIPOFF, *et al.* 1993. Thrombin regulates tissue factor and thrombomodulin mRNA level and activities in human saphenous vein endothelial cells by distinct mechanisms. J. Biol. Chem. **268:** 421–429.
37. OETH, P.A., G.C.N. PARRY, C. KUNSCH, *et al.* 1994. Lipopolysaccharide induction of tissue factor gene expression in monocytic cells is mediated by binding of c-Rel/p65 heterodimers. Mol. Cell. Biol. **14:** 3772–3781.
38. LOCKWOOD, C.J., Y. NEMERSON, G. KRIKUN, *et al.* 1993. Steroid-modulated stromal cell tissue factor expression: a model for the regulation of endometrial hemostasis and menstruation. J. Clin. Endocrinol. Metab. **77:** 1014–1019.
39. LOCKWOOD, C.J., G. KRIKUN, C. PAPP, *et al.* 1994. Biological mechanisms underlying RU 486 clinical effects: inhibition of endometrial stromal cell tissue factor content. J. Clin. Endocrinol. Metab. **79:** 786–790.
40. IRWIN, J.C., W.H. UTIAN & R.L. ECKERT. 1991. Sex steroids and growth factors differentially regulate the growth and differentiation of cultured human endometrial stromal cells. Endocrinology **129:** 2385–2392.
41. CARPENTER, G. 1987. Receptor for epidermal growth factor and other polypeptide mitogens. Annu. Rev. Biochem. **56:** 881–914.
42. TANG, P., P.A. STECK & A. YUNG. 1997. The autocrine loop of TGFα/EGFR and brain tumors. J. Neurol. Oncol. **35:** 303–314.
43. RIESE II, D.J. & D.F. STERN. 1998. Specificity within the EGF family/ErbB receptor family signaling network. BioEssays **20:** 41–48.
44. LOCKWOOD, C.J., G. KRIKUN, R. RUNIC, *et al.* 2000. Progestin–epidermal growth factor regulation of tissue factor expression during decidualization of human endometrial stromal cells. J. Clin. Endocrinol. Metab. **85:** 297–301.
45. LOCKWOOD, C.J. 2001. Regulation of plasminogen activator inhibitor1 expression during decidualization of human endometrial stromal cells. Am. J. Obstet. Gynecol. **184:** 798–805.

46. IMAI, T., H. KURACHI, K. ADACHI, et al. 1995. Changes in epidermal growth factor receptor and levels of its ligands during menstrual cycle in human endometrium. Biol. Reprod. **52:** 928–938.
47. WANG, D.P., S. FUJI, I. KONISHI, et al. 1992. Expression of c-erbB-2 protein and epidermal growth factor receptor in normal tissues of the female reproductive tract and in the placenta. Virchows Arch. [A] **420:** 385–393.
48. KRIKUN, G., F. SCHATZ, N. MACKMAN, et al. 1998. Transcriptional regulation of the tissue factor gene by progestins in human endometrial stromal cells. J. Clin. Endocrinol. Metab. **83:** 926–930.
49. MACKMAN, N. 1997. Regulation of the tissue factor gene. Thromb. Haemost. **78:** 747–754.
50. KRIKUN, G., F. SCHATZ, N. MACKMAN, et al. 2000. Regulation of tissue factor gene expression in human endometrium by transcription factors Sp1 and Sp3. Molec. Endocrinol. **14:** 393–400.
51. RUNIC, R., F. SCHATZ, L. KREY, et al. 1997. Alterations in endometrial stromal cell tissue factor protein and messenger ribonucleic acid expression in patients experiencing abnormal uterine bleeding while using Norplant-2 contraception. J. Clin. Endocrinol. Metab. **82:** 1983–1988.

Design and Conduct of Clinical Trials in Hormone Replacement Therapy

CHRISTIAN F. HOLINKA

PharmConsult, New York, New York 10013, USA

ABSTRACT: Postmenopausal hormone replacement therapy represents an area of outstanding importance in preventive medicine that greatly affects personal well-being as well as public health. The number of women living in the United States who are 50 years or older has been estimated at nearly 50 million.[1] Many of those women are likely to be eligible for postmenopausal hormone replacement, which may consist either of estrogen replacement therapy (ERT) in women without a uterus or, more frequently, estrogen/progestin combination therapy (HRT) in women with a uterus. This chapter first presents an overview of general regulatory requirements pertaining to the design and conduct of clinical studies in support of marketing approval for a drug product. These requirements include, but are not restricted to, studies in HRT. The chapter next discusses the design and conduct of clinical trials in support of marketing approval for the indications: treatment of moderate to severe vasomotor symptoms and vulvovaginal atrophy; prevention of osteoporosis; and protection by adjunctive progestin against estrogen-induced endometrial hyperplasia/cancer in women with a uterus. Finally, data related to the potential cardioprotective action of HRT and its protection against Alzheimer's disease and colon cancer are discussed.

KEYWORDS: hormone replacement therapy; estrogen replacement therapy; preventive medicine; clinical trial design

REGULATION OF DRUG DEVELOPMENT

The Investigational New Drug Application

Before the initiation of clinical trials in the United States, a sponsor must submit an Investigational New Drug Application (IND) to the Food and Drug Administration (FDA). This application is based on a successful preclinical development program that includes the evaluation of a drug's toxic and pharmacologic effects *in vitro* and *in vivo* in laboratory animals. The IND is not an application for marketing approval. Legally, it represents a request for exemption from the federal statute that forbids unapproved drugs from being shipped in interstate commerce. Its principal scientific purpose is a detailed presentation of data to show that a potential new compound exhibits biological activity, that it is reasonably safe for initial use in human trials, and that it justifies commercial development. Such documentation includes data from three broad areas: animal pharmacology and toxicology studies that sup-

Address for correspondence: Christian F. Holinka, PharmConsult, P.O. Box 1544, New York, New York 10013-1544. Voice: 212-727-8156; fax: 212-352-1566.
holinka@worldnet.att.net

port reasonable safety for initial testing in humans; information pertaining to the composition of the compound, its manufacture, stability, and controls used for manufacturing the drug substance and drug product; and clinical protocols. The protocols for initial clinical studies must be sufficiently detailed to allow an assessment of safety in the early exposure of humans to the investigational compound. Information on the qualification of the investigators, usually physicians, who oversee the administration of the experimental compound must be included in the IND.

During the IND review process by the FDA's Center for Drug Evaluation and Research (CDER), the medical reviewer evaluates the potential overall clinical development plan and, specifically, the initial clinical trial protocol(s) to determine that the study participants are not exposed to unnecessary risks and that the study design will provide data relevant to the safety (and effectiveness) of the drug. Federal regulations require that the initial (Phase 1) studies are reviewed almost exclusively for safety. During the 30-day protocol review process, CDER decides whether patients would be exposed to unnecessary risks, or whether the data submitted in the IND are insufficient to make such a decision. If CDER does not notify the sponsor within 30 days, the trial may proceed as submitted. Alternatively, the sponsor is notified that the study has been placed on clinical hold, and the reasons for this decision are provided. Once an IND is approved, the sponsor is required to submit annual safety updates for all studies conducted under that IND.

In addition to commercial INDs submitted primarily by pharmaceutical companies with the goal to obtain marketing approval for a new product, there is a broad category of noncommercial INDs, including Emergency Use INDs and Treatment INDs. The latter are intended to make promising new drugs available as early as possible to desperately ill patients and to those who suffer from immediately life-threatening diseases.

The New Drug Application

A New Drug Application (NDA) submitted to the FDA by a commercial sponsor is an extensive file in support of marketing approval for a new drug. In addition to clinical data from Phase 1 to Phase 3 studies documenting the safety and efficacy of a new drug, the NDA presents a broad spectrum of information, which includes drug chemistry, manufacturing and control data; nonclinical pharmacology and toxicology data; human pharmacology and pharmacokinetics data; methods of statistical evaluation; the proposed labeling; patent information; and all relevant publications reported in the professional literature. The FDA reviewers of each area prepare a written evaluation that presents their conclusions and their recommendations on the application. The FDA division director or office director evaluates the reviews and recommendations and decides on the action. An action letter is issued containing one of three decisions: the NDA is approved; is approvable pending additional requirements; or is nonapprovable; the letter also presents a justification for each recommendation. The process from the submission of an NDA to its approval usually takes up to one year.

The Institutional Review Board and Informed Consent

Before the recruitment of subjects, each study must be reviewed by an Institutional Review Board (IRB) to ensure the rights and welfare of study volunteers, both before and during their participation in the trial, and to ascertain that volunteers are fully informed about the purpose and the potential risks of the study. To ensure a complete and adequate review of research protocols and activities commonly performed at research institutions, IRBs must be composed of at least five persons of varying backgrounds.

Before entering a study, the volunteer must sign an informed consent form, written in clearly understandable language, which states that the participation in the trial is voluntary and that the subject may refuse to participate and may withdraw from the trial at any time without penalty. The consent form must include a statement on reasonably expected benefits and reasonably foreseeable risks or inconvenience to the subject.

Research Protocols

Each clinical study must be fully defined in a protocol, including a statement on the objective and design of the study, estimated subject numbers, exclusion and inclusion criteria to ensure proper subject selection consistent with the objectives of the study, active treatment periods, drug dosages, and the type of control groups. The protocol must further contain a clear description of the outcomes under investigation and a statistical plan for their analysis; it must describe the means of ensuring the safety of the study participants, such as physical examination, laboratory tests, and other measures to monitor potential adverse effects and minimize the risk to study participants.

PHASES OF CLINICAL TRIALS

The study of a previously untested drug is generally divided into three distinct, although sometimes overlapping, phases. Regarding hormone replacement therapy (HRT), neither estrogens nor progestins represent previously untested drugs, and, therefore, Phase 1 studies should not be necessary, unless new molecular entities are under development. The need for Phase 2 studies may vary and depend on the estrogen/progestin under investigation. In Phase 1, an investigational new drug is initially introduced in humans after appropriate preclinical trials. The closely monitored studies are designed to determine the metabolic and pharmacologic actions of the drug and its metabolism, and to monitor side effects associated with increasing doses; these studies are usually, but not always, conducted in healthy volunteers rather than in patients for whom the drug may eventually be indicated. Phase 1 studies may require between 20 and 80 subjects. Their results are expected to yield sufficient information about the drug to permit the design of well-controlled scientific Phase 2 trials.

Phase 2 of drug development includes early, well-controlled trials, usually requiring several hundred subjects with the disease or condition for which the drug is proposed to be indicated. Phase 2 studies usually provide for the administration of the experimental drug at various dose levels. They are designed to obtain safety information and preliminary efficacy data, including some information on the lowest effective dose.

Phase 3 studies are large safety and efficacy trials designed on the basis of Phase 2 study results. Phase 3 studies are conducted in support of the indication for the experimental drug in the patient population for which the drug is targeted. The detailed analysis of efficacy and safety data from Phase 3 studies represents a major part of the NDA.

CLINICAL TRIALS IN HORMONE REPLACEMENT THERAPY

Design of Clinical Trials: Treatment of Vasomotor Symptoms and Vulvovaginal Atrophy

To collect data for marketing approval of an HRT product for the indication of treatment of vasomotor symptoms, United States regulatory authorities require two Phase 3 studies in highly symptomatic postmenopausal women who experience at least seven to eight moderate to severe hot flushes a day. These are randomized, double-blind studies monitoring vasomotor symptoms over a treatment period of at least three months on the basis of daily recordings of subjectively evaluated hot flushes, perspiration, and waking episodes. One study should be placebo controlled.[2] The second study may compare symptoms at the end of treatment with those at baseline, or with those observed during parallel treatment with an approved comparator drug. Vaginal responses to estrogen are evaluated by the maturation index, that is, shifts in epithelial cells of the lateral vaginal wall from immature (parabasal) to mature (superficial) cells.

Hormone Replacement Therapy and the Prevention of Osteoporosis

Osteoporosis, a pathophysiological condition characterized by diminished bone mass, deteriorating bone architecture, and subsequent skeletal fractures, represents a global public health problem of major proportions. The morbidity and mortality associated with osteoporotic fractures are expected to rise worldwide as life expectancy increases and the world population grows from the current six billion to about 8.3 billion by 2025. Apart from the detrimental consequences on quality of life and increased mortality, the annual cost related to complications from osteoporosis is formidable; it was estimated at $13.8 billion in the United States for 1995.

Although men lose bone mass at approximately the same rate following the attainment of peak bone mineral density (BMD), bone loss in women increases dramatically after menopause or ovariectomy. During their lifetimes, women lose about 50% of their trabecular and 30% of their cortical bone. By comparison, men lose about 30% trabecular and 20% cortical bone. The adverse consequences of this accelerated bone loss are compounded by the fact that bone mass in women after the age of 50 is only about two-thirds that of men. A 50-year-old woman has an estimated 15% chance of suffering from a hip fracture during her remaining life.

It is now well known that estrogen replacement therapy prevents bone loss and reduces the incidence of vertebral and hip fractures.[3] A randomized trial of HRT with fractures as the outcome showed a significant reduction in hip and arm fractures in nonosteoporotic, early postmenopausal women during an average follow-up of 4.3 years.[4]

In addition to prevention, promising results in the treatment of osteoporosis have also been reported.[5] Beneficial effects are not restricted to a given type of estrogen, for example, estradiol or conjugated estrogens, nor are they limited to a specific route of administration. Oral as well as transdermal therapy has been found to be effective, whereas treatment with injectable estrogen or implantable estrogen pellets is not recommended.[6] Treatment of patients with established osteoporosis with 0.625 mg/day conjugated equine estrogens (CEE) for two years resulted in significant increases of vertebral bone mass,[7] and transdermal therapy with 0.1 mg 17β-estradiol (E_2) for one year in a double-blind, randomized, placebo-controlled study produced significant increases in BMD in the lumbar spine, mid-radius, and femoral trochanter and yielded a lower vertebral fracture rate.[8] Transdermal E_2 at the low dose of 0.05 mg/day produced increases in vertebral and proximal femur BMD comparable to those observed in the 0.625 mg/day CEE group after 12 to 18 months of treatment,[9] and these favorable changes persisted up to three years of follow-up.[10]

In another study, treatment with transdermal E_2 over the range of 0.025 to 0.1 mg/day produced dose-dependent increases in BMD of the lumbar spine and bone mineral content of the mid-radius; the lowest dose resulted in significant increases at both sites after two years.[11] Treatment for 18 months with oral E_2 at doses of 0.5 mg, 1.0 mg, and 2.0 mg significantly increased spinal trabecular BMD at all doses, including 0.5 mg/day.[12] Similarly, treatment with esterified estrogens (0.3, 0.625, or 1.25 mg/day) for two years produced significant BMD increases in the lumbar spine over the whole range, including the low dose of 0.3 mg/day.[13] These results indicate that bone is highly sensitive to estrogen replacement, even at very low doses.

Although data on the effects of adjunctive progestin are limited, the combination is considered to be probably at least as effective as estrogen therapy.[14]

Design of Clinical Trials: Prevention of Osteoporosis

To document the efficacy of estrogen in the prevention of postmenopausal osteoporosis, one 24-month, double-blind, placebo-controlled clinical Phase 3 trial is required, which should contain three estrogen strengths to identify the lowest effective dose. At least 50 subjects should be randomized to each treatment group.

Bone mineral density, measured by dual-energy x-ray absorptiometry (DEXA), is recognized as the primary efficacy outcome, while changes in biochemical bone markers may serve as supportive information or, when obtained in Phase 2 studies, to identify preliminarily the appropriate doses for Phase 3 studies. Two DEXA measurements should be obtained before start of treatment and thereafter at appropriate intervals, usually every six months. The lumbar spine and the proximal femur are the most relevant skeletal sites to evaluate BMD in HRT studies, but forearm measurements should also be included.[15] Typical effects of HRT on BMD of two skeletal sites are illustrated in FIGURE 1 for oral and transdermal estrogen therapy.[10]

For women with contraindications to hormonal products, effective alternatives to HRT, such as bisphosphonate therapy,[16] are available for the prevention and treatment of postmenopausal osteoporosis.

Effects of Hormone Replacement Therapy on the Endometrium

The untoward postmenopausal physiologic changes (e.g., hot flushes, bone loss) are related to estrogen depletion after the menopause and, consequently, the objective of replacement therapy is the replenishment of estrogen. However, in women

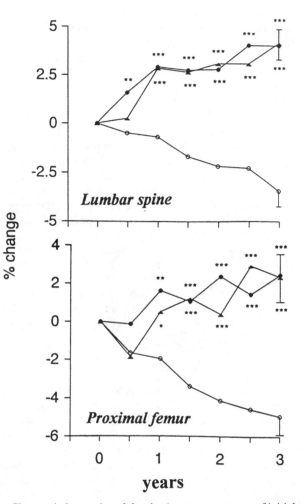

FIGURE 1. Changes in bone mineral density (mean percentages of initial values) in the lumbar spine and proximal femur in response to estrogen treatment. *Open circles*: untreated; *filled circles*: transdermal 17β–estradiol, 0.05 mg/day; *filled triangles*: oral conjugated equine estrogens, 0.625 mg/day. (From Hillard.[10] Reprinted by permission from *Osteoporosis International*.)

with a uterus, adjunctive progestin is indicated to protect against estrogen-induced endometrial cancer. Adjunctive progestin therapy is not appropriate for hysterectomized women.

It was first recognized over 50 years ago that hyperestrogenic states may be associated with endometrial hyperplasia and that hyperplasia may progress to endometrial cancer.[17] Starting in the 1970s, epidemiologic data increasingly showed an association between unopposed estrogen treatment and endometrial adenocarcinoma.[18,19] A number of studies subsequently revealed that the addition of progestins to estrogen therapy substantially reduced the risk of endometrial cancer.[20–22] Three large, population-based, case-control studies estimated the relative risk (RR) in subjects receiving various regimens of estrogen/progestin combination therapy.[23–25] No increased risk was found with use of continuous combined estrogen/progestin[24,25] or, in one study, with sequential regimens that added progestin for at least 10 days each month.[24] In contrast, the other study reported that the addition of progestin for 10 to 21 days was not fully protective; this regimen lowered the RR to 1.3 (95% CI = 0.8, 2.2) in subjects exposed for fewer than 5 years, compared to the fourfold risk observed with unopposed estrogen; with treatment for longer than 5 years, the RR increased to 2.5 (95% CI = 1.1, 5.5).[23] The third study reported a RR of 2.9 (95% CI = 1.8, 4.6) with cyclic regimens (progestin addition for fewer than 16 days, usually for 10 days) used for 5 years or longer. Continuous combined therapy reduced the RR to 0.2 (95% CI = 0.1, 0.8) in that study.[25]

Although there is consensus on the substantial reduction of estrogen-related endometrial cancer risk by adjunctive progestin,[26] quantitative data from a prospective, well-controlled study are needed to identify the optimal regimen and evaluate the extent of protection following long-term HRT use.

Unopposed Estrogen and Endometrial Hyperplasia

Results from several large clinical trials that also contained an unopposed estrogen treatment arm[27–30] are summarized in TABLE 1. These data, as well as those from smaller studies on estrogen-only treatment shown in TABLE 2,[31,32] indicate that estrogen-induced hyperplasia is related to treatment duration as well as dose. Following unopposed estrogen therapy, the incidence of hyperplasia increased with the length of treatment: it rose from 7% to 20%, respectively, after 6 and 12 months of treatment with 0.625 mg CEE in the Woodruff study, and from 20.4% to 28.8%, respectively, after 12 and 24 months of treatment with 0.625 mg esterified estrogens (ESE) in the Notelovitz 1997 study. The cumulative hyperplasia incidence of 62.2% reported in the PEPI study at the end of three years was distributed evenly across the 3-year period.

Treatment with ESE over a dose range of 0.3 mg to 1.25 mg for two years (TABLE 2) revealed a dose-dependent relationship in addition to the treatment-duration effect. The incidence following one year of treatment with 0.625 mg ESE (20.4%) is comparable to that after one year of 0.625 mg CEE therapy (20%) shown in TABLE 1.

These results are consistent with those of two earlier, smaller studies. One of those reported a hyperplasia incidence of 32% in subjects exposed to 1.25 mg CEE (or equivalent doses of other estrogens) for a mean period of 15.8 months and an incidence of 18% in subjects exposed to half that dose.[33] The other study found 15% and 30% hyperplasia after treatment with 0.625 mg CEE for one-half and one year, respectively; and it found 17% and 57% hyperplasia after treatment with 1.25 mg CEE for one-half or one year, respectively.[34] In both studies, the regimens included a drug-free period of 5 to 7 days per monthly cycle. A duration- as well as dose-dependent increase in the incidence of hyperplasia was also reported in a large clinical trial after treatment with ethynyl estradiol in the range of 1 to 10 μg.[35]

Dose-dependent hyperplasia rates were also observed with E_2 treatment in the range of 0.5 mg to 2.0 mg (TABLE 2), although these data should be viewed with caution because of the small numbers. It is noteworthy, however, that hyperplasia in that

TABLE 1. **Incidence of endometrial hyperplasia following treatment with unopposed estrogen, and its prevention by adjunctive progestin**

Study	Regimen estrogen/progestin (mg)		Follow-up (years)	Hyperplasias/ biopsies	Hyperplasia incidence (%)
Woodruff, 1994[27]	CE/MPA	0.625/ 0	0.5	21/298	7
		0.625/2.5 continuous	0.5	1/295	<1
		0.625/5.0 continuous	0.5	0/291	0
		0.625/5.0 cyclic	0.5	1/293	<1
		0.625/10.0 cyclic	0.5	0/292	0
	CE /MPA	0.625/0	1.0	57/283	20
		0.625/2.5 continuous	1.0	2/279	<1
		0.625/5.0 continuous	1.0	0/274	0
		0.625/5.0 cyclic	1.0	3/277	1
		0.625/10.0 cyclic	1.0	0/272	0
PEPI, 1996[28]	Placebo		3.0	2/119	1.7
	CE/MPA	0.625/0	3.0	74/119	62.2
		0.625/2.5 continuous	3.0	1/120	<1
		0.625/10.0 cyclic	3.0	6/118	5.1
	CE/P	0.625/200 cyclic	3.0	6/120	5.0
Corson, 1999[29]	E$_2$/NGM	1/0	1.0	74/265	28
		1/0.030	1.0	16/260	6
		1/0.090	1.0	0/242	0
		1/0.180	1.0	0/243	0
Kurman, 2000[30]	E$_2$/NETA	1/0	1.0	36/246	14.6
		1/0.1	1.0	2/249	<1
		1/0.25	1.0	1/251	<1
		1/0.5	1.0	1/241	<1

study was observed after the short treatment period of three months. Likewise, a short period of estrogen action in the induction of hyperplasia is suggested by a study that found a 14% (4/29 subjects) hyperplasia incidence after treatment with E$_2$ for 70–72 days.[36] However, the interpretation of the results from this study is complicated by treatment with adjunctive progestin in a prior cycle and by escalating doses of E$_2$.

The hyperplasia incidence in the unopposed estrogen groups of the PEPI study was 62.2%, compared to 1.7% in the placebo group. It was made up of 27.7% simple, 22.7% complex, and 11.8% atypical hyperplasia. One case of adenocarcinoma was reported in the placebo group of the PEPI study, and one case each in the unopposed 0.625 CEE group and in the 0.625 mg CEE + 10 mg cyclic MPA group in the Woodruff study.

TABLE 2. Dose and duration effect on the incidence of endometrial hyperplasia following treatment with unopposed esterified estrogens or estradiol

Study		Treatment (mg)	Follow-up	Hyperplasias/ biopsies	Hyperplasia incidence (%)
Notelovitz, 1997[31]	Placebo		1 yr	1/60	1.7
	ESE	0.3	1 yr	1/59	1.7
		0.625	1 yr	12/59	20.4
		1.25	1 yr	26/60	43.3
	Placebo		2 yr	1/60	1.7
	ESE	0.3	2 yr	1/59	1.7
		0.625	2 yr	17/59	28.8
		1.25	2 yr	32/60	53.3
Notelovitz, 2000[32]	Placebo		3 mo	0/19	0
	E_2	0.5	3 mo	1/18	6
		1.0	3 mo	4/27	15
		2.0	3 mo	3/10	30

A study following up 43 women with a uterus for an average of 3.2 years reported 45% hyperplasia,[37] an incidence somewhat lower than that observed in the PEPI study after 3 years. This difference may in part be due to the smaller size of the study or to different review processes (up to three pathologists reviewed slides in the PEPI study). It may also be related to the definition of the threshold for hyperplasia. Some pathologists consider anovulatory persistent proliferative endometrium not distinct from hyperplasia but rather its earliest morphologic manifestation.[34]

Data from studies that reported hyperplastic changes by type suggest that the relative rate of atypical hyperplasia increases with length of exposure to unopposed estrogen: After 3 months of treatment, no atypical hyperplasia was found among 7 cases; after one year of treatment, 2 of 36 hyperplasia cases (5.6%) were atypical in the Kurman study, and 18 of 74 cases (10.8%) were atypical in the Corson study. After 3 years of exposure, 14 of 74 cases (18.9%) were atypical in the PEPI study. Although these numbers are small and must be interpreted accordingly, they suggest a progression toward the more severe type of hyperplasia with increasing length of estrogen exposure.

No endometrial carcinoma was found after three years of exposure to unopposed estrogen in the PEPI study. The absence of cancer is unexpected in light of a report that the relative risk (RR) of endometrial cancer increases by five times in women who had used unopposed estrogen for three years or longer.[21] Another report showed an increase in RR by 2.2 and 2.7 times after exposure for more than 3 years to conjugated estrogens and estradiol, respectively,[20] and a meta-analysis of HRT and endometrial cancer estimated a threefold increase in endometrial cancer risk with unopposed estrogen treatment for 1 to 5 years.[26] The absence of cancer following three years of unopposed estrogen treatment in the PEPI study may reflect the relatively small number of subjects studied, that is, 98 women completed the 3-year follow-up visit.

Protective Effects of Adjunctive Progestin

As illustrated in TABLE 1, different types of adjunctive progestins (medroxyprogesterone acetate, norethindrone acetate, norgestimate) protected against estrogen-induced hyperplasia in several large, well-controlled clinical trials. The table suggests a dose–response relationship in the protective effect in the Woodruff study that was significant ($p < 0.001$) in the Corson study.

Clinical Trials: Endometrial Protection Studies

For marketing approval of an HRT product, regulatory authorities in the United States[2] and Europe[38] accept endometrial hyperplasia as the only valid endpoint in clinical trials designed to evaluate the efficacy of adjunctive progestin to protect against endometrial cancer, although it is likely that not all types of hyperplasia are precursors of cancer[39] and not all cancers are estrogen-dependent.[40,41]

Endometrial protection studies are large, prospective, double-blinded, randomized clinical trials extending over a 1-year treatment period and studying several hundred subjects in each treatment arm. Specific guidance for the study design is available from the Center for Drug Evaluation and Research of the FDA[2] as well as from the European Agency for the Evaluation of Medicinal Products.[38]

Endometrial protection studies are required to document the lowest effective progestin dose that prevents the excess risk of endometrial cancer associated with a specific ERT regimen. In addition to the combination estrogen/progestin treatment arms, one arm of unopposed estrogen at the dose intended for the combination therapy is included in the study.[2] The estrogen-only arm serves as a positive control to measure the hyperplasia-inducing potential of the estrogen type and dose intended for the final HRT product. The principal outcome of the study is hyperplasia (versus its absence). The type of hyperplasia or the varieties of nonhyperplastic endometrial tissues are not considered major endpoints for regulatory purposes.

Histologic samples are evaluated for the presence of hyperplasia by two independent gynecologic pathologists blinded to treatment and to each other's diagnosis. In cases of discordance among the two readers, a third pathologist, also blinded, serves as adjudicator. In those cases, the majority diagnosis is considered final.

Design of Clinical Trials: Safety Assessments

In addition to efficacy, thorough safety evaluations are an essential part of all clinical trials. Strict inclusion/exclusion criteria are applied to determine a volunteer's eligibility for study participation. These criteria are intended to ensure the safety of the study participants, but also to achieve entry characteristics consistent with the evaluation of efficacy. Standard safety assessments in HRT studies include physical and gynecologic examinations, mammography, pap smear, laboratory tests (including hematology, chemistry, and urinalysis). Women with a uterus are closely monitored for endometrial hyperplasia. Prolonged vaginal bleeding in women receiving unopposed estrogen may suggest the presence of hyperplasia, and a biopsy may be indicated in cases of severe or prolonged bleeding. Depending on the type of study, additional metabolic parameters, such as lipid profiles, coagulation factors, or carbohydrate metabolism–related parameters, are frequently evaluated in HRT studies because of potential beneficial or adverse effects of hormones on those parameters.

All treatment-emergent adverse events, whether or not related to the investigational drug, are recorded throughout the study. An adverse event is considered serious if it is fatal or immediately life-threatening, requires or prolongs inpatient hospitalization, causes permanent or significant disability, is the result of an overdose, is a congenital abnormality or cancer, or requires medical or surgical intervention to prevent permanent sequelae.

HORMONE REPLACEMENT THERAPY AND CARDIOPROTECTION

The abject consequences of cardiovascular disease, its associated morbidity and mortality, and the numbers of affected individuals are enormous, and any protective intervention reducing cardiovascular pathology can therefore be expected to result in substantial benefits for large numbers of people.[42] Cardiovascular disease, including stroke, is the major cause of death in the United States. In 1997, 43% of all deaths of women in the United States were due to cardiovascular disease. A 50-year-old woman has a 46% lifetime probability of developing heart disease and a 31% probability of dying from it.[14]

Based on strong and consistent data from a large number of observational studies, estrogen has long been considered to protect against heart disease. Benefits were reported both in primary and secondary prevention, suggesting an estimated reduction of cardiovascular accidents by 50% in current users.[43] The relative risk of death from all-cause mortality as well as from cardiovascular disease was also reduced in estrogen users.[44] Although most studies examined the effects of estrogen alone, the data available on combined estrogen/progestin therapy did not suggest any impairment of the protective estrogen effect on cardiovascular risk. FIGURE 2 presents results from early observational studies showing a substantial reduction in the RR of coronary heart disease (CHD) associated with estrogen treatment.

A large body of additional data has since accumulated in support of the cardioprotective effect of estrogen. In the Nurses' Health Study, the RR of major heart disease in the follow-up of 59,337 women for up to 16 years was estimated to be 0.45 (95% CI = 0.34, 0.60) for current users of oral CEE. After adjustment for cardiovascular risk factors, the RR was 0.60 (95% CI = 0.43, 0.83). The RR of 0.60 in current users increased to 0.69 in women who had discontinued estrogen therapy less than three years earlier, and approached 1.0 after 10 years of discontinuation. The adjusted RR among women who took estrogen with progestin was 0.39 (95% CI = 0.19, 0.78).[45]

Notwithstanding the strong and consistent information from observational studies, we should be cautioned against considering these data derived from nonrandomized studies definitive because of various biases inherent to observational studies, such as the potential influence of selection bias, recall bias, and other confounding factors.

The Human Estrogen/Progestin Replacement Study

The enthusiasm about the cardioprotective effects of HRT has been dampened as the data from the first large, prospective, blinded, randomized placebo-controlled secondary prevention trial, the Heart and Estrogen/Progestin Replacement Study

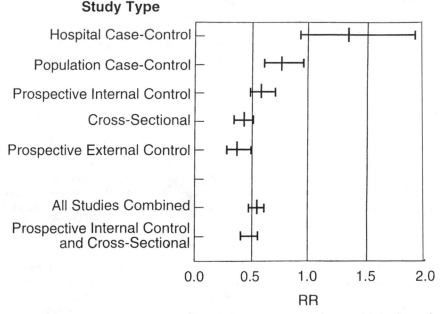

FIGURE 2. Summary of studies showing relative risks and 95% confidence intervals of coronary heart disease associated with estrogen treatment. (From Sullivan.[77] Reprinted by permission from *British Journal of Obstetrics and Gynaecology.*)

(HERS), became available. The study randomized postmenopausal women with established coronary disease to 0.625 mg CEE plus 2.5 mg MPA daily or to placebo. The primary outcome was nonfatal myocardial infarction or death from CHD. The follow-up period of the 2,763 subjects (mean age 66.7 years) enrolled in the study (active treatment = 1,380; placebo = 1,383) averaged 4.1 years. The incidence of myocardial infarction and coronary death was comparable in the treatment (172 cases) and placebo groups (176 cases). The RR was 0.99 (CI = 0.80, 1.22), thus indicating that treatment with CEE/MPA did not reduce the overall rate of CHD in women with established coronary disease. The data also revealed a statistically significant time trend, showing more CHD events in the hormone group than in the placebo group in year 1, and fewer events in years 4 and 5. This lack of a cardioprotective effect occurred despite favorable changes in lipid patterns usually associated with cardioprotection. After one year of treatment, LDL levels had decreased by 11%, and HDL had increased by 10% compared to placebo. Hormone treatment was associated with more thromboembolic events and a greater incidence of gallbladder disease than was placebo.[46]

These results have elicited numerous published critical comments in an effort to reconcile the apparent discrepancies between the positive association of HRT and cardioprotection reported consistently in observational studies and its absence in HERS. It was noted that HERS had compromised its initial estimates of statistical power, that enrollment rates were not linear but skewed toward the end of the recruitment phase, that the follow-up period was shorter than originally planned, and that the CHD incidence observed in the placebo group was significantly lower than had been anticipated in planning the study. It was also pointed out that the mean age of the study population was higher than that of most other HRT studies and that, unlike HERS, the majority of other studies have focused on primary prevention in healthier women. It was also noted that the observational studies had used either estrogen alone or in combination with sequentially administered adjunctive progestin and that any effect of continuous adjunctive progestin remained to be examined. Finally, the possibility was considered that MPA may have specific properties not common to other progestins, as suggested by experiments in monkeys, where MPA,[47] but not progesterone,[48] antagonized the inhibitory effects of estrogen on coronary artery atherosclerosis.

The Estrogen Replacement and Atherosclerosis Trial

Recently, the data from the second prospective, randomized, blinded clinical study evaluating the effects of HRT in women with established heart disease, the Estrogen Replacement and Atherosclerosis (ERA) trial, have become available. The study randomized 309 women (mean age 65.8 years) with previously diagnosed coronary artery disease to one of three treatment arms: 0.625 mg CEE, 0.625 mg CEE plus 2.5 mg MPA, or placebo. Unlike the HERS, the ERA study contained an arm of unopposed estrogen and thus allowed researchers to dissect the specific effects of adjunctive progestin. The primary outcome of the study was the development of new coronary lesions or the progression of established lesions, as determined by quantitative coronary angiography. The women were followed up for an average of 3.2 years. Neither estrogen alone nor estrogen/progestin combination therapy affected the incidence of new lesions or the progression rate of established lesions when compared to placebo. Nevertheless, as in HERS, favorable changes in lipid patterns consistent with cardioprotection were observed.[37]

As has been pointed out,[1] caution should be applied in generalizing these results for several reasons, including the observation that angiographically measured lesions may not be a valid endpoint for the evaluation of the course of CHD.[49]

As in HERS, the study population in the ERA trial was relatively old, and the follow-up period was relatively short. The authors noted that atherosclerosis and aging are associated with impaired endothelial function and that older women with established coronary disease may therefore be less likely to benefit from hormonal interventions, as suggested by animal data showing that the ability of estrogen to prevent cholesterol accumulation in the vessel walls requires a healthy endothelium.[50]

FUTURE PERSPECTIVES

The effectiveness of estrogen in the treatment of vasomotor symptoms and vulvovaginal atrophy and in the prevention of osteoporosis has been well established, and the lowest effective doses have been identified for different estrogens. Likewise, the protective action of adjunctive progestin against estrogen-induced endometrial hyperplasia has been documented in a number of large clinical trials, with the underlying assumption that the protection against hyperplasia, observed in these trials for up to three years, is a valid surrogate endpoint for the long-term protection of adjunctive progestin against endometrial cancer. Short of a large prospective clinical trial, careful and coordinated surveys of post-approval safety reports are in order to support this assumption.

The current system of using endometrial hyperplasia of any type as a marker for potential endometrial cancer needs revision. It has been shown that atypical hyperplasia, rather than simple or complex hyperplasia, is likely to progress to cancer,[39,51] but it is doubtful that every case of atypical hyperplasia will advance to cancer. Clearly, further work is needed to identify precancerous lesions with reliable precision.[52]

A major concern relates to long-term continuance of HRT. It has been estimated that in the United States approximately 100,000 women discontinue hormonal treatment every month.[53] A frequent reason for noncompliance is unacceptable bleeding. The continued development of estrogen/progestin regimens to minimize bleeding should therefore be encouraged. Promising in this regard are the favorable bleeding patterns reported for tibolone, a steroidal compound exhibiting both estrogenic and progestogenic properties, thus obviating the need for adjunctive progestin.[54]

The fear of breast cancer is another reason for discontinuing HRT or declining HRT as an option. The currently available information on the HRT-related breast cancer incidence is derived from studies that frequently lacked adequate statistical power or contained methodological inadequacies. Nevertheless, these data for the most part suggest a small, duration-related increase in breast cancer risk associated with estrogen replacement therapy. Data on breast cancer risk specifically associated with adjunctive progestin treatment are limited.[55] In one of several meta-analyses, the relative risk was estimated to be 1.35 (floated CI = 1.21, 1.49) after HRT use for five years or longer.[56]

Clearly, quantitative information on the incidence of HRT-related breast cancer from prospective, randomized trials is needed. The Women's Health Initiative (WHI) study, a randomized trial started in 1992 and targeted for completion in 2007, will include breast cancer as an outcome, to be followed up for a period of about nine years in an estimated 27,500 women treated with 0.625 mg/day CEE or 0.625 mg/day CEE plus 2.5 mg/day MPA for women with a uterus or placebo.

Information on breast cancer will also be collected in another large trial: the Women's International Study of Long-Duration Oestrogen after Menopause (WISDOM), which is currently being conducted in the United Kingdom and 11 other countries. The trial has a targeted enrollment of 34,000 subjects to receive 0.625 mg/day CEE with or without 2.5 mg MPA/day (depending on the presence of a uterus) or placebo over a period of approximately 10 years.[57]

Both the WHI and WISDOM studies will also assess the effects of HRT on the primary prevention of cardiovascular disease (CVD). Two other studies will yield data on secondary prevention of CVD, The Western Connecticut Estrogen for Prevention of Stroke Trial (WEST; $n = 650$) and the Estrogen in the Prevention of Reinfarction Trial (ESPRIT; $n = 2,000$). Of the three ongoing studies with angiographic endpoints, two will evaluate the effects of CEE plus MPA: the Estrogen and Bypass Graft Atherosclerosis Regression Trial (EAGAR, $n = 200$) and the Women's Atherosclerosis Vitamin/Estrogen Trial (WAVE; $n = 400$). The third study, the Women's Estrogen/Progestin Lipid Lowering Heart Atherosclerosis Trial (WELLHART), will assess the effects of estradiol (E_2). The study contains three treatment arms: 1.0 mg/day E_2; 1.0 mg/day E_2 plus 5.0 mg/day MPA (added cyclically) for women with a uterus, or placebo. These controlled trials will yield a wealth of data with regard to

CEE and MPA. A remaining challenge for future studies pertains to the effects of other estrogens and progestins.

Selective Estrogen Receptor Modulators

Intensive research efforts are currently directed at compounds with selective, tissue-specific estrogen activities. These substances with estrogen agonist/antagonist properties are collectively known as selective estrogen receptor modulators (SERMs). The SERMs have been considered a promising alternative to HRT, and raloxifene, a SERM with bone-sparing activity[58,59] and minimal, if any, estrogenic effects on the endometrium,[59,60] has been approved for the prevention and treatment of osteoporosis in postmenopausal women.

When used as hormone replacement therapy, a SERM ideally would exert estrogen agonist functions where needed, for example, in the skeletal, cardiovascular, and central nervous systems and liver, while acting as an estrogen antagonist in endometrium and breast. Raloxifene, as an example, has estrogen-antagonist effects on breast[61] and uterus,[59,62] while acting as an estrogen agonist on bone[58,59] and possibly on cardiovascular risk factors.[60]

Although thorough efficacy and safety studies have been conducted, which resulted in the approval of raloxifene for the prevention and treatment of postmenopausal osteoporosis, little information is available on its cardiovascular effects. A large study, the Raloxifene Use for the Heart (RUTH) trial, was initiated in mid-1998 to assess the effects of raloxifene in postmenopausal women with a high risk for coronary heart disease. The study, conducted in 26 countries, has a planned enrollment of 10,000 women with documented cardiovascular disease. The primary outcome is nonfatal myocardial infarction and coronary death. The trial will terminate when 1,669 primary endpoint events have occurred.

Phytoestrogens

The potential of estrogenic plant products, the phytoestrogens, in hormone replacement therapy has recently received attention and deserves to be further explored,[63] in particular with regard to cardiovascular benefits.[64,65] Dietary supplementation with soy isoflavones, a major class of phytoestrogens, enhanced coronary vascular reactivity in atherosclerotic monkeys.[66] In a double-blinded, randomized study of postmenopausal women, dietary supplementation with soy protein significantly alleviated vasomotor symptoms[67] and produced vaginal maturation.[68] However, studies on the effects of isoflavones on lipids showed variable effects. By current consensus, isoflavones have some physiologic effects, but extensive clinical trials are needed before specific recommendations can be made regarding increased consumption of foods or supplements that contain high amounts of isoflavones.[69]

Alzheimer's Disease and Colon Cancer

Clinical research in support of currently nonapproved indications for HRT represents a major challenge for the future, as exemplified by two diseases—Alzheimer's disease and colon cancer. Although Alzheimer's disease affects both men and women, the majority of afflicted persons are women. There is evidence to suggest that HRT may reduce the risk, delay the onset, and slow the progression of Alzheimer's

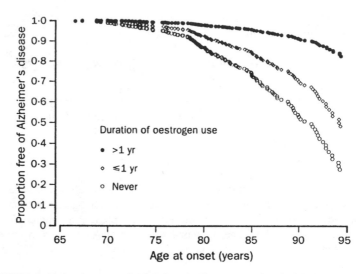

FIGURE 3. Delay in onset of Alzheimer's disease associated with the duration of estrogen use. (From Tang.[70] Reprinted with permission from *Lancet*.)

disease (FIG. 3).[70,71] However, the observations to date are based on small studies of low validity and sometimes conflicting results. Large-scale prospective studies are in order.

Interesting, but as yet inconclusive observations suggest a protective effect of HRT against colorectal cancer.[72] An analysis of a subpopulation of subjects (422,373 postmenopausal women) participating in the large, prospective Cancer Prevention Study II (CPS-II) found a significantly decreased risk of fatal colon cancer in ERT users (RR = 0.71; 95% CI = 0.61, 0.83). The risk reduction was strongest among current users (RR = 0.55; 95% CI = 0.40, 0.76), and there was a significant trend of decreased risk with increasing years of use among all users.[73] A meta-analysis of observational study data reported a substantial reduction in colon cancer risk (RR = 0.67; 95% CI = 0.59, 0.77) in recent users but not in those who had ever been users. The RR of death from colon cancer in that study was 0.72 (95% CI = 0.64, 0.81). There was no association between rectal cancer and HRT.[74] Another meta-analysis found a reduced risk of colon cancer (RR = 0.80; 95% CI = 0.74, 0.86) and rectal cancer (RR = 0.81; 95% CI = 0.72, 0.92) in those who had ever been users and a RR of 0.66 (95% CI = 0.59, 0.74) in current users.[75] Finally, a recent case-control study, which was published after the two meta-analyses, found a decreased risk in colon cancer (RR = 0.6; 95% CI = 0.4, 1.0) among recent users and a RR of 0.5 (95% CI = 0.3, 0.9) with long duration (>5 years). No association between HRT and rectal cancer risk was found.[76]

Research on a possible association between HRT and colorectal cancer is at an early stage. Colorectal cancer is the fourth most common cancer, and the second cause of cancer death in the United States. In view of the magnitude of this public health problem, and encouraged by the presently available data from observational studies, the hypothesis of a protective effect of HRT should be tested in an adequately sized, randomized prospective study.

CONCLUSION

During the last decade, extensive knowledge has accumulated regarding the benefits and risks of HRT, and large prospective studies have been initiated that will contribute further information obtained under controlled conditions. Additional prospective, randomized, blinded studies are needed to document potential benefits of HRT that may have major positive consequences for public health, including, but not restricted to, cardioprotection, Alzheimer's disease, and colon cancer. Despite their enormous cost, their long duration, and large study populations, there is no substitute for controlled clinical trials to evaluate the full potential of HRT as preventive medicine.

REFERENCES

1. NABEL, E.G. 2000. Coronary heart disease in women—an ounce of prevention. N. Engl. J. Med. **343:** 572–574.
2. U.S. DEPARTMENT OF HEALTH AND HUMAN SERVICES, FOOD AND DRUG ADMINISTRATION. 1997. Guidance for Clinical Evaluation of Combination Estrogen/Progestin-Containing Drug Products Used for Hormone Replacement Therapy of Postmenopausal Women. Food and Drug Administration. Rockville, MD.
3. LINDSAY, R. 1996. The menopause and osteoporosis. Obstet. Gynecol. **87:** 16S–19S.
4. KOMULAINEN, M.H., H. KRÖGER, M.T. TUPPURAINEN, *et al.* 1998. HRT and Vit D in prevention of non-vertebral fractures in postmenopausal women: a 5 year randomized trial. Maturitas **31:** 45–54.
5. CHRISTIANSEN, C. 1999. Treatment of osteoporosis. *In* Treatment of the Postmenopausal Woman. R.A. Lobo, Ed.: 315–328. Lippincott Williams & Wilkins. Philadelphia, PA.
6. LUFKIN, E.G. & S.J. ORY. 1994. Relative value of transdermal and oral estrogen therapy in various clinical situations. Mayo Clin. Proc. **69:** 131–135.
7. LINDSAY, R. & J.F. TOHME. 1990. Estrogen treatment of patients with established postmenopausal osteoporosis. Obstet. Gynecol. **76:** 290–295.
8. LUFKIN, E.G., H.W. WAHNER, W.M. O'FALLON, *et al.* 1992. Treatment of postmenopausal osteoporosis with transdermal estrogen. Ann. Int. Med. **117:** 1–9.
9. STEVENSON, J.C., M.P. CUST, K.F. GANGAR, *et al.* 1990. Effects of transdermal versus oral hormone replacement therapy on bone density in spine and proximal femur in postmenopausal women. Lancet **336:** 265–269.
10. HILLARD, T.C., S.J. WHITCROFT, M.S. MARSH, *et al.* 1994. Long-term effects of transdermal and oral hormone replacement therapy on postmenopausal bone loss. Osteop. Int. **4:** 341–348.
11. FIELD, C.S., S.J. ORY, H.W. WAHNER, *et al.* 1993. Preventive effects of transdermal 17β-estradiol on osteoporotic changes after surgical menopause: a two-year placebo-controlled trial. Am. J. Obstet. Gynecol. **168:** 114–121.
12. ETTINGER, B., H.K. GENANT, P. STEIGER & P. MADVIG. 1992. Low-dosage micronized 17β-estradiol prevents bone loss in postmenopausal women. Am. J. Obstet. Gynecol. **166:** 479–488.
13. GENANT, H.K., J. LUCAS, S. WEISS, *et al.* 1997. Low-dose esterified estrogen therapy. Arch. Intern. Med. **157:** 2609–2615.
14. GRADY, D., S.M. RUBIN, D.B. PETITTI, *et al.* 1992. Hormone therapy to prevent disease and prolong life in postmenopausal women. Ann. Int. Med. **117:** 1016–1037.

15. DIVISION OF METABOLISM AND ENDOCRINE DRUG PRODUCTS. FOOD AND DRUG ADMINISTRATION. 1994. Draft Guidelines for Preclinical and Clinical Evaluation of Agents Used in the Prevention or Treatment of Postmenopausal Osteoporosis. CLIN 04/ 01/94. Food and Drug Administration. Rockville, MD.
16. ROSSINI, M., D. GATTI, S. GIRARDELLO, et al. 2000. Effects of two intermittent alendronate regimens in the prevention or treatment of postmenopausal osteoporosis. Bone 27: 119–122.
17. GUSBERG, S.B. 1947. Precursors of corpus carcinoma: estrogens and adenomatous hyperplasia. Am. J. Obstet. Gynecol. 54: 905–927.
18. ZIEL, H. & W. FINKLE. 1975. Increased risk of endometrial carcinoma among users of conjugated estrogens. N. Engl. J. Med. 293: 1167–1170.
19. HULKA, B. 1980. Effect of exogenous estrogens on postmenopausal women: the epidemiologic evidence. Obstet. Gynecol. Surv. 35: 389–399.
20. PERSSON, I., H-O. ADAMI, L. BERGKVIST, et al. 1989. Risk of endometrial cancer after treatment with oestrogens alone or in conjunction with progestogens: results of a prospective study. Br. Med. J. 298: 147–151.
21. VOIGT, L.F., N.S. WEISS, J. CHU, et al. 1991. Progestagen supplementation of exogenous oestrogens and risk of endometrial cancer. Lancet 338: 274–277.
22. ZIEL, H.K., W.D. FINKLE & S. GREENLAND. 1998. Decline in incidence of endometrial cancer following increase in prescriptions for opposed conjugated estrogens in a prepaid health plan. Gynecol. Oncol. 68: 253–255.
23. BERESFORD, S.A.A., N.S. WEISS, L.F. VOIGT & B. MCNIGHT. 1997. Risk of endometrial cancer in relation to use of oestrogen combined with cyclic progestagen therapy in postmenopausal women. Lancet 349: 458–461.
24. PIKE, M.C., R.K. PETERS, W. COZEN, et al. 1997. Estrogen–progestin replacement therapy and endometrial cancer. J. Natl. Cancer Inst. 89: 1110–1116.
25. WEIDERPASS, E., H-O. ADAMI, J.A. BARON, et al. 1999. Risk of endometrial cancer following estrogen replacement with and without progestins. J. Natl. Cancer Inst. 91: 1131–1137.
26. GRADY, D., T. GEBRETSADIK, K. KERLIKOWSKE, et al. 1995. Hormone replacement therapy and endometrial cancer risk: a meta-analysis. Obstet. Gynecol. 85: 304–313.
27. WOODRUFF, J.D. & J.H. PICKAR FOR THE MENOPAUSE STUDY GROUP. 1994. Incidence of endometrial hyperplasia in postmenopausal women taking conjugated estrogens (Premarin) with medroxyprogesterone acetate or conjugated estrogens alone. Am. J. Obstet. Gynecol. 170: 1213–1223.
28. THE WRITING GROUP FOR THE PEPI TRIAL. 1996. Effects of hormone replacement therapy on endometrial histology in postmenopausal women. J. Am. Med. Soc. 275: 370–375.
29. CORSON, S.L., R.M. RICHART, P. CAUBEL & P. LIM. 1999. Effect of a unique constant-estrogen, pulsed-progestin hormone replacement therapy containing 17β-estradiol and norgestimate on endometrial histology. Int. J. Fertil. 44: 279–285.
30. KURMAN, R.J., J.C. FÉLIX, D.F. ARCHER, et al. 2000. Norethindrone acetate and estradiol-induced endometrial hyperplasia. Obstet. Gynecol. 96: 373–379.
31. NOTELOVITZ, M., R.E. VARNER, R.W. REBAR, et al. 1997. Minimal endometrial proliferation over a two-year period in postmenopausal women taking 0.3 mg of unopposed esterified estrogens. Menopause 4: 80–88.
32. NOTELOVITZ, M. & J.H. MATTOX. 2000. Suppression of vasomotor and vulvovaginal symptoms with continuous oral 17β-estradiol. Menopause 7: 310–317.
33. WHITEHEAD, M.I. 1978. The effects of oestrogens and progestogens on the postmenopausal endometrium. Maturitas 1: 87–98.
34. GELFAND, M.M. & A. FERENCZY. 1989. A prospective 1-year study of estrogen and progestin in postmenopausal women: effects on the endometrium. Obstet. Gynecol. 74: 398–402.
35. SPEROFF, L., J. ROWAN, J. SYMONS, et al. 1996. The comparative effect on bone density, endometrium, and lipids of continuous hormones as replacement therapy (CHART Study). J. Am. Med. Soc. 276: 1397–1403.

36. BOERRIGTER, P.J., P.H.M. VAN DER WEIJTER, J.P.A. BANK, et al. 1996. Endometrial response in estrogen replacement therapy quarterly combined with a progestogen. Maturitas **24:** 63–71.
37. HERRINGTON, D.M., D.M. REBOUSSIN, K. BRIDGET BROSNIHAN, et al. 2000. Effects of estrogen replacement on the progression of coronary-artery atherosclerosis. N. Engl. J. Med. **343:** 522–529.
38. THE EUROPEAN AGENCY FOR THE EVALUATION OF MEDICINAL PRODUCTS. COMMITTEE FOR PROPRIETARY MEDICINAL PRODUCTS. 1997. Points to Consider for Hormone Replacement Therapy. London, U.K.
39. KURMAN, R.J., P.F. KAMINSKI & H.J. NORRIS. 1985. The behavior of endometrial hyperplasia. A long-term study of "untreated" hyperplasia in 170 patients. Cancer **56:** 403–412.
40. DELIGDISCH, L. & C.F. HOLINKA. 1986. Progesterone receptors in two groups of endometrial carcinoma. Cancer **57:** 1385–1388.
41. DELIGDISCH, L. & C.F. HOLINKA. 1987. Endometrial carcinoma: two diseases? Cancer Detect. Prev. **10:** 237–246.
42. HOLINKA, C.F. 1994. Aspects of hormone replacement therapy. Ann. N.Y. Acad. Sci. **734:** 271–284.
43. BARRETT-CONNOR, E. 1996. The menopause, hormone replacement, and cardiovascular disease: the epidemiologic evidence. Maturitas **23:** 227–234.
44. HENDERSON, B.E., A. PAGANINI-HILL & R.K. ROSS. 1991. Decreased mortality in users of estrogen replacement therapy. Ann. Intern. Med. **151:** 75–78.
45. GRODSTEIN, F., M.J. STAMPFER, J.E. MANSON, et al. 1996. Postmenopausal estrogen and progestin use and the risk of cardiovascular disease. N. Engl. J. Med. **335:** 453–461.
46. HULLEY, S., D. GRADY, T. BUSH, et al. FOR THE HEART AND ESTROGEN/PROGESTIN REPLACEMENT STUDY (HERS) RESEARCH GROUP. 1998. Randomized trial of estrogen plus progestin for secondary prevention of coronary heart disease in postmenopausal women. J. Am. Med. Assoc. **280:** 605–613.
47. ADAMS, M.R., T.C. REGISTER, D.L. GOLDEN, et al. 1997. Medroxyprogesterone acetate antagonizes inhibitory effects of conjugated equine estrogens on coronary artery atherosclerosis. Arterioscler. Thromb. Vasc. Biol. **17:** 217–221.
48. ADAMS, M.R., J.R. KAPLAN, S.B. MANUCK, et al. 1990. Inhibition of coronary artery atherosclerosis by 17β-estradiol in ovariectomized monkeys. Arteriosclerosis **10:** 1051–1057.
49. BROWN, B.G., X.Q. ZHAO, D.E. SACCO & J.J. ALBERS. 1993. Lipid lowering and plaque regression: new insights into prevention of plaque disruption and clinical events in coronary disease. Circulation **87:** 1781–1791.
50. HOHN, P., H.L. ANDERSEN, M.R. ANDERSEN, et al. 1999. The direct antiatherogenic effect of estrogen is present, absent, or reversed, depending on the state of the arterial endothelium: a time course study in cholesterol clamped rabbits. Circulation **100:** 1727–1733.
51. FERENCZY, A. & M. GELFAND. 1989. The biologic significance of cytologic atypia in progestogen-treated endometrial hyperplasia. Am. J. Obstet. Gynecol. **160:** 126–131.
52. MUTTER, G.L. 2000. Endometrial intraepithelial neoplasia (EIN): will it bring order to chaos? Gynecol. Oncol. **76:** 287–290.
53. ANONYMOUS. 1998. Achieving long-term continuance of menopausal ERT/HRT: consensus opinion of the North American Menopause Society. Menopause **5:** 69–76.
54. DÖREN M., A. RÜBIG, H.J.T. COELINGH BENNINK & W. HOLZGREVE. 1999. Impact on uterine bleeding and endometrial thickness: Tibolone compared with continuous combined estradiol and norethisterone acetate replacement therapy. Menopause **6:** 299–306.
55. ROSS, R.K. & L. BERNSTEIN. 1999. Influence of sex hormones on breast cancer risk and mortality. In Treatment of the Postmenopausal Woman. R.A. Lobo, Ed.: 487–495. Lippincott Williams & Wilkins. Philadelphia.
56. COLLABORATIVE GROUP ON HORMONAL FACTORS IN BREAST CANCER. 1997. Breast cancer and hormone replacement therapy: collaborative reanalysis of data from 51 epi-

demiological studies of 52 705 women with breast cancer and 108 411 women without breast cancer. Lancet **350:** 1047–1059.

57. HOLINKA, C.F. & J.H. PICKAR. 1999. Clinical studies in hormone replacement therapy. *In* Treatment of the Postmenopausal Woman. R.A. Lobo, Ed.: 629–635. Lippincott Williams & Wilkins. Philadelphia.

58. LUFKIN, E.G., M.D. WHITAKER, T. NICKELSEN, *et al.* 1998. Treatment of established postmenopausal osteoporosis with raloxifene: a randomized trial. J. Bone Min. Res. **13:** 1747–1754.

59. DELMAS, P.D., N.H. BJARNASON, B.H. MITLAK, *et al.* 1997. Effects of raloxifene on bone mineral density, serum cholesterol concentrations, and uterine endometrium in postmenopausal women. N. Engl. J. Med. **337:** 1641–1647.

60. GUZZO, J.A. 2000. Selective estrogen receptor modulators—a new age of estrogens in cardiovascular disease? Clin. Cardiol. **23:** 15–17.

61. CUMMINGS, S.R., S. ECKERT, K.A. KRUEGER, *et al.* 1999. The effect of raloxifene on risk of breast cancer in postmenopausal women. J. Am. Med. Soc. **281:** 2189–2197.

62. BOSS, S.M., W.J. HUSTER, J.A. NEILD, *et al.* 1997. Effects of raloxifene hydrochloride on the endometrium of postmenopausal women. Am. J. Obstet. Gynecol. **177:** 1458–1464.

63. THAM, D.M., C.D. GARDNER & W.L. HASKELL. 1998. Potential health benefits of dietary phytoestrogens: a review of clinical, epidemiological, and mechanistic evidence. J. Clin. Endocrinol. Metab. **83:** 2223–2235.

64. MARSH, J.D. 2000. Phytoestrogens and vascular therapy. J. Am. Coll. Cardiol. **35:** 1986–1987.

65. WROBLEWSKI LISSIN, L. & J.P. COOKE. 2000. Phytoestrogens and cardiovascular health. J. Am. Coll. Cardiol. **35:** 1403–1410.

66. HONORÉ, E.K., J.K. WILLIAMS, M.S. ANTHONY & T.B. CLARKSON. 1997. Soy isoflavones enhance coronary vascular reactivity in atherosclerotic female macaques. Fertil. Steril. **67:** 148–154.

67. ALBERTAZZI, P., F. PANSINI, G. BONACCORSI, *et al.* 1998. The effect of dietary soy supplementation on hot flushes. Obstet. Gynecol. **91:** 6–11.

68. WILCOX, G., M.L. WAHLQUIST, H.G. BURGER & G. MEDLEY. 1990. Oestrogenic effects of plant foods in postmenopausal women. Br. Med. J. **301:** 905–906.

69. ANONYMOUS. 2000. The role of isoflavones in menopausal health: consensus opinion of the North American Menopause Society. Menopause **7:** 215–229.

70. TANG, M-X., D. JACOBS, Y. STERN, *et al.* 1996. Effect of oestrogen during menopause on risk and age at onset of Alzheimer's disease. Lancet **348:** 429–432.

71. KAWAS, C., S. RESNICK, A. MORRISON, *et al.* 1997. A prospective study of estrogen replacement therapy and the risk of developing Alzheimer's disease: The Baltimore Longitudinal Study of Aging. Neurology **48:** 1517–1521.

72. STAMPFER, M.J, & F. GRODSTEIN. 1999. Colorectal cancer: does postmenopausal estrogen use reduce the risk? Menop. Manage. **8:** 8–10.

73. CALLE, E.E., H.L. MIRACLE-MCMAHILL, M.J. THUN & C.W. HEATH, JR. 1995. Estrogen replacement therapy and risk of fatal colon cancer in a prospective cohort of postmenopausal women. J. Natl. Cancer Inst. **87:** 517–523.

74. NANDA, K., L.A. BASTIAN, V. HASSELBLAD & D.L. SIMEL. 1999. Hormone replacement therapy and the risk of colorectal cancer: a meta-analysis. Obstet. Gynecol. **93:** 880–888.

75. GRODSTEIN, F., P.A. NEWCOMB & M.J. STAMPFER. 1999. Postmenopausal hormone therapy and the risk of colorectal cancer: a review and meta-analysis. Am. J. Med. **106:** 574–582.

76. PRIHARTONO, N., J.R. PALMER, C. LOUIK, *et al.* 2000. A case-control study of use of postmenopausal female hormone supplements in relation to the risk of large bowel cancer. Cancer Epidemiol. Biomarkers Prev. **9:** 443–447.

77. SULLIVAN, J.M. 1996. Hormone replacement therapy and cardiovascular disease: the human model. Br. J. Obstet. Gynaecol. **103(Suppl. 13):** 59–67.

Endocrine and Paracrine Regulation of Endometrial Angiogenesis

ROBERT N. TAYLOR,[a] DAN I. LEBOVIC,[a,b] DANIELA HORNUNG,[a,c] AND MICHAEL D. MUELLER[a,d]

[a]*Center for Reproductive Sciences, Department of Obstetrics, Gynecology and Reproductive Sciences, University of California, San Francisco, California 94143-0556, USA*

[b]*University of Michigan, School of Medicine, Ann Arbor, Michigan 48109, USA*

[c]*University of Tübingen, Tübingen, Germany*

[d]*University of Berne, Berne, Switzerland*

ABSTRACT: The human endometrium is a complex tissue comprised of different cell types, including epithelial, stromal, inflammatory, perivascular, and blood vessel cells. The hormonal receptivity and distribution of these cell populations change during the menstrual cycle. Cyclical endometrial growth is dependent on its ability to regenerate a vascular capillary network, which grows in parallel with the proliferation and differentiation of the endometrial lining. Natural hormonal effects on the endometrium and endocrine manipulation of this tissue, in response to the use of exogenous steroid therapies, can affect endometrial capillary proliferation and function, leading to clinical abnormalities of uterine bleeding. We propose that the regulation of endometrial angiogenesis is mediated indirectly via complex interactions among cell types. Our laboratory has focused on a prototypical member of the angiogenic proteins, vascular endothelial growth factor (VEGF)-A. In this paper we present data demonstrating that VEGF-A expression in normal endometrial epithelial and stromal cells and in Ishikawa adenocarcinoma cells is increased by an ovarian steroid, estradiol. Infiltrating immune cells, particularly polymorphonuclear granulocytes, also are sources of VEGF-A. In inflammatory conditions involving the endometrium (e.g., endometriosis), a proinflammatory cytokine, IL-1β, can mediate neoangiogenesis by inducing VEGF-A gene transcription. Thus, endometrial vascularization is effected by both endocrine and paracrine pathways.

KEYWORDS: cytokines; steroids; uterus; VEGF

INTRODUCTION

Endometrial angiogenesis, as with neovascularization in other sites, requires the sprouting of new capillaries from preexisting vessels. This complex process involves the proteolytic degradation of extracellular matrix, the proliferation and migration of endothelial cells, and ultimately the formation of patent capillary tubules supply-

Address for correspondence: Robert N. Taylor, M.D., Ph.D., Director, Center for Reproductive Sciences, University of California, San Francisco, San Francisco, CA 94143-0556. Voice: 415-476-4556; fax: 415-753-3271.

rtaylor@socrates.ucsf.edu

ing the growing endometrium. Few normal adult tissues are as dynamic as the human endometrium, whose thickness grows up to 10-fold each month after menstrual desquamation. The precise regulation of its vascularization, critical to endometrial perfusion, embryonic implantation, and survival of the species, is understood poorly. Many growth factors and cytokines have been shown to exert chemotactic, mitogenic, or inhibitory activity on endothelial cells, smooth muscle cells, and pericytes and to participate in angiogenic processes either directly or indirectly. As angiogenesis occurs when the balance of local factors promoting vascular growth exceeds the action of vascular inhibitors, several different regulatory mechanisms are possible. In this paper we focus on the upregulation of a prototypical angiogenic factor, vascular endothelial growth factor (VEGF)-A, as a key mediator of neovascularization.

Several pleiotropic growth factors (e.g., basic FGF, PDGF, TGF-β, and interleukin [IL]-6) have been shown to exert angiogenic activities.[1] By contrast, the 43-kD, dimeric, heparin-binding glycoprotein VEGF-A is specifically mitogenic for endothelial cells,[2] and VEGF receptors are restricted primarily to endothelial and trophoblast cells. Five molecular species of VEGF-A have been identified to date (VEGF$_{121}$, VEGF$_{145}$, VEGF$_{165}$, VEGF$_{189}$, and VEGF$_{201}$), each named for the length of its amino acid sequence. The different mature proteins arise via alternative splicing of a single primary mRNA transcript. The dominant VEGF-A mRNA transcripts expressed by human endometrium and primary human endometrial cells encode the VEGF$_{165}$[3] and VEGF$_{121}$[4] proteins.

Cyclical vascular changes within the primate endometrium were first documented in the classical experiments of Markee.[5] Heterotopic transplants of rhesus endometrium into the anterior chamber of the eye could be observed directly in this model. The functionalis layer of endometrium is supplied by an end-arteriole, referred to as the spiral arteriole. Each arteriole is responsible for the perfusion of ~4–7 mm^2 of endometrium. These vessels, unlike the radial and basal arteries that feed them, are highly sensitive to ovarian steroids. The endometrial vascular architecture changes throughout the menstrual cycle, paralleling growth of the supporting epithelium and stroma. From days 0–25, there is a gradual increase in branching and coiling of spiral arterioles, corresponding to an increase in the length and coiling of endometrial glands. A decade later, in their landmark article, Noyes and colleagues[6] reported effects of enhanced vascular permeability and perivascular edema during the human endometrial cycle, providing further evidence that steroids from the ovary orchestrate vascular responses in normal endometrium. Beginning in the late proliferative phase, under the influence of ovarian estradiol production, a complex subepithelial capillary plexus develops in the cycling endometrium.[7] The capillary endothelial cells also acquire mitogenic activity, evidenced by [^{3}H]thymidine incorporation in tissue explants obtained at this cycle phase.[8] More recent morphometric evaluations of endometrial vessel formation indicate significant variation in endothelial cell proliferation within different regions of the uterus. Samples from hysterectomy specimens show that the endothelial cell proliferation index is significantly elevated in functionalis compared with basalis layer vessels.[9]

In the last decade it has become apparent that some steroid hormone actions on uterine tissues are not direct but are effected by paracrine mediators such as cytokines and growth factors.[10] Cytokines are key mediators of intercellular communication within the immune system and can exert proliferative, cytostatic, chemoattractant, or differentiative effects on the surrounding endometrium. The current studies sought to evaluate the potential mechanisms of VEGF-A gene regulation vis-à-vis the neovascularization of normal endometrium and endometriotic implants. The *in vitro* models used in the following experiments were designed to test hormone and cytokine responses of cells from the endometrial functionalis layer. Primary cell cultures were derived from Pipelle biopsy material, which yields predominantly superficial endometrial glands and stroma. Transfected Ishikawa cell models were designed to approximate the ovarian steroid receptor phenotype of functionalis epithelium, which differs from that of the underlying basalis zones.[11]

MATERIALS AND METHODS

Subjects and Specimens

Normally menstruating women undergoing laparoscopy for various indications were recruited. Women who had taken oral contraceptives, hormonal supplements, or gonadotropin-releasing hormone (GnRH) analogs over the previous 3 months were excluded. Control subjects were identified at laparoscopy for tubal sterilization or for assessment of pelvic pain in whom no visible evidence of pelvic pathology was found. Subjects with endometriosis were identified when laparoscopy revealed the presence of classical or atypical endometriotic lesions. Clinical staging of endometriosis followed the revised modification of the American Fertility Society scoring system, as described.[12] Endometrial biopsies and resection of endometriotic ovarian cysts were performed with the patient under anesthesia. All subjects provided written informed consent under a protocol approved by the Committee on Human Research at the University of California, San Francisco.

Immunohistochemistry

Endometrial tissue specimens were fixed for 24 hours in Histochoice MB (Amresco, Solon, OH), paraffin embedded, and cut in serial sections of 8 μm. Sections were stained with a rabbit polyclonal anti-human VEGF-A antiserum (Santa Cruz Antibodies, Santa Cruz, CA) at a concentration of 10 μg/ml using the Vectastain Elite ABC kit (Vector Laboratories, Burlingame, CA). Negative controls for immunostaining were performed using normal rabbit serum at the identical protein concentration (10 μg/ml), as described previously.[13] Immunostaining for polymorphonuclear granulocytes was performed using mouse monoclonal antibodies against human neutrophil elastase (2 μg/ml, Zymed, So. San Francisco, CA). Negative controls for immunostaining were performed using an irrelevant, isotype-specific mouse monoclonal antibody (anti-synaptophysin) at the identical protein concentration (2 μg/ml), as described previously.[14,15] The chromagen signal was enhanced with $NiSO_4$ using the Liquid Diaminobenzidine-Black Substrate kit (Zymed, South San Francisco, CA).

Establishment of Human Endometrial Cell Cultures

The techniques for isolation and culture of human endometrial and endometriotic stromal cells *in vitro* were described in detail elsewhere.[12] Briefly, follicular phase endometrial biopsies from control women were used to prepare cultures of normal endometrial cells, and endometriotic ovarian cysts were used as the source of endometriotic cells. The specimens were minced, digested with collagenase, and serially filtered through narrow gauge sieves with apertures of 38–105 μm to trap the glandular epithelium. Stromal cells were plated and allowed to adhere to plastic cellculture dishes for 30 minutes, at which time contaminating epithelial and blood cells and tissue debris were rinsed free. Epithelial cells were backwashed from the cell sieves and plated onto Matrigel-coated culture wells. Stromal cells were subcultured twice to eliminate contamination by immunocytes. All experiments were performed with cells at passage zero (epithelium) or two (stroma), within 14 days of initial isolation. Under these conditions the primary cells retain estrogen receptor (ER) mRNA and protein.[12,16] Purity of the epithelial and stromal cell populations was confirmed by positive immunostaining for cytokeratin and vimentin, respectively, using specific mouse anti-human monoclonal antibodies.[12]

Polarized Endometrial Epithelial Cell Cultures

In some experiments, human proliferative phase endometrial epithelial cells were grown under polarizing conditions.[17] Primary endometrial epithelial cells were prepared from biopsies, as described above, and plated onto polyethylene terephthalate Transwell culture inserts with a pore size of 0.4 μm (Becton Dickinson, Lincoln Park, NJ). The cells were cultured in MEM-α reconstituted with 10% fetal calf serum (FCS), nucleosides, essential amino acids, 100 U/ml penicillin G, and 100 μg/ ml streptomycin.

Steroid and Cytokine Treatment

Prior studies documented the presence of ER-α and ER-β mRNA and functional ER proteins in endometrial stromal cells cultured in $vitro$.[16] Confluent cultures of endometrial stromal cells and Ishikawa adenocarcinoma cells were incubated overnight in low-serum medium (phenol red–free MEM-α supplemented with 2.5% dextran-charcoal stripped FBS, nucleosides, antibiotics, and nonessential amino acids) and exposed to 10 or 100 nM E_2 or vehicle (ethanol) control for an additional 24 hours. The latter concentration was used in Ishikawa cells transfected with the human ER-α cDNA (HEO), as this construct carries a point mutation that renders the K_d ~70% higher than that of the wild-type ER.[18]

Similar experiments were performed in primary endometrial stromal cells using 10 ng/ml IL-1β (R&D Systems, Minneapolis, MN) or 100 ng/ml tumor necrosis factor (TNF)-α and interferon (IFN)-γ (Sigma Chemical Co., St. Louis, MO). All the cytokines were recombinant human proteins, to which the endometrial stromal cells were exposed for up to 24 hours. These doses previously were shown to optimally induce IL-6[19] and RANTES (regulated on activation, normal T-cell expressed and secreted)[20] expression in primary endometrial stromal cell cultures.

Quantification of VEGF-A Protein and mRNA

At the end of each experiment, conditioned media were aspirated and centrifuged to pellet floating cells, and the supernatants were assayed for secreted $VEGF_{165}$ using a sensitive sandwich ELISA developed at Genentech, Inc. (South San Francisco, CA).[13] The cells were lysed in TriZOL reagent (Gibco-BRL, Gaithersburg, MD), and total RNA was isolated and subjected to formaldehyde gel electrophoresis. Northern blotting with random-primed [α-^{32}P]dCTP-labeled VEGF and glyceraldehyde-3-phosphate dehydrogenase (GAPDH) cDNA probes was performed as described.[15] In some experiments with Ishikawa cells, semiquantitative reverse transcription-polymerase chain reaction (RT-PCR) assays were used to estimate the concentration of VEGF-A mRNA relative to GAPDH mRNA.[15] Actinomycin D, an inhibitor of DNA-dependent RNA synthesis, was used at a concentration of 5 μg/ml to prove that mRNA accumulation was the result of transcriptional, rather than post-transcriptional, control.[21]

Quantification of VEGF-A Gene Promoter Activity

VEGF-A promoter-luciferase reporter constructs were designed as described[22] and contained 2.3 kb of the human VEGF-A gene promoter upstream of firefly luciferase cDNA in the pGL2 reporter vector (Promega, Minneapolis, MN). These plasmids were transiently transfected into primary endometrial epithelial and stromal cells and into Ishikawa adenocarcinoma cells by calcium phosphate precipitation, lipofection, and electroporation, respectively, as described.[22]

Data Analysis and Statistics

The data are expressed as the mean ± SEM. Paired Student's *t* tests were used. Statistical significance was accepted at $p < 0.05$ for two-tailed analyses.

RESULTS

Immunohistochemical staining of endometrial biopsy specimens from normal women revealed both epithelial and stromal expression of VEGF-A, as we and others reported previously.[13,23] Typically, the epithelial staining pattern was more prominent, with secretory vacuoles showing concentrated VEGF-A protein (FIG. 1A). Endometrial stromal cells were labeled more diffusely for VEGF-A, with an appearance suggestive of extracellular matrix localization of the protein (FIG. 1A). Isolated round cells within the endometrial stroma (arrow) and endometrial vessels (arrowhead) also were stained brightly by the anti-VEGF-A antiserum (FIG. 1A). These cells were identified as polymorphonuclear granulocytes by their intense reaction with human neutrophil elastase antibodies in adjacent sections (FIG. 1B). Double immunoenzymatic labeling techniques, described elsewhere, proved that the same cells coexpressed human neutrophil elastase and VEGF-A.[15]

Monolayers of primary endometrial epithelial cells were established in bicameral chambers.[20] The development of high electrical resistance (868 ± 53 Ω/cm^2, mean ± SD) and the establishment of a gradient of [^{125}I]ovalbumin added to the upper chamber of the epithelial cell–lined Transwell inserts verified the integrity of the polarized endometrial epithelial monolayer. In these cells we noted a fivefold higher ratio of apical to basal VEGF secretion ($p < 0.05$). By contrast, directional secretion of a soluble isoform of fibronectin was not statistically different in the same cells (FIG. 2).

Other *in vitro* models were established to investigate the regulation of VEGF-A mRNA and protein in these cells. Endometrial stromal cells cultured in the presence

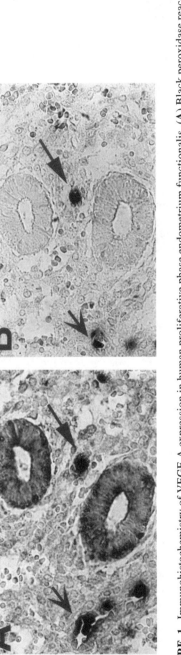

FIGURE 1. Immunohistochemistry of VEGF-A expression in human proliferative phase endometrium functionalis. (**A**) Black peroxidase reaction denotes VEGF-A protein present predominantly in endometrial glands and more diffusely in endometrial stroma cells. Isolated round cells within blood vessels (*arrowhead*) and in the stroma (*arrow*) also demonstrated intense VEGF-A immunostaining. (**B**) Labeling with anti-human neutrophil elastase in adjacent sections demonstrated that the intravascular (*arrowhead*) and stromal (*arrow*) VEGF-A–positive cells are polymorphonuclear granulocytes.

TABLE 1. Estradiol effects on VEGF mRNA accumulation in endometrial cells

Cell type	Hormone treatment	VEGF mRNA (arbitrary units)
Endometrial stromal cells	Control (0.1% ethanol)	1.0
	10 nM E$_2$	3.1 ± 1.8[a]
Ishikawa cells	Control	1.0
	100 nM E$_2$	1.1 ± 0.5
Ishikawa cells transfected with ER-α	Control	1.0
	100 nM E$_2$	2.0 ± 0.2[a]

[a]$p < 0.05$ (paired Student's t test).

of 10 nM E$_2$, to mimic the endocrine milieu of the late proliferative phase, showed an increase in VEGF-A mRNA accumulation (3.1-fold increase; TABLE 1). Ishikawa cells expressed basal levels of VEGF-A mRNA, but these did not change after exposure to up to 100 nM E$_2$. However, following transfection with physiological concentrations of functional human ER-α (HEO, ~20,000 receptors/cell), treatment with 100 nM E$_2$ caused a 2.0-fold stimulation in steady-state levels of VEGF-A transcripts (TABLE 1[15]).

Exposure of normal endometrial stromal cells to IL-1β had no effect on steady-state VEGF transcript concentrations (TABLE 2) and failed to increase VEGF secretion by these cells. Likewise, treatment of the stromal cells with TNF-α and IFN-γ for 24 hours failed to induce VEGF protein secretion.[21] By contrast, endometriotic stromal cells, derived from ovarian endometrioma tissue, manifested a three- to four-fold upregulation of VEGF-A mRNA accumulation and protein secretion after exposure to IL-1β. The former effect was blocked by preincubation with actinomycin D, an inhibitor of mRNA synthesis, indicating a transcriptional mechanism of action.

Direct transcriptional regulation of the VEGF-A gene was examined by transfecting VEGF-A promoter-luciferase vectors into primary endometrial epithelial and stromal cells by calcium phosphate precipitation and lipofection, respectively. Reporter plasmids containing 2.3 kb of the human VEGF-A gene promoter were tested in primary endometrial epithelial and stromal cells and in the Ishikawa adenocarci-

TABLE 2. Cytokine effects on VEGF mRNA accumulation in endometrial cells

Cell type	Hormone treatment	VEGF mRNA (arbitrary units)	VEGF secreted (pg/ml)
Endometrial stromal cells	Control	1.0	64 ± 34
	0.6 nM IL-1β	0.8 ± 0.1	45 ± 7
Endometriosis stromal cells	Control	1.0	162 ± 93
	0.6 nM IL-1β	2.6 ± 0.2[a]	671 ± 470[a]

[a]$p < 0.05$ (paired Student's t test).

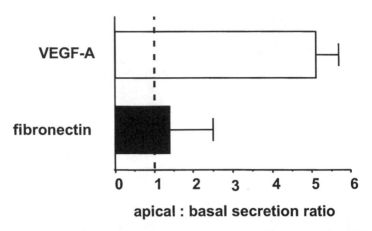

FIGURE 2. Vectorial secretion of VEGF-A from polarized endometrial epithelial cells. VEGF-A was secreted preferentially into the apical compartment of Transwell chambers (*open histogram*), whereas fibronectin secretion (*closed histogram*) was similarly distributed into the apical and basal chambers.

noma cell line.[22] Treatment with 10 nM E_2 induced a three- to fourfold activation of the promoter in both endometrial epithelial and stromal cells (FIG. 3, histograms 1 and 2). Transfection of the same construct into Ishikawa adenocarcinoma cells failed to respond to E_2 at concentrations up to 100 nM (FIG. 3, histogram 3). However, co-transfection of vectors expressing functional human ER-α, restored E_2 responsiveness of the VEGF-A gene promoter (FIG. 3, histogram 4).

DISCUSSION

Although changes in endometrial capillary proliferation and permeability are modulated during the ovarian cycle and with exogenous steroids, endothelial cells *per se* may not be direct targets of classical ER (α) or progesterone receptor-mediated effects. Receptors for these steroids are present in human uterine artery smooth muscle, but have not been identified convincingly in endothelium *in situ*.[24,25] Using the highly sensitive reverse transcriptase-PCR approach, we[26] and others[27] were unable to detect either ER-α or ER-β mRNAs in human umbilical vein endothelium. However, functional evidence of ER-mediated gene activation and gel mobility shift assays have been reported by some investigators using these cells.[28] Nuclear progesterone receptors have been reported in murine endothelial cells[29] and human endometrial endothelium.[30] In general, however, it is believed that ovarian steroid effects on angiogenesis are mediated indirectly via the paracrine actions of prostaglandins or polypeptide growth factors derived from nearby endometrial epithelial or stromal cells.

Findings in the current study confirm previous results from ourselves[13] and others[31] that VEGF-A gene expression is upregulated in isolated human endometrial cells by E_2. This endocrine milieu models that observed in the late proliferative

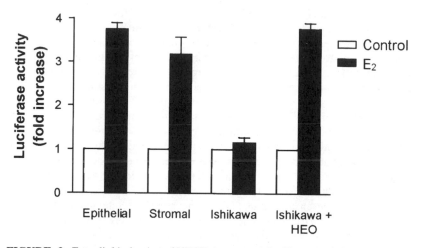

FIGURE 3. Estradiol induction of VEGF-A promoter-luciferase activity in primary endometrial epithelial cells, primary endometrial stromal cells, and nontransfected and ER-α-transfected (HEO) Ishikawa adenocarcinoma cells.

phase of the menstrual cycle. Estrogens upregulate VEGF mRNA and protein production in uterine tissues and cells. If similar results are confirmed in endometriotic tissues, these studies support the obligatory role of estrogen on endometriosis implants[32] and the observation that downregulating doses of GnRH analogues, which diminish circulating E_2 levels, also decrease the size and vascularity of endometriosis lesions.[33] However, while microvascular growth and VEGF-A expression are temporally correlated within the endometrium, a clear correlation between VEGF intensity and markers of endothelial cell proliferation is disputed.[34] It is likely that coexpression of other angiogenic factors and substrates (e.g., basic FGF, VEGF receptors, or angiopoietins) also are required for full vascularization of this tissue.

The apical localization *in situ* and secretion *in vitro* of VEGF-A remain a curious observation. We have proposed that this angiogenic factor also may affect blastocyst function. Hemochorial placentation, such as that observed in human pregnancy, is associated with the development of an endothelial-like phenotype of trophoblastic cells.[35] Invasive first trimester human cytotrophoblasts and cultured choriocarcinoma cells both express the flt-1 and KDR receptors for VEGF-A.[36] Hence, endometrial luminal VEGF-A may provide a trophic signal to the implanting human blastocyst.

Using the same *in vitro* cell model, we failed to observe effects of IL-1β (IL-1β), TNF-α, and IFN-γ on VEGF expression in normal endometrial stromal cells, despite the known actions of all three cytokines on other bioactive proteins (e.g., IL-6[19] and RANTES[20]). However, we did observe that cytokines can increase VEGF-A mRNA and protein expression in stromal cells derived from endometriotic lesions. Thus, proinflammatory cytokines are mediators of neovascularization in endometriotic implants.

It is unlikely that ovarian steroids are direct mediators of endometrial angiogenesis. Most investigators have failed to identify detectable levels of classical estrogen (α) or progesterone (A and B) receptors in endometrial vascular endothelial cells.[25,37] However, in some recent reports, immunohistochemistry and RT-PCR demonstrated estrogen and progesterone receptor expression in human endometrial endothelial cells.[29,30] In the latter study, progesterone-receptor complexes were reported to inhibit mitotic activity of endothelial cells. Further studies will be needed to clarify whether some endothelial cells have direct ovarian steroid responses.

The cloned human VEGF gene promoter consists of 2.4 kb of DNA upstream from the transcription start site and a long 5′ untranslated region.[38] Initiation of VEGF mRNA synthesis is modulated by sequence-specific consensus sites that bind transcriptional control factors. Analyses of the primary sequence of the VEGF promoter reveal several common response elements, including: AP-1, AP-2, and hypoxia-induced enhancer sequences in this gene.[39–43]

Although no consensus palindromic estrogen response element (ERE) sequence exists in the 2.4-kb VEGF promoter, E_2 treatment increases VEGF mRNA as early as 1 hour after hormone administration, suggesting a direct regulation of VEGF gene transcription.[13] VEGF gene expression also has been shown to be regulated rapidly by E_2 in the rat uterus.[44] We recently identified a functional variant ERE about 1.5 kb 5′ to the transcription initiation site of the human gene promoter,[22] and Hyder and colleagues[44] reported an estrogen-dependent element in the 3′ untranslated region of the VEGF-A gene.

Estrogen-receptor complexes classically bind as dimers to consensus, 13-bp palindromic EREs.[45] Although few natural genes contain perfect palindromic EREs, ER complexes also can activate components of the AP-1 complex (e.g., c-fos and c-jun)[46] or bind imperfect EREs if a GATA-6 sequence is present nearby.[39] As described herein, IL-1β can upregulate VEGF in endometriotic stromal cells and has been demonstrated in other cell types.[47] It has been postulated that this cytokine effect is mediated via NFκB motifs located in the VEGF promoter.[48] This hypothesis is under examination currently in our laboratory.

In summary, we propose that endocrine and paracrine modulation of endometrial angiogenesis is mediated via transcriptional upregulation of VEGF-A gene expression in endometrial stromal and epithelial cells. VEGF-A is an angiogenic factor of hierarchical importance, particularly in the uterus, where it responds to multiple stimuli. Steroids, cytokines, and chemokines, by virtue of their recruitment of VEGF-A–producing inflammatory cells, allow fine-tuning of endometrial vascularization. Interruption of single or multiple pathways within this complex network should provide therapeutic opportunities for the amelioration of vascular abnormalities associated with endometrial disorders such as endometriosis and dysfunctional uterine bleeding.

ACKNOWLEDGMENTS

These studies were supported by National Institutes of Health Grants HD33238 (RNT) and HD08517 (DIL), the Deutsche Forschungsgemeinschaft Ho-1832/2-1 (DH), and the Swiss National Science Foundation (MDM). The authors thank Dale Leitman, Evelyn Garrett, Mary Matli and Victor Chao (UCSF), and Napoleone Ferrara and Gloria Meng (Genentech, So. San Francisco) for their generous assistance with this project and Julia Qi-Turner for preparing the manuscript.

REFERENCES

1. FOLKMAN, J.& M. KLAGSBURN. 1987. Angiogenic factors. Science **235:** 442–447.
2. FERRARA, N. *et al.* 1992. Molecular and biological properties of the vascular endothelial growth factor family of proteins. Endocrine Rev. **13:** 18–32.
3. TORRY, D.S. *et al.* 1996. Vascular endothelial growth factor expression in cycling human endometrium. Fertil. Steril. **66:** 72–80.
4. HUANG, J.C., D. Y. LIU & M.Y. DAWOOD. 1998. The expression of vascular endothelial growth factor isoforms in cultured human endometrial stromal cells and its regulation by 17beta-oestradiol. Mol. Hum. Reprod. **4:** 603–607.
5. MARKEE, J. 1940. Menstruation in intraocular endometrial transplants in the rhesus monkey. Contrib. Embryol. **177:** 221–308.
6. NOYES, R.W., A.T. HERTIG & J. ROCK. 1950. Dating the endometrial biopsy. Fertil. Steril. **1:** 3–25.
7. FANGER, H. & B.E. BARKER. 1961. Capillaries and arterioles in normal endometrium. Obstet. Gynecol. **17:** 543–550.
8. FERENCZY, A., G. BERTRAND & M. GELFAND. 1979. Proliferation kinetics of human endometrium during the normal mentrual cycle. Am. J. Obstet. Gynecol. **133:** 859–867.
9. ROGERS, P.A., F. LEDERMAN & N. TAYLOR. 1998. Endometrial microvascular growth in normal and dysfunctional states. Hum. Reprod. Update **4:** 503–508.
10. NELSON, K. *et al.* 1991. Epidermal growth factor replaces estrogen in the stimulation of female genital-tract growth and differentiation. Proc. Natl. Acad. Sci. USA **88:** 21–25.
11. KAISERMAN-ABRAMOF, I. & H. PADYKULA. 1989. Angiogenesis in the postovulatory primate endometrium: the coiled arteriolar system. Anat. Rec. **224:** 479–489.
12. RYAN, I., E. SCHRIOCK & R. TAYLOR. 1994. Isolation, characterization and comparison of human endometrial and endometriosis cells *in vitro*. J. Clin. Endocrinol. Metab. **78:** 642–649.
13. SHIFREN, J. *et al.* 1996. Ovarian steroid regulation of vascular endothelial growth factor in the human endometrium: implications for angiogenesis during the menstrual cycle and in the pathogenesis of endometriosis. J. Clin. Endocrinol. Metab. **81:** 3112–3118.
14. HORNUNG, D. *et al.* 1997. Immunolocalization and regulation of the chemokine RANTES in human endometrial and endometriosis tissues and cells. J. Clin. Endocrinol. Metab. **82:** 1621–1628.
15. MUELLER, M.D. *et al.* 2000. Neutrophils infiltrating the endometrium express vascular endothelial growth factor: potential role in endometrial angiogenesis. Fertil. Steril. **74:** 107–112.
16. BRANDENBERGER, A.W. *et al.* 1999. Oestrogen receptor (ER)-α and ER-β isoforms in normal endometrial and endometriosis-derived stromal cells. Mol. Hum. Reprod. **5:** 651–655.
17. WANG, G.M.J. & S.R. GLASSER. 1996. Effects of tamoxifen and ICI 164384 on protein synthesis and vectorial secretion in polarized rat uterine epithelial cells. J. Steroid Biochem. Mol. Biol. **58:** 307–317.
18. TORA, L.M.A., D. METZGER, M. PONGLIKITMONGKOL, *et al.* 1989. The cloned human oestrogen receptor contains a mutation which alters its hormone binding properties. EMBO J. **8:** 1981–1986.
19. TSENG, J. *et al.* 1996. Interleukin-6 secretion *in vitro* is up-regulated in ectopic and eutopic endometrial stromal cells from women with endometriosis. J. Clin. Endocrinol. Metab. **81:** 1118–1122.
20. HORNUNG, D., J.-L. VIGNE & R.N. TAYLOR. 1998. RANTES derived from normal endometrial and endometriosis stromal cells has altered bio- to immunoactivity. J. Soc. Gynecol. Invest. **5:** 18.

21. LEBOVIC, D.I. *et al.* 2000. Induction of an angiogenic phenotype in endometriotic stromal cell cultures by interleukin-1beta. Mol. Hum. Reprod. **6:** 269–275.
22. MUELLER, V.J., A. MINCHENKO, D.I. LEBOVIC, *et al.* 2000. Regulation of vascular endothelial growth factor (VEGF) gene transcription by estrogen receptors alpha and beta. Proc. Natl. Acad. Sci. USA **97:** 10972–10977.
23. DONNEZ, J. *et al.* 1998. Vascular endothelial growth factor (VEGF) in endometriosis. Hum. Reprod. **13:** 1686–1690.
24. PERROT-APPLANAT, M. *et al.* 1988. Immunocytochemical demonstration of estrogen and progesterone receptors in muscle cells of uterine arteries in rabbits and humans. Endocrinology **123:** 1511–1519.
25. TAYLOR, R.N. *et al.* 1999. Ovarian steroids and angiogenesis. *In* Understanding and Managing Endometriosis. A. Lemay & R. Maheux, eds.: 131–137. Parthenon. London.
26. BAKER, V.L. *et al.* 1997. Human umbilical vessels and cultured umbilical vein endothelial and smooth muscle cells lack detectable protein and mRNA encoding estrogen receptors. J. Soc. Gynecol. Invest. **4:** 316–324.
27. JENSEN, I. *et al.* 1998. Human umbilical vein endothelial cells lack expression of the estrogen receptor. Endothelium **6:** 9–21.
28. KIM-SCHULZE, S. *et al.* 1996. Expression of an estrogen receptor by human coronary artery and umbilical vein endothelial cells. Circulation **94:** 1402–1407.
29. VAZQUEZ, F., J.C. RODRIGUEZ-MANZANEQUE, J.P. LYDON, *et al.* 1999. Progesterone regulates proliferation of endothelial cells. J. Biol. Chem. **274:** 2185–2192.
30. IRUELA-ARISPE, M., C.A. DIGLIO & E.H. SAGE. 1991. Modulation of extracellular matrix proteins by endothelial cells undergoing angiogenesis in vitro. Arterioscler. Thromb. **11:** 805–815.
31. SMITH, S. 1998. Angiogenesis, vascular endothelial growth factor and the endometrium. Hum. Reprod. Update **4:** 509–519.
32. DIZEREGA, G., D. BARBER & G. HODGEN. 1980. Endometriosis: role of ovarian steroids in initiation, maintenance, and suppression. Fertil. Steril. **33:** 649–653.
33. SCHRIOCK, E. *et al.* 1985. Treatment of endometriosis with a potent agonist of gonadotropin-releasing hormone (nafarelin). Fertil. Steril. **44:** 583–588.
34. GARGETT, C.E. *et al.* 1999. Lack of correlation between vascular endothelial growth factor production and endothelial cell proliferation in the human endometrium. Hum. Reprod. **14:** 2080–2088.
35. DAMSKY, C.H. & S.J. FISHER. 1998. Trophoblast pseudo-vasculogenesis: faking it with endothelial adhesion receptors. Curr. Opin. Cell Biol. **5:** 660–666.
36. CHARNOCK-JONES, D.S. *et al.* 1994. Vascular endothelial growth factor receptor localization and activation in human trophoblast and choriocarcinoma cells. Biol. Reprod. **51:** 524–530.
37. PERROT-APPLANAT, M., M. DENG, H. FERNANDEZ, *et al.* 1994. Immunohistochemical localization of estradiol and progesterone receptors in human uterus throughout pregnancy: expression in endometrial blood vessel. J. Clin. Endocrinol. Metab. **78:** 216–224.
38. TISCHER, E. *et al.* 1991. The human gene for vascular endothelial growth factor: multiple protein forms are encoded through alternative exon splicing. J. Biol. Chem. **266:** 11947–11954.
39. DAVIS, D.L. & J.B.E. BURCH. 1996. The chicken vitellogenin II gene is flanked by a GATA factor-dependent estrogen response unit. Mol. Endocrinol. **10:** 937–944.
40. GARRIDO, C., S. SAULE & D. GOSPODAROWICZ. 1993. Transcriptional regulation of vascular endothelial growth factor gene expression in ovarian bovine granulosa cells. Growth Factors **8:** 109–117.
41. KLEIN-HITPAß, L. *et al.* 1988. A 13 bp palindrome is a functional estrogen responsive element and interacts specifically with estrogen receptor. Nucl. Acids Res. **16:** 647–663.
42. VON DER AHE, D. *et al.* 1985. Glucocorticoid and progesterone receptors bind to the same sites in two hormonally regulated promoters. Nature **313:** 706–709.
43. WELTER, J.F. *et al.* 1995. Fos-related Antigen (Fra-1), junB, and junD activate human involucrin promoter transcription by binding to proximal and distal AP1 sites to

mediate phorbol ester effects on promoter activity. J. Biol. Chem. **270:** 12614–12622.

44. HYDER, S.M. *et al.* 2000. Identification of functional estrogen response elements in the gene coding for the potent angiogenic factor vascular endothelial growth factor. Cancer Res. **60:** 3183–3190.

45. KUMAR, V. & P. CHAMBON. 1988. The estrogen receptor binds tightly to its responsive element as a ligand-induced homodimer. Cell **55:** 145–156.

46. PAECH, K. *et al.* 1997. Differential ligand activation of estrogen receptors ERalpha and ERbeta at AP1 sites. Science **277:** 1508–1510.

47. RYUTO, M. *et al.* 1996. Induction of vascular endothelial growth factor by tumor necrosis factor alpha in human glioma cells. Possible roles of SP-1. J. Biol. Chem. **271:** 28220–28228.

48. ROYDS, J.A. *et al.* 1998. Response of tumour cells to hypoxia: role of p53 and NFkB. Mol. Pathol. **51:** 55–61.

Endometrial Quality in Infertile Women with Endometriosis

ANTONIO PELLICER,[a–c] JOSÉ NAVARRO,[a] ERNESTO BOSCH,[a]
NICOLÁS GARRIDO,[a] JUAN A. GARCIA-VELASCO,[a]
JOSÉ REMOHÍ,[a,b] AND CARLOS SIMÓN[a,b]

[a]Instituto Valenciano de Infertilidad, Valencia 46020, Spain

[b]Department of Pediatrics, Obstetrics and Gynecology, Valencia University School of Medicine, Valencia, Spain

[c]Hospital Universitario Dr. Peset, Valencia, Spain

ABSTRACT: Several analyses in our infertility (IVF) and oocyte donation programs were carried out to gain clinical knowledge of the factors involved in the etiology of endometriosis-associated infertility. We first compared the IVF outcomes in women with tubal infertility and endometriosis. The results indicated that patients with endometriosis had a poorer IVF outcome in terms of reduced pregnancy rate per cycle, per transfer, and reduced implantation rate per embryo replaced. We then evaluated embryo development *in vitro* in women with and without endometriosis who underwent IVF and embryo replacement 72 hours after oocyte retrieval. We observed that compared to controls, patients with endometriosis had a significantly reduced number of blastomeres per embryo as well as an increased incidence of arrested embryos *in vitro*. In subsequent studies we compared fertility parameters in patients receiving donor oocytes. We noted that when donor oocytes came from patients without known endometriosis, embryo development and implantation rates were similar in patients with and without endometriosis. However, when the results of oocyte donation were classified according to the nature of the oocytes donated, patients who received embryos derived from oocytes from women with endometriotic ovaries showed a significantly reduced implantation rate compared to the controls. Taken together, these observations suggest that IVF in patients with endometriosis may be related to alterations within the oocyte, which, in turn, result in embryos of lower quality with a reduced ability to implant.

KEYWORDS: embryo quality; endometrium; endometriosis; infertility; oocyte donation

INTRODUCTION

The link between endometriosis and infertility when there is no mechanical alteration of the reproductive organs is a controversial issue. Prospective studies on the prevalence of endometriosis in women undergoing laparoscopy have shown that endometriotic lesions are more frequent in women with pelvic and abdominal pain, in-

Address for correspondence: Dr. Antonio Pellicer, Instituto Valenciano de Infertilidad, Guardia Civil 23, Valencia.46020, Spain. Voice: (34) 963624399; fax: 34-96-3694735.
apellicer@interbook.net

fertility, or dysfunctional uterine bleeding than in those requesting tubal sterilization.[1] A study showed that women presenting with endometriotic lesions at laparoscopy who were treated by surgery had higher pregnancy rates than did those managed expectantly.[2]

The mechanism of infertility associated with nonsevere endometriosis is poorly understood. Many factors have been suggested, such as altered folliculogenesis,[3] ovulatory dysfunction,[4] hyperprolactinemia,[5] luteal phase defect,[6] accelerated ovum transport,[7] sperm phagocytosis,[8] impaired fertilization,[9-11] embryotoxicity against early embryonic development,[12,13] and defective implantation.[14-16]

INFERTILITY IN PATIENTS WITH ENDOMETRIOSIS

Some pathophysiologic questions have been answered, taking into account that the processes of follicular development, fertilization, embryo development, and implantation can now be screened in IVF cycles. However, the data are highly controversial. Some investigators have reported poorer outcome with IVF in patients with endometriosis than in those with infertility of other etiologies.[9-11,14-17] Others have reported favorable results in endometriosis,[18-22] at least as good as those in women with tubal infertility. Two main mechanisms have been proposed to explain the detrimental influence of endometriosis on fertility: (1) *poor oocyte quality*, resulting in decreased fertilization rates,[9-11,17,23-26] and (2) *defective implantation capacity* of the embryos, especially in severe endometriosis.[4,14-16,27,28]

A study was undertaken to investigate the subfertile status of 59 women (96 cycles) with different degrees of endometriosis compared with a control group of 78 women (96 cycles) with tubal infertility.[27] The number of oocytes retrieved and the fertilization rates were no different between groups. Similarly, the total number of embryos transferred in each group was comparable. Interestingly, a statistically significant decrease in pregnancy rate per cycle (not shown) (12.5% vs. 34.4%; p <0.0004), pregnancy per transfer (15.1% vs. 37.3%; p <0.002), and implantation rate (5.8% vs. 13.4%; p <0.003) was observed in patients with endometriosis compared to women with tubal infertility (FIG. 1).

In a retrospective analysis,[29] the quality of embryos derived from 36 women with endometriosis was compared with embryos from 34 women with tubal infertility. The number of blastomeres and the degree of fragmentation were established after 48 and 72 hours in culture. Embryo blockage was considered when embryos presented 1 to 2 blastomeres 72 hours after oocyte retrieval.[30] No differences were noted between groups in age, number of oocytes retrieved, number fertilized, and mean number of blastomeres after 48 hours. However, after 72 hours there was a significant (p <0.04) decrease in the number of blastomeres in women with endometriosis compared to those with tubal infertility (5.4 ± 0.1 vs. 6.1 ± 0.3, respectively). Similarly, a significant (p <0.05) increase was noted in the percentage of arrested embryos in the endometriosis group compared with the tubal infertility group (57.4 ± 2.3; 45.2 ± 5.8, respectively). Our observations have been confirmed by other investigators who employed videocameras to record zygote formation and embryo development *in vitro,* showing that the percentage of aberrant forms was higher in patients with endometriosis than in others.[31]

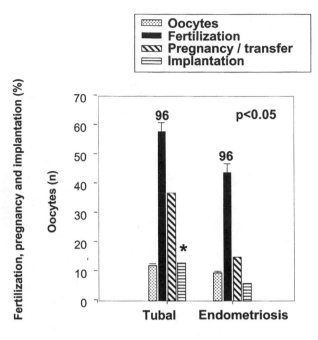

FIGURE 1. Infertility outcome comparing endometriosis and tubal infertility. Numbers on the top of each column represent the cycles performed. Adapted from reference 27.

Based on our results, implantation was significantly impaired in women with endometriosis. The quality of the embryos replaced was probably responsible for this finding. To gain more insight, we addressed this issue by analyzing the results of our oocyte donation program.

OOCYTE DONATION IN PATIENTS WITH ENDOMETRIOSIS

Oocyte donation is a therapeutic option for women with premature ovarian failure, low responders to conventional controlled ovarian stimulation, and those with severe endometriosis with repeated IVF program failure. This therapeutic strategy provides an interesting model to investigate the reproductive outcome in women with endometriosis, because it is possible to compare women who received fresh oocytes from nonendometriotic women with those receiving oocytes from women with endometriosis.

We retrospectively analyzed the results of our oocyte donation program.[27] One hundred seventy-eight embryo transfers were performed in 141 women divided into three groups: (1) women with premature ovarian failure ($n = 54$), (2) women with a low response to controlled ovarian stimulation ($n = 77$), and (3) women with endometriosis ($n = 10$) who underwent oocyte donation because of a low response. A

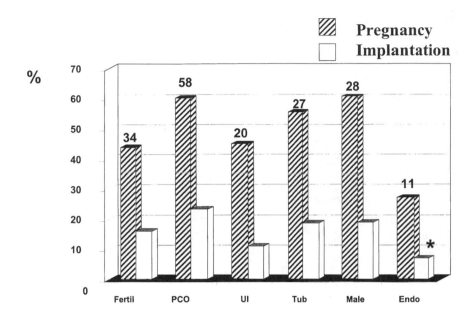

FIGURE 2. Oocyte donation outcome according to the origin of the donated oocytes. Numbers on the top of each column represent the cycles performed. PCO, polycystic ovary; UI, unexplained infertility; Tub, tubal disease; *p <0.05. Adapted from reference 27.

similar number of embryos was replaced in each group. No difference was noted among groups in the pregnancy rate per woman, per cycle, or per implantation.

We also analyzed the outcome of oocyte donation according to the origin of the donated oocytes.[27] We were able to compare the ability of embryos to implant in women with tubal infertility, in male infertility, in ovulation disorders, in fertile women simultaneously undergoing tubal ligation, and in patients with endometriosis. No differences were noted among groups in pregnancy rates per transfer. However, implantation rates (7.0%) were significantly (p <0.05) lower in recipients who received oocytes from women with endometriosis (FIG. 2).

To eliminate the inherent bias of the retrospective model, we designed a prospective study in which three groups were established:[32] Group 1 ($n = 44$), donors and recipients without signs of endometriosis; Group 2 ($n = 14$), donors with endometriosis who donated oocytes to recipients without the disease; and Group 3 ($n = 16$), donors without endometriosis who donated oocytes to recipients with the disease. Impairment of pregnancy rates per transfer ($p = 0.08$) was observed in Group 2 (28.6%) compared to the other two groups (61.4% for Group 1 and 60.0% for Group 3), despite the similar number of embryos that were replaced. A significant (p <0.05) decrease in implantation rates was noted also in Group 2 (6.8%) compared to Groups 1 (20.1%) and 3 (20.8%), confirming that embryos derived from the ovaries of women with endometriosis display a reduced ability to implant. Our observations were confirmed in a previous study showing that the presence of large endometriomas in

TABLE 1. Infertility outcome in recipients of sibling oocytes with and without stage III–IV endometriosis[a]

	Study group		
	Endometriosis (III–IV)	Control	p value
Patients (n)	25	33	
Cycles (n)	25	33	
Age[a]	35.0 ± 3.4	38.5 ± 4.9	0.004
Oocytes donated (n)[a]	7.8 ± 1.6	7.7 ± 1.9	NS
Embryos transferred (n) [a]	4.0 ± 0.7	4.1 ± 1.2	NS
Good quality embryos transferred (n)[a]	3.6 ± 0.2	3.7 ± 0.1	NS
Implantation (%)	15/101 (14.8)	22/137 (16.0)	NS
Pregnancies (n and %)	10 (40.0)	15 (45.5)	NS
Miscarriage (%)	3 (30.0)	4 (26.0)	NS
Live births (%)	7 (28.0)	9 (27.2)	NS

[a]Values are mean ± SD. NS, not significant.
Source: Reprinted from Diaz et al.[34] with permission.

women undergoing ovum donation is not a factor against successful implantation and pregnancy.[33]

We also designed a prospective matched case-control study to evaluate the impact of severe endometriosis on IVF outcome in women receiving oocytes from the same donor.[34] Fifty-eight recipients were included in the study. Twenty-five patients diagnosed by laparoscopy to have stage III–IV endometriosis (Group I) and 33 women free of the disease (Group II) were included. On the day of retrieval, oocytes from a single donor were randomly donated to recipients in both groups. Comparison of the reproductive outcome addresses how this disease affects fertility. Implantation in recipients of sibling oocytes was not affected by stage III–IV endometriosis as compared to results in controls, indicating that endometriosis does not alter endometrial receptivity (TABLE 1).

Our results therefore show that women with severe endometriosis undergoing hormonal replacement therapy are as likely to conceive as are controls, suggesting that uterine receptivity is not impaired. The question still to be answered is whether these observations hold in natural cycles in which GnRH analogs and HRT are not employed. It is possible that GnRH and HRT treatments affect the endometrial milieu, and this is why in ovum donation endometriosis does reduce fertility. In fact, it was shown that treatment with GnRH analog for several months in patients with endometriosis improved pregnancy rates in IVF.[35]

The poor IVF outcome in advanced stages of endometriosis may be related to the reduced number of retrieved oocytes, leading to the reduced number of selected embryos available to be transferred. A strong body of evidence indicates that embryo morphology correlates with implantation rates and IVF success. Thus, the better the embryo selection, the better the IVF outcome, despite the presence of endometriosis.

This adds credibility to our hypothesis that endometriosis does not affect implantation, even when severe, and that the poor outcome observed in these patients is more likely due to oocyte and embryo alterations. Whether this is the result of a direct effect of endometriosis on folliculogenesis remains to be determined. Given the contemporary methods of endometrial preparation for the transfer of embryos derived from donor eggs, any potential negative effect of severe endometriosis on the uterine environment is undetectable.

ALTERED ENDOMETRIAL ENVIRONMENT IN WOMEN WITH ENDOMETRIOSIS

Despite the accumulated clinical evidence that implantation is not affected, at least in women with endometriosis undergoing ovum donation treated with GnRH analogs and HRT, other investigators have provided data that the endometrial environment is different in women with endometriosis. In keeping with this concept, we first showed an altered endometrial milieu, employing mouse embryos as the experimental model.[13] Embryo development up to the blastocyst stage was impaired when serum from patients with endometriosis was added to the culture medium. Corticosteroids reversed this effect. Similar results were obtained by Damewood *et al.*[12] However, when we applied this concept to women treated with corticosteroids during the luteal phase of the IVF cycle, we were unable to reproduce the results (unpublished observations).

Subsequently, Lessey *et al.*[36] demonstrated that coexpression of the $\alpha 1$, $\alpha 4$, and $\beta 3$ integrins in the endometrium only occurs during the embryonic "implantation window," and it is possible to use this pattern of integrin expression as a marker of endometrial receptivity. They found that women with endometriosis showed defective expression of the $\alpha v \beta 3$ integrin.[37] First, in a retrospective study of 268 endometrial biopsies considered "in phase" based on traditional histologic criteria, they showed that absence of $\alpha v \beta 3$ integrin expression was correlated with the presence of endometriosis. Using a second approach, they addressed a prospective and double blind study of 89 endometrial biopsies that were taken before diagnostic laparoscopy. They proved that most women with abnormal $\alpha v \beta 3$ integrin expression had endometriosis stage I or II. Based on these results, $\alpha v \beta 3$ integrin expression could be a useful marker of mild endometriosis. However, other investigators did not confirm these findings.[38,39] In a recent clinical prospective study, Lessey *et al.*[40] concluded that inmmunohistochemical criteria based on epithelial endometrial expression during the menstrual cycle cannot substitute for traditional histologic dating criteria of the endometrium.

Moreover, there are other potential biochemical and morphologic markers that need to be further explored. Considerable evidence in the literature indicates that localized eutopic endometrium (EUE) and localized ectopic endometrium (EEE) obtained from women with endometriosis are clearly different from the endometrium of women without the disease. This theory is based on the following three concepts. (1) EEE does not go through the characteristic endometrial cyclic changes, probably because steroid receptor expression in the EEE is clearly different from the distribution in EUE.[41,42] (2) In contrast to normal endometrium, EEE and EUE express aromatase enzyme activity and consequently have the capacity to produce estrogen.

This altered function may explain the ability of the EEE to implant in the peritoneal surface and further grow through paracrine and autocrine mechanisms.[43] (3) There are intrinsic differences between normal endometrium and EEE and EUE with respect to cytokine production and/or regulation.[44,45]

Other molecules were recently studied in women with endometriosis. ICAM-1 (intercellular adhesion molecule-1) levels in endometrial stromal cell cultures were higher in cells isolated from uteri of women with endometriosis.[46] It is unclear if high levels of ICAM-1 are an inherent property of endometriotic cells or simply a consequence of the immune and inflammatory events linked with endometriosis. Cadherins,[47] trophinin and tastin,[48] and CD44[49] have been identified in the endometrium. However, their role during implantation is unclear. The level of IGFBP-1 (insulin-like growth factor binding protein-1) is elevated in the peritoneal fluid of women with endometriosis,[50] and its binding to the alpha $5/\beta1$ integrin by means of its Arg-Gly-Asp sequence has been described.[51] This protein could act through an autocrine mechanism to modify the action of endometrial implants.

We recently performed a prospective study to assess pinopod formation in women with and without endometriosis undergoing oocyte donation.[52] We found no differences between the two groups. This suggests that the endometrium of women with endometriosis is able to develop an adequate response to the HRT in terms of uterine receptivity as evaluated by pinopod formation.

Altered endometrial contractility has been described to occur in the uterus of women with endometriosis. Altered contractility is suggested to compromise normal sperm transport and contribute to reduced fertility in these patients.[53] However, further prospective studies should be designed to directly test endometrial contractibility in women with endometriosis.

REFERENCES

1. MAHMOOD, T.A. & A.A. TEMPLETON. 1991. Folliculogenesis and ovulation in infertile women with mild endometriosis. Hum. Reprod. 6: 227–231.
2. MARCOUX, S., R. MAHEUX, S. BÉRUBÉ, et al. 1997. Laparoscopic surgery in infertile women with minimal or mild endometriosis. N. Engl. J. Med. 337: 217–222.
3. TUMMON, I.S., V.M. MACLIN, D. RADWANSKA, et al. 1988. Occult ovulatory dysfunction in women with minimal endometriosis or unexplained infertility. Fertil. Steril. 50: 716–20.
4. DMOWSKI, W.P., E. RADWANSKA, Z. BINOR, et al. 1986. Mild endometriosis and ovulatory dysfunction: effect of danazol treatment on success of ovulation induction. Fertil. Steril. 46: 784–789.
5. MUSE, K., E.A. WILSON & M.J. JAWAR. 1982. Prolactin hyperstimulation in response to thyrotropin-releasing hormone in patients with endometriosis. Fertil. Steril. 38: 419–422.
6. GRANT, A. 1966. Additional sterility factors in endometriosis. Fertil. Steril. 17: 514–519.
7. CROXATO, H.B., M.-E. ORTIZ, E. GUILOFF, et al. 1978. Effect of 15(S)-15-methyl prostaglandin F2a on human oviductal motility and ovum transport. Fertil. Steril. 30: 408–414.
8. SOLDATI, G., A. PIFFARETTI-YAÑEZ, A. CAMPANA, et al. 1989. Effect of peritoneal fluid on sperm motility and velocity distribution using objective measurements. Fertil. Steril. 52: 113–119.
9. MAHADEVAN, M.M., A.O. TROUNSON & J.F. LEETON. 1983. The relationship of tubal blockage, infertility of unknown cause, suspected male infertility, and endometriosis to success of in vitro fertilization and embryo transfer. Fertil. Steril. 40: 755–762.
10. WARDLE, P.G., P.A. FOSTER, J.D. MITCHELL, et al. 1986. Endometriosis and IVF: effect of prior therapy. Lancet 1: 276–277.

11. WARDLE, P.G., E.A. MCLAUGHLIN, A. MCDERMOTT, *et al.* 1985. Endometriosis and ovulatory disorder:reduced fertilisation in vitro compared with tubal and unexplained infertility. Lancet **2:** 236–239.
12. DAMEWOOD, M.D., J.S. HESLA, W.D. SCHLAFF, *et al.* 1990. Effect of serum from patients with minimal to mild endometriosis on mouse embryo development *in vitro.* Fertil. Steril. **54:** 917–920.
13. SIMÓN, C., E. GÓMEZ, A. MIR, *et al.* 1992. Glucocorticoid treatment decreases sera embryotoxicity in endometriosis patients. Fertil. Steril. **58:** 284–289.
14. YOVICH, J.L., J.M. YOVICH, A.I. TUVIK, *et al.* 1985. *In-vitro* fertilization for endometriosis. Lancet **2:** 552.
15. MATSON, P.L. & J.L. YOVICH. 1986. The treatment of infertility associated with endometriosis by in vitro fertilization. Fertil. Steril. **46:** 432–434.
16. O'SHEA, R.T., C. CHEN, T. WEISS, *et al.* 1985. Endometriosis and *in-vitro* fertilization. Lancet **2:** 723.
17. PAL, L., J.L. SHIFREN, K.B. ISAACSON, *et al.* 1998. Impact of varying stages of endometriosis on the outcome of in vitro fertilization-embryo transfer. J. Assist. Reprod. Genet. **15:** 27–31.
18. GEBER, S., T. PARASCHOS, G. ATKINSON, *et al.* 1995. Results of IVF in patients with endometriosis: the severity of the disease does not affect outcome, or the incidence of miscarriage. Hum. Reprod. **10:** 1507–1511.
19. JONES, H.W., JR., A.A. ACOSTA, M.C. ANDREWS, *et al.* 1984. Three years of *in vitro* fertilization at Norfolk. Fertil. Steril. **42:** 826–834.
20. OLIVENNES, F., D. FELDBERG, H.C. LIU, *et al.* 1995. Endometriosis: a stage by stage analysis-the role of in vitro fertilization. Fertil. Steril. **64:** 392–398.
21. OEHNINGER, S., A.A. ACOSTA, D. KREINER, *et al.* 1988. *In vitro* fertilization and embryo transfer (IVF/ET): an established and succesful therapy for endometriosis. J. In Vitro Fertil. Embryo Transfer **5:** 249–256.
22. FIVNAT (French In Vitro National): French national IVF registry: analysis of 1986 to 1990 data. 1993. Fertil. Steril. **59:** 587–595.
23. CAHILL, D.J., P.G. WARDLE, L.A. MAILE, *et al.* 1997. Ovarian dysfunction in endometriosis-associated and unexplained infertility. J. Assist. Reprod. Genet. **14:** 554–557.
24. BERGENDAL, A., S. NAFFAH, C. NAGY, *et al.* 1998. Outcome of IVF in patients with endometriosis in comparison with tubal factor infertility. J. Assist. Reprod. Genet. **15:** 530–534.
25. HULL, M.G., J.A. WILLAIMS, B. RAY, *et al.* 1998. The contribution of subtle oocyte or sperm dysfunction affecting fertilization in endometriosis-associated or unexplained infertility: a controlled comparison with tubal infertility and use of donor spermatozoa. Hum. Reprod. **13:** 1825–1830.
26. MILLS, M.S., H.A. EDDOWES, D.J. CAHILL, *et al.* 1992. A prospective controlled study of in-vitro fertilization, gamete intra-Fallopian transfer and intrauterine insemination combined with superovulation. Hum. Reprod. **7:** 490–494.
27. SIMÓN, C., A. GUTIERREZ, A. VIDAL, *et al.* 1994. Outcome of patients with endometriosis in assisted reproduction: results from *in vitro* fertilization and oocyte donation. Hum. Reprod. **9:** 725–729.
28. ARICI, A., E. ORAL, O. BUKULMEZ, *et al.* 1996. The effects of endometriosis on implantation: results from the Yale University *in vitro* fertilization and embryo transfer programme. Fertil. Steril. **65:** 603–607.
29. PELLICER, A., N. OLIVEIRA, A. RUIZ, *et al.* 1995. Exploring the mechanism(s) of endometriosis-related infertility: an analysis of embryo development and implantation in assisted reproduction. Hum. Reprod. **10** (Suppl. 2): 91–97.
30. CLAMAN, P., D.R. ARMANT, M.M. SEIBEL, *et al.* 1987. The impact of embryo quality and quantity on implantation and the establishment of viable pregnancies. J. in Vitro Fertil. Embryo Transfer **4:** 218–221.
31. BRIZEK, C.L., S. SCHLAFF, V.A. PELLEGRINI, *et al.* 1995. Increased incidence of aberrant morphological phenoptypes in human embryogenesis: an association with endometriosis. J. Assist. Reprod. Genet.**12:** 106–112.

32. PELLICER, A., N. OLIVEIRA, A. GUTIERREZ, et al. 1994. Implantation in endometriosis: Lessons learned from IVF and oocyte donation. In Progress in Endometriosis. P. Spinola & E.M. Coutinho, eds. :177–183. Parthenon Publ. Group. Casterton-Hill.

33. SUNG, L., T. MUKHERJEE, T. TAKESHIGE, et al. 1997. Endometriosis is not detrimental to embryo implantation in oocyte recipients. J. Assist. Reprod. Genet. **14:** 152–156.

34. DÍAZ, I., J. NAVARRO, L. BLASCO, et al. 2000. Impact of stages III–IV of endometriosis on recipients of sibling oocytes. Matched case-control study. Fertil Steril. **74:** in press.

35. MARCUS, S.F. & R.G. EDWARDS. 1994. High rates of pregnancy after long-term down-regulation of women with severe endometriosis. Am. J. Obstet. Gynecol. **171:** 812–817.

36. LESSEY, B.A., A.J. CASTELBAUM, C.A. BUCK, et al. 1994. Further characterization of endometrial integrins during the menstrual cycle and in pregnancy. Fertil. Steril. **62:** 497–506

37. LESSEY, B.A., A.J. CASTELBAUM, S.W. SAWIN, et al. 1994. Aberrant integrin expression in the endometrium of women with endometriosis. J. Clin. Endocrinol. Metab. **79:** 643–649.

38. BRIDGES, J., A. PRENTICE, W. ROCHE, et al. 1994. Expression of integrin adhesion molecules in endometrium and endometriosis. Br. J. Obstet. Gynaecol. **101:** 696–700.

39. HILL, L. & P. ROGERS. 1998. Endometrial vascular and glandular expression of integrins alpha (v) beta 3 in women with and without endometriosis. Hum. Reprod. **13:** 1030–1035.

40. LESSEY, B.A., A.J. CATELBAUM, L. WOLF, et al. 2000. Use of integrins to date the endometrium. Fertil. Steril. **73:** 779–787.

41. JÄNNE, O., A. KOUPPILA, E. KOKKO, et al. 1981. Estrogen and progestin receptors in endometriosis lesions: comparison with endometrial tissue. Am. J. Obstet. Gynecol. **141:** 562.

42. VAZQUEZ, G., F. CORNILLIE & I. BROSENS. 1984. Peritoneal endometriosis: scanning electron microscopy and histology of minimal pelvic endometriotic lesions. Fertil. Steril. **42:** 696–703

43. NOBLE, L., E. SIMPSON, A. JOHNS, et al. 1996. Aromatase expression in endometriosis. J. Clin. Endocrinol. Metab. **81:** 174–179.

44. HORNUNG, D., I. RYAN, V. CHAO, et al. 1997. Immunolocalization and regulation of the chemokine RANTES in human endometrial and endometriosis tissues and cells. J. Clin. Endocrinol. Metab. **82:** 1621–1628.

45. IWABE, T., T. HARADA, T. TSUDO, et al. 1998. Pathogenetic significance of increased levels of interleukin-8 in the peritoneal fluid of patients with endometriosis. Fertil. Steril. **69:** 924–930.

46. SOMIGLIANA, E., P. VIGANO, B. GAFURRI, et al. 1996. Human endometrial stromal cells as a source of soluble intercellular adhesion molecules (ICAM)-1 molecules. Hum. Reprod. **10:** 1571–1578.

47. VAN DER LINDEN, P., A. DE GOEIJ, G. DUNSELMAN, et al. 1995. Expression of cadherins and integrins in human endometrium throughout the menstrual cycle. Fertil. Steril. **63:** 1210.

48. FUKUDA, M., T. SATO, J. NAKAYAMA, et al. 1995. Trophinin and tastin, a novell cell adhesion molecule complex with potential involvement in embryo implantation. Genes Dev. **9:** 1199–1210.

49. YAEGASHI, N., N. FUJITA, A. YAJIMA, et al. 1995. Menstrual cycle dependent expression of CD44 in normal endometrium. Hum. Pathol. **26:** 862–865.

50. TASKIN, O., L. GIUDICE, R. MANGAL, et al. 1996. Insulin growth factor binding proteins in peritoneal fluid of women with minimal and mild endometriosis. Hum. Reprod. **11:** 1741–1746.

51. JONES, J., A. GOCKERMAN, W. BUSBY, et al. 1993. Insulin like growth factor binding protein-1 stimulated cell migration and bind to the alpha 5/b1 integrin by means of tis Arg-Gly-Asp sequence. Proc. Natl. Acad. Sci. USA **90:** 10553–10557.

52. GARCÍA-VELASCO, J., C. SIMON, G. ARDILES, et al. 1998. Assesment of endometrial response to HRT using the detection of pinopods in women with endometriosis undergoing oocyte donation (abstr.). Fertil. Steril. **70:** S242.

53. DE VRIES, K., E. LYONS, G. BALLARD, et al. 1990. Contractions of the inner third of the myometrium. Am. J. Obstet. Gynecol. **162:** 679–682.

Endometrial Anomalies in Women with Endometriosis

KATHY L. SHARPE-TIMMS

Departments of Obstetrics and Gynecology and Animal Sciences; Division of Ob/Gyn Research; and MU Hospital and Clinics Assisted Reproduction Laboratories, University of Missouri-Columbia, Columbia, Missouri 65212, USA

ABSTRACT: Endometriotic lesions are defined by extrauterine growth of endometrial glands and stroma. Retrograde menstruation with subsequent attachment, invasion, and neovascularization are believed to give rise to the endometriotic lesions. As most women exhibit some degree of retrograde menstruation, some other unidentified factor(s) must render certain women susceptible to attachment and growth of ectopic endometrial tissue. A variety of theories have been proposed to account for this susceptibility, including genetic predisposition, aberrant immunological response, and an altered peritoneal environment. Ectopic endometriotic lesions are histologically similar to their putative eutopic precursors, yet significant biochemical differences exist between these two tissues. Less information is available regarding differences between eutopic endometrium from women with or without endometriosis. This report describes anomalies in structure, proliferation, immune components, adhesion molecules, proteolytic enzymes and inhibitors, steroid and cytokine production and responsiveness, and gene expression and protein production that have been identified in eutopic endometrium from women with endometriosis.

KEYWORDS: endometrium; endometriosis; endometrial anomalies

INTRODUCTION

Endometriosis is defined as extrauterine growth of endometrial glands and stroma. Although the ectopic endometriotic lesions are histologically similar to their putative eutopic precursors, significant biochemical differences between these two tissues have been identified (TABLE 1).[1]

Evidence is now accumulating which suggests that eutopic endometrium from women with endometriosis has some fundamental differences compared to eutopic endometrium from women without endometriosis. These include a variety of anomalies in structure, proliferation, immune components, adhesion molecules, proteolytic enzymes and inhibitors, steroid and cytokine production and responsiveness, and gene expression and protein production (TABLE 2). To date, however, some of the data in the literature are contradictory and mandate further investigation. Ultimately,

Address for correspondence: Dr. Kathy L. Sharpe-Timms, Department of Obstetrics and Gynecology, 1 Hospital Drive N625 HSC, University of Missouri-Columbia, Columbia, MO 65212. Voice: 573-882-7937. Fax: 573-882-9010.
timmsk@health.missouri.edu

TABLE 1. Qualitative and quantitative differences between endometriotic lesions and eutopic endometrium

Anomaly	Description in endometriotic lesions	References
Steroid hormone responsiveness & receptor content	• Less hormonally regulated than eutopic endometrium and heterogeneous content and altered cyclic pattern of expression of steroid receptors	Vierikko et al.;[63] Lechner et al.;[64] Megela et al.;[65] Bergqvist et al.;[66] Bergqvist & Ferno;[67] Nisolle et al.;[68] Howell et al.;[69] Jones et al.[70]
Growth factor responsiveness and receptor content	• Diminished response to EGF	Haining et al.;[71] Prentice et al.;[72] Huang & Yeh;[73] Mellor & Thomas[74]
	• Fibroblast growth factor similar to eutopic endometrium	Ferriani et al.[75]
	• Increased expression of GM-CSF in the secretory stage	Sharpe-Timms et al.[76]
	• Increased INF g mRNA and receptors	Klein et al.[77]
	• Deficiency of IL-1 receptor antagonist	Sahakian et al.[78]
Protein production	• Synthesize and secrete more CA 125	Kobayashi et al.[79]
	• Lack of estrogen regulation of complement component 3	Isaacson et al.[80,81]
	• Significant expression of ENDO-I = endometriotic haptoglobin	Sharpe-Timms et al.[82–85] & Piva and Sharpe-Timms[86]
Expression of enzymes and their inhibitors	• Higher levels of cathepsin D	Bergqvist et al.[87]
	• Continuous expression of several MMPs	Osteen et al.[88] & Cox et al.[89]
	• Overexpression of TIMPs in vitro	Sharpe-Timms et al.[90,91]
	• High levels of uPA	Fernandez-Shaw et al.[92]

these differences lend credence to the possibility the eutopic endometrium from women with endometriosis is innately aberrant and plays an important role in the pathogenesis and pathophysiologies associated with endometriosis. Additional insight into such differences may be used in the development of less invasive methods of diagnosis or novel therapeutic or preventive approaches for this enigmatic disorder.

ENDOMETRIAL ANOMALIES IN WOMEN WITH ENDOMETRIOSIS

Most women undergoing laparoscopy during menses exhibit some degree of retrograde menstruation.[2] However, some other unidentified factor or factors render certain women susceptible to attachment, growth, and persistence of ectopic endometrial tissue in the peritoneal cavity. A variety of theories have been proposed to account for this susceptibility and include genetic predisposition,[3] aberrant immunologic response,[4] and an altered peritoneal environment.[5] As noted previously, significant biochemical differences have been described between eutopic endometrium and ectopic endometriotic lesions,[1] yet until recently, surprisingly little information

TABLE 2. Endometrial anomalies in eutopic endometrium from women with endometriosis

Anomaly	Description	References
Structure	• Increased heterogeneity in surface epithelium, reduced glandular and stromal mitoses, basal vacuolated cells • Reduced endometrial thickness	Fedele et al.[6] Shapiro et al.[7]
Proliferation	• Increased numbers of proliferating endometrial epithelial, stromal, and endothelial cells • No differences in endometrial cell proliferative activity	Wingfield et al.[8] Kruitwagen et al.[10] & Jurgensen et al.[9]
Apoptosis	• Impaired spontaneous apoptosis. • No significant difference in apoptosis or Bcl-2	Gebel et al.[11] Jones et al.[12]
Immune components	• Increased secretion of complement component C3 • No difference in presence of C3 or C4 • Presence of endometrial antigens of MW 60 and 66 kDa of the IgG class • Decreased mitogenicity for autologous lymphocytes • Trend for fewer T-suppressor/cytotoxic (CD8$^+$) cells and endometrial granulated lymphocytes but more T-helper/inducer (CD4$^+$) cells, CD68$^+$cells and CD16$^+$ cells • No difference in defined stromal leukocyte subpopulations • Increased numbers of CD45$^+$, CD43$^+$, and CD3$^+$ intraepithelial leukocytes • Increased resistance to the cytotoxic effect of heterologous lymphocytes • Increased expression of heat shock protein 27	Isaacson et al.[18] Bartosik et al.[17] Odukoya et al.[19] Helvacioglu et al.[20] Klentzeris et al.[21] Jones et al.[22] Bulmer et al.[23] Oosterlynck et al.[26] Ota et al.[27] & Nip et al.[28]
Cell adhesion molecules	• Lack of αv3 expression on endometrial epithelium • No difference in endometrial epithelial αv3 expression • Increased expression of β-1 integrins and E-cadherin on endometrial glandular epithelium	Lessey et al.[32,33] Hii and Rogers[34] Ota and Tanaka[31]
Proteases and their inhibitors	• Aberrant production of matrix metalloproteinases (MMPs) and their inhibitors, the tissue inhibitor of metalloproteinases (TIMPs)	Osteen et al.[36] & Sharpe-Timms et al.[35]
Steroid and cytokine production and responsiveness	• Expression of aromatase P450 • No difference in estrogen nor progesterone receptor expression • Increased secretion of hepatic growth factor • Elevated production of IL-6 • Elevated responsiveness to IL-1 and IL-6 • Increased production of MCP-1	Noble et al.[46] & Kitawaki et al.[47] Nisolle et al.[48] & Jones et al.[22] Sugawara et al.[49] Tseng et al.[50] Tseng et al.[50] & Piva and Sharpe-Timms[51] Akoum et al.[52] & Jolicoeur et al.[53]

TABLE 2. Endometrial anomalies in eutopic endometrium from women with endometriosis (*Continued*)

Anomaly	Description	References
Protein production and gene expression	• Increased production of CA-125 • Absence of the mid-luteal rise in eutopic endometrial HOX gene expression • Increased production of de novo synthesized endometriotic haptoglobin	McBean et al.[54] Taylor et al.[55] Sharpe-Timms et al.[57,62] & Piva and Sharpe-Timms[58]

was available regarding differences between eutopic endometrium from women with and those without endometriosis. The following information provides details of the potential significance of eutopic endometrial anomalies that may be central to the pathogenesis and/or pathophysiologies of this disorder.

Structure

Structural and ultrastructural defects in preovulatory endometrium from women with minimal or mild endometriosis have been identified by light, scanning, and transmission electron microscopic studies (FIG. 1).[6] These analyses revealed heterogeneity of the endometrial surface epithelium in 77% of patients with endometriosis and in 16% of the non-endometriosis controls. Glandular and stromal mitoses, basal vacuolated cells, and the ciliated to nonciliated cell ratio were significantly reduced in the endometriosis group compared with the controls. Whereas further studies are needed to clarify the role of these observed endometrial anomalies, these data suggest that a primary endometrial factor may be involved in the pathogenesis of infertility in patients with minimal or mild endometriosis. Clinical observation study showing inadequate endometrial thickness in women with endometriosis undergoing superovulation and intrauterine insemination as compared to women with other diagnoses undergoing the same protocols support these observations of structural anomalies.[7]

Proliferation

Wingfield and co-workers[8] described increased *in vivo* proliferation of endometrial epithelial, stromal, and endothelial cells in women with endometriosis. Immunohistochemical analyses performed on fixed tissue sections detected proliferation of both endothelial cells (anti-CD43) and endometrial epithelial and stromal cells (antiproliferating cell nuclear antigen or anti-PCNA). The PCNA antigen peaks in the S (DNA synthesis) phase of the cell cycle. Staining differences were quantified by a combined score of the fraction of cells staining and the intensity of the staining. They concluded elevated endometrial cell proliferation could lead to enhanced ability of clumps of endometrial cells that reach the peritoneal cavity through retrograde menstruation to implant, induce an angiogenic response, and thus survive outside the uterus.

Alternatively, Jurgensen and associates,[9] who immunohistochemically studied frozen endometrial tissues with an antibody against Ki-S3 (an epitope of the Ki-67

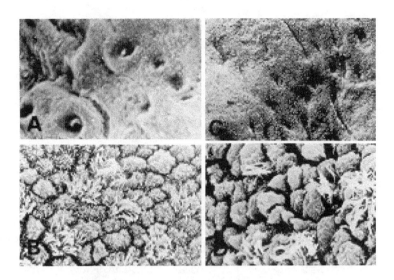

FIGURE 1. Heterogeneity of the endometrial surface in women with endometriosis as demonstrated by scanning electron microscopy. (**A**) Preovulatory stage endometrial surface in control subject shows normal development of nonciliated cells. Glandular ostia are uniformly circular (SEM 400x). (**B**) Secretory stage endometrial surface in control subject shows cells with thick bunches of cilia surrounded by cells with dense coverings of microvilli (SEM 5,000x). (**C**) Preovulatory stage endometrial surface in woman with mild endometriosis shows surface heterogeneity with irregularly distributed glandular lumina (SEM 200x). (**D**) Secretory stage endometrial surface in woman with mild endometriosis shows nonciliated cells of irregular form. Ciliated cells are scant and have incomplete ciliogenesis. (Adapted from Fedele *et al.* 1990. Fertil. Steril. **53:** 991–992.)

antigen), found no significant differences in endometrial cell proliferation between women with and those without endometriosis. This antibody recognized cells in G1 (postmitotic phase), S (DNA synthesis), G2 (pre-mitotic phase), and M (mitosis), but not G0 (proliferating resting or terminal phase) of the cell cycle. Staining differences were quantified by comparing separate scores for the fraction of cells staining and the staining intensity.

The disparities in the findings of these two studies may be attributed to differences in patient populations, technical details including tissue processing and antibodies chosen for staining, or method used for data analysis. Others have failed to show any enhanced proliferation of endometrial cells harvested from the peritoneal fluid of women with and those without endometriosis.[10] These studies, however, were performed *in vitro* and may have lacked paracrine influence from entities in the peritoneal cavity. Ultimately, further studies will have to be performed to resolve the differences between these observations and to determine if aberrant endometrial cell proliferation contributes to the pathogenesis of endometriosis. It is also possible that altered endometrial proliferation may interfere with embryo implantation and thus contribute to the infertility and increased risk of miscarriage associated with endometriosis. This too remains to be proven.

Apoptosis

Gebel *et al.*[11] reported that among women with endometriosis, the percentage of sloughed endometrial cells undergoing apoptosis was greatly reduced, implying that the number of surviving cells that enter the peritoneal cavity is greater in women who develop endometriosis. A commercially available cell death ELISA kit, reportedly a highly sensitive and specific assay for apoptosis, was used. Conversely, Jones and colleagues[12] reported that neither apoptosis nor expression of Bcl-2 (a cell surface receptor associated with triggering apoptosis) was elevated in these tissues. The later studies, however, used the dUTP nick-end labeling TUNEL assay that measures fragmented DNA but cannot determine between apoptotic and necrotic cells. Others have confirmed that Bcl-2 expression is not different in these tissues from women with endometriosis.[13]

Another possible explanation offered for the inappropriate transduction of the apoptotic signal in endometrium from women with endometriosis is that the second messenger that triggers apoptosis in endometrium from healthy women actually triggers cellular proliferation in women with endometriosis.[11] Ceramide, a metabolite of sphingomyelin, may mediate these two apparently contradictory activities.[14] Precedence has been set for such contradictory response in the endometrium, as the proliferation of endometrium from normal healthy controls is suppressed by tumor necrosis factor-α (TNF-α), whereas proliferation of endometrium from patients with endometriosis is enhanced by TNF-α.[15]

Immune Components

The role of the immune system in endometriosis has been studied extensively. Yet, whether immune anomalies are a cause or a result of endometriosis has not been resolved. Nonetheless, numerous immune anomalies have been identified in women with this disorder. The following information describes anomalous immune components that have been observed in association with the eutopic endometrium.

Weed and Arquembourg[16] first described deposition of complement component C3 in endometrial glandular epithelial cells of women with endometriosis. Subsequently, it was discovered that C3 synthesis and secretion by early proliferative endometrium of patients with minimal endometriosis was significantly greater than that of patients with no endometriosis or patients with severe endometriosis.[17,18] It is possible that the known biological functions of C3 may play a role in the pathogenesis or pathophysiologies associated with endometriosis. C3 could exert these effects via opsonization for phagocyte (macrophage) activation, stimulation of prostaglandin synthesis from a variety of cell types, platelet aggregation and thrombin release, or activation of other components of the complement system.

The presence of endometrial antigens of MW 60 and 66 kDa of the IgG class has been observed in approximately 50% of patients with endometriosis.[19] It remains unclear whether these represent a pathologically distinct subgroup of such patients.

Autologous lymphocyte and eutopic endometrial cells from women with and those without endometriosis were cocultured to observe lymphocyte proliferation.[20] A diminished proliferative response of lymphocytes from women with endometriosis was noted. Yet, as these same lymphocytes were stimulated by phytohemagglutinin (PHA) in a simultaneous assay, it was determined that the diminished proliferative response of lymphocytes from women with endometriosis was probably not the consequence of an intrinsic lymphocyte abnormality. It was hypothesized that a fundamental defect in endometriosis may reside within the eutopic endometrial cells.

Endometrial leukocyte populations have been studied in women with endometriosis. Although not statistically different, a trend was observed for fewer T-suppressor/cytotoxic (CD8[+]) cells and endometrial granulated lymphocytes but more T-helper/inducer (CD4[+]) cells, CD68[+] cells, and CD16[+] cells in the endometrium of women with endometriosis.[21] Additional studies of specific endometrial cell types found no difference in defined stromal leukocyte subpopulations[22] yet increased numbers of CD45[+], CD43[+], and CD3[+] intraepithelial leukocytes[23] when comparing eutopic endometrium from women with endometriosis with that of controls. While providing semiquantitative information about the leukocyte populations in these tissues, these studies have not provided data about the functional differences of endometrial leukocytes between the two groups. It is possible that although leukocyte numbers were not significantly different, leukocyte subpopulations may differ in their activational status. Activated immune cells produce cytokines that could be either beneficial or detrimental to the processes of embryo implantation or the disease pathogenesis in the case of endometriosis.[24,25]

The role of natural killer (NK) cells in the decreased cellular immunity of women with endometriosis has been investigated.[26] NK activity (K562-assay) and cytotoxicity against autologous endometrial cells were both decreased in women with endometriosis and correlated with the severity of the disease. It was concluded that the decreased cytotoxicity to endometrial cells in women with endometriosis was mainly due to a defect in NK activity, but it was also partially because of a resistance of the eutopic endometrium to NK cytotoxicity.

A number of heat shock proteins are expressed constitutively in mammalian organs. They are also synthesized in response to a variety of physical and chemical stimuli such as heat shock, steroids, and oxidative damage. Studies also suggest that heat shock proteins are involved directly or indirectly with the immune system through antigen processing, antigen presentation, or peptide binding. Certain T cells can recognize heat shock proteins as specific antigens, and as such, heat shock proteins may serve as ligands of T cells. Ota and coworkers[27] found a significant increase in expression of heat shock protein 27 (hsp 27) in eutopic endometrium from patients with endometriosis and adenomyosis compared with controls regardless of menstrual cycle stage. The increase in intracellular hsp 27 was implicated in the immune response mediated by macrophages and or T cells in endometriosis. Furthermore, as Danazol treatment reduced the expression of hsp 27, it was speculated that this protein might participate in the activation process of estrogen. Clinically, eutopic endometrial expression of hsp 27 has been associated with unexplained infertility in association with endometriosis.[28]

Recently, we observed that macrophages residing in the functionalis zone of the endometrium are intensely immunoreactive with anti-human haptoglobin antibody (Sharpe-Timms, unpublished data; FIG. 2). We hypothesize that de novo synthesized, extrahepatic, endometrial haptoglobin inhibits macrophage phagocytic function in endometrial functionalis sloughed at menses. As with a reduction in apoptosis, this implies that more viable endometrial cells may reach the peritoneal cavity and establish themselves as endometriotic lesions. Additional information about the role of endometriosis-associated haptoglobin is provided at the end of this manuscript.

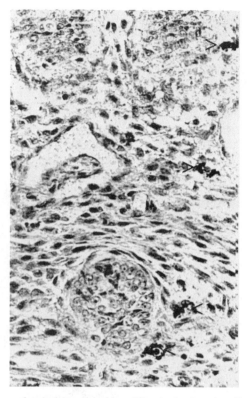

FIGURE 2. Macrophages (*arrowheads*) residing in the functionalis zone of endometria of women with endometriosis are intensely immunoreactive with antihuman haptoglobin antibody. We hypothesize that de novo synthesized, extrahepatic, endometrial haptoglobin inhibits macrophage phagocytic function in endometrial functionalis sloughed at menses.[84,85]

Cell Adhesion Molecules

Integrins are a family of cell adhesion molecules that function in both cell-cell and cell substratum adhesion. The integrins promote cell attachment to proteins within the extracellular matrix (ECM) and potentiate cell migration and invasion. Some cases of integrin attachment to the ECM require tyrosine kinase receptor-mediated signaling, whereas others do not. It appears that cytokine receptors and adhesion molecules may cooperate functionally to promote cell motility and perhaps invasion.[29] Integrins, in particular αvβ3 and of αvβ5, have also been shown to form cell surface complexes with matrix metalloproteinases to facilitate matrix degradation and motility, thereby facilitating directed cellular invasion.[30]

Many members of the integrin family are expressed by the endometrium throughout the menstrual cycle. For example, increased expression of β-1 integrins and E-cadherin has been observed on endometrial glandular epithelium.[31] The expression of αvβ3 by endometrial epithelium is coincident with the period of uterine receptivity.[32] Expression of cell adhesion molecules reportedly differs in the eutopic endometrium of women with endometriosis. The absence of αvβ3 expression on endometrial epithelium of women with endometriosis is notable.[33] Others have failed to detect cycle-specific expression of this integrin;[34] yet, evidence suggests differences in technical approach account for these negative findings.

We recently showed that $\alpha v\beta3$ colocalizes and forms a complex with MMP-2 and that $\alpha v\beta5$ colocalizes and forms complexes with both MMP-2 and MMP-3 on the luminal epithelial surface of eutopic human endometrium.[35] This suggests interactions between endometrial integrins and MMPs that may coordinate cell adhesion, migration, invasion, and targeted proteolytic endometrial remodeling, thereby facilitating embryo implantation. Hence, lack of $\alpha v\beta3$ expression by the eutopic endometrium during the period of uterine receptivity in women with endometriosis may be associated with decreased cycle fecundity due to defects in uterine receptivity.

Proteases and Their Inhibitors

Aberrant production of matrix metalloproteinases (MMPs) and their inhibitors, the tissue inhibitor of metalloproteinases (TIMPs), have been associated with endometriosis and eutopic endometrium.[36–39] The MMPs serve to break down all components of the extracellular matrix (ECM) and thereby participate in both normal and pathological tissue remodeling. Under normal conditions, MMP expression is highly regulated by steroid hormones and growth factors.[40] MMPs participate in monthly endometrial remodeling during the menstrual cycle, trophoblast invasion, and decidualization.[41–44] Expression of several members of the MMP family by endometrium of women with endometriosis is miss-regulated and may contribute to the establishment of the ectopic endometriotic lesions in the peritoneal cavity.[36,39,45]

As just described, the MMPs may form complexes with integrin cell adhesion molecules to localize protease activity and facilitate directed cell migration. The TIMPs serve to control this migration. We have shown that women with endometriosis have significantly less TIMP-1 in their peritoneal fluid than do women without endometriosis.[38] Whereas endometriotic lesions and endometrial tissues have been shown to produce TIMP-1,[1,37,46] it remains to be resolved if TIMP-1 production is altered in eutopic endometrium from women with endometriosis.

Steroid and Cytokine Production and Responsiveness

Various anomalies in steroid and cytokine production and responsiveness have been reported in eutopic endometrium in women with endometriosis. A variety of molecular and protein techniques have been used to demonstrate that both endometriotic lesions and eutopic endometrium from women with endometriosis contain transcripts for P450 aromatase.[46,47] Aromatase P450 acts in the conversion of C19 steroids to estrogens in various tissues including the ovary and placenta, but not the normal endometrium from controls. It was concluded that aromatase expression by eutopic endometrium may be related to the capability of these tissues to implant on peritoneal surfaces. As the estrogen and progesterone receptor status of eutopic endometrium from women with and without endometriosis does not vary,[22,48] the unique ability to produce estrogen in eutopic endometrium from women with endometriosis may serve to selectively promote their growth in ectopic locations.

Cytokine production has been shown to be divergent when comparing ectopic and eutopic endometrium.[1] Recently, differences in cytokine production have been rec-

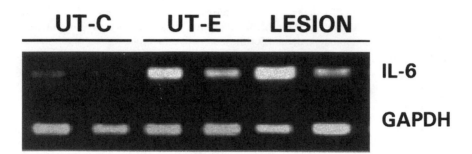

FIGURE 3. Interleukin-6 (IL-6) expression relative to the housekeeping gene GAPDH. Eutopic endometrial stromal cells from women with endometriosis (UT-E) and endometriotic lesions (Lesions) produce significantly more IL-6 than do eutopic endometrial stromal cells from women without endometriosis (UT-C) as measured by RT-PCR.

ognized between eutopic endometrium from women with and that from women without endometriosis. For example, the secretion of hepatic growth factor was upregulated in the stromal cells of these tissues from patients with endometriosis.[49] As hepatic growth factor is considered to be involved specifically in the regeneration or reconstruction of various tissues, it may be involved in the pathogenesis of endometriosis. Eutopic endometrial stromal cells from women with endometriosis also produce significantly more interleukin-6 (IL-6; FIG. 3) and demonstrate an elevated responsiveness to both IL-1 and IL-6.[50,51] This differential cytokine expression and responsiveness also support the hypothesis that eutopic endometrium from women with endometriosis has intrinsic quantitative differences compared to eutopic endometrium from women without this disorder.

Incubation of endometrial epithelial cells from women with and those without endometriosis with IL-1β or tumor necrosis factor-α (TNF-α) demonstrated an increased production of monocyte chemotactic protein-1 (MCP-1) by eutopic endometrial epithelial cells from women with the disorder.[52,53] Upregulated production of MCP-1 in the peritoneal cavity may contribute to the local inflammatory processes taking place in the peritoneal cavity. MCP-1 may also serve as an effector cell mediator in the pathogenesis and pathophysiology of endometriosis.

PROTEIN PRODUCTION AND GENE EXPRESSION

CA 125, a cell surface, high molecular weight glycoprotein identified by monoclonal antibody OC-125, is expressed in tissues derived from embryonic coelomic epithelium such as endometrium, endocervix, fallopian tubes, peritoneum, pleura, and pericardium. CA 125 is also expressed by many epithelial cancers, and elevated CA 125 serum levels have been associated with gynecologic and nongynecologic malignancies but primarily ovarian carcinoma. Serum concentrations of CA 125 are elevated in most women with endometriosis. McBean and Brumstead[54] evaluated eutopic endometrium as a potential source of the elevated serum concentrations in women with moderate to severe endometriosis. When compared with controls, the

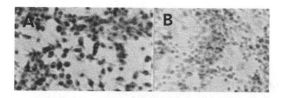

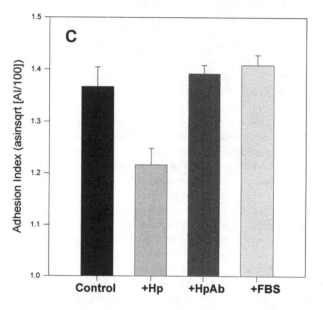

FIGURE 4. Endometriosis-associated haptoglobin binds to peritoneal macrophages and alters their function. (**A**) Significantly more macrophages isolated from the peritoneal fluid of women with endometriosis, as compared to (**B**) women without this disorder, immunohistochemically stain for haptoglobin. (**C**) Adhesion, the first step in the phagocytic process, is decreased when peritoneal macrophages from women *without* endometriosis are incubated with haptoglobin, an effect that can be reversed by the addition of antihuman haptoglobin antibody and is not observed by the addition of serum proteins (FBS, fetal bovine sera without haptoglobin).

endometrium of women with endometriosis secreted two to four times more CA-125 in both the early and late luteal stages of the menstrual cycle. Thus, eutopic endometrial CA-125 production represents a potential source of the elevated serum levels of CA-125 seen in these women.

Examples of differential gene expression and protein production by eutopic endometrium from women with endometriosis are emerging in the literature. Recently, Taylor and co-workers[55] demonstrated a lack in the midluteal rise in eutopic endometrial HOX gene expression in women with endometriosis. HOXA10 and

HOXA11 are homeobox genes that function as transcription factors essential to embryonic development and regulation of endometrial development in the adult during the course of the menstrual cycle. Aberrant HOX gene expression suggests that altered development of the endometrium at the molecular level may contribute to the etiology of infertility in patients with endometriosis.

Our laboratory has shown that endometriotic lesions synthesize and secrete a unique form of extrahepatic haptoglobin.[56–59] Production of endometriotic haptoglobin is significantly enhanced by IL-6.[51] Both endometriotic haptoglobin mRNA expression and protein localization are dramatically increased in established endometriotic lesions, and interestingly, are greater in eutopic endometrium from women with endometriosis than women without this disorder.[59] Recently, some nontraditional biological functions for haptoglobin functions including immunomodulatory properties and angiogenic activity have been reported.[60,61]

We have shown that significantly more of the macrophages isolated from the peritoneal fluid of women with endometriosis compared to women without this disorder bind haptoglobin, which subsequently alters macrophage function (FIG. 4).[62] Adherence, the first step in the phagocytic process, is decreased when endometriotic haptoglobin is bound to peritoneal macrophages, while paradoxically IL-6 production is upregulated in these same haptoglobin-bound macrophages.[62] Endometriotic haptoglobin can also increase proliferation of endothelial cells and elicits neovascularization (Sharpe-Timms, unpublished data). Hence, differential expression of haptoglobin by eutopic endometrium from women with endometriosis may explain why although most women have retrograde menstruation, only some develop this disease. We hypothesize that haptoglobin-expressing endometrial cells can avoid phagocytosis by peritoneal macrophages, stimulate macrophages to produce cytokines that promote additional endometriotic haptoglobin production by the ectopic endometrial cells, and allow establishment and growth of endometrial tissue in the peritoneal cavity. Overall, these data offer insight into the biochemical mechanisms associated with the endometriotic disease process, which may be used to develop novel methods to restore immune function and to block the establishment of ectopic endometrial tissue growth in the peritoneal cavity.

SUMMARY

A variety of anomalies in structure, proliferation, immune components, adhesion molecules, proteolytic enzymes and inhibitors, steroid and cytokine production and responsiveness, and gene expression and protein production occur in eutopic endometrium from women with endometriosis. Some of the data in the literature are contradictory and mandate further investigation. Ultimately, these differences lend credence to the possibility that eutopic endometrium from women with endometriosis is innately aberrant and possibly central to the pathogenesis and pathophysiologies associated with endometriosis. Additional insight into such differences may be used in the development of less invasive methods of diagnosis or novel therapeutic or preventive approaches for this enigmatic disorder.

REFERENCES

1. SHARPE-TIMMS, K.L. 1997. Basic research in endometriosis. Obstet. Gynecol. Clin. N. Am. **24:** 269–290.
2. HALME, J., M.G. HAMMOND, J.F. HULKA, et al. 1984. Retrograde menstruation in healthy women and in patients with endometriosis. Obstet. Gynecol. **64:** 151–154.
3. LAMB, K., R.G. HOFFMAN & T.R. NICHOLS. 1986. Family trait analysis: a case-control study of 43 women with endometriosis and their best friends. Am. J. Obstet. Gynecol. **154:** 596–601.
4. DMOWSKI, W.P. & D.P. BRAUN. 1997. Immunologic aspects of endometriosis. In Endometrium and Endometriosis. M.P. Diamond & K.G. Osteen, eds. **25:** 174–184. Blackwell Science. Malden, MA.
5. ARICI, A. & E. ORAL. 1997. The peritoneal environment in endometriosis. In Endometrium and Endometriosis. M.P. Diamond & K.G. Osteen, eds. **24:** 161–173. Blackwell Science. Malden, MA.
6. FEDELE, L., M. MARCHINI, S. BIANCHI, et al. 1990. Structural and ultrastructural defects in preovulatory endometrium of normo-ovulating infertile women with minimal or mild endometriosis. Fertil. Steril. **53:** 989–993.
7. SHAPIRO, D.B., S.J. WALSH, C. ALGERT, et al. 1995. Endometrial thickness in women with endometriosis or unexplained infertility undergoing superovulation with intrauterine insemination. J. Soc. Gynecol. Invest. **2:** 367.
8. WINGFIELD, M., A. MACPHERSON, D.L. HEALY, et al. 1995. Cell proliferation is increased in the endometrium of women with endometriosis. Fertil. Steril. **64:** 340–346.
9. JURGENSEN, A., L. METTLER, N. VOLKOV, et al. 1996. Proliferative activity of the endometrium throughout the menstrual cycle in infertile women with and without endometriosis. Fertil. Steril. **66:** 369–375.
10. KRUITWAGEN, R.F.P., L.G. POELS, W.N.P. WILLEMSEN, et al. 1991. Endometrial epithelial cells in peritoneal fluid during the early follicular phase. Fertil. Steril. **55:** 297–303.
11. GEBEL, H.M., D.P. BRAUN, A. TAMBUR, et al. 1998. Spontaneous apoptosis of endometrial tissue is impaired in women with endometriosis. Fertil. Steril. **9:** 1042–1047.
12. JONES, R.K., R.F. SEARLE & J.N. BULMER. 1998. Apoptosis and bcl-2 expression in normal human endometrium, endometriosis and adenomyosis. Hum. Reprod. **13:** 3496–3502.
13. WATANABE, H., H. KANZAKI, S. NARUKAWA, et al. 1997. Bcl-2 and Fas expression in eutopic and ectopic human endometrium during the menstrual cycle in relation to endometrial cell apoptosis. Am. J. Obstet. Gynecol. **176:** 360–368.
14. KOLESNICK, R. & Z. FUK. 1995. Cermide: a signal for apoptosis or mitogenesis? J. Exp. Med. **181:** 1949–1952.
15. BRAUN, D.P., H.M. GEBEL, A. MURIANA, et al. 1992. Differential endometrial cell proliferation in response to peripheral blood monocytes, peritoneal macrophages, and macrophage-derived cytokines in patients with endometriosis [abstr.]. Am. Fertil. Soc. P-057. New Orleans, LA.
16. WEED, J.C. & P.C. ARQUEMBOURG. 1980. Endometriosis: can it produce an autoimmune response resulting in infertility? Clin. Obstet. Gynecol. **23:** 885–893.
17. BARTOSIK, D., I. DAMJANOV, R.R. VISCARELLO & J.A. RILEY. 1987. Immunoproteins in the endometrium: clinical correlates of the presence of complement fractions C3 and C4. Am. J. Obstet. Gynecol. **156:** 11–15.
18. ISAACSON, K.B., M. GALMAN, C. COUTIFARIS, et al. 1990. Endometrial synthesis and secretion of complement component-3 by patients with and without endometriosis. Fertil. Steril. **53:** 836–841.
19. ODUKOYA, O.A., N. WHEATCROFT, A.P. WEETMAN, et al. 1995. The prevalence of endometrial immunoglobulin G antibodies in patients with endometriosis. Hum. Reprod. **10:**1214–1219.
20. HELVACIOGLU A., S. AKSEL & R.D. PETERSON. 1997. Endometriosis and autologous lymphocyte activation by endometrial cells. Are lymphocytes or endometrial cell defects responsible? J. Reprod. Med. **42:** 71–75.

21. KLENTZERIS, L.D., J.N. BULMER, D.T. LIU & L. MORRISON. 1995, Endometrial leukocyte subpopulations in women with endometriosis. Eur. J. Obstet. Gynecol. Reprod. Biol.**63:** 41–47.
22. JONES, R.K., J.N. BULMER & R.F. SEARLE. 1995. Immunohistochemical characterization of proliferation oestrogen receptor and progesterone receptor expression in endometriosis: comparison of eutopic and ectopic endometrium with normal cycling endometrium. Hum. Reprod. **10:** 3272–3279.
23. BULMER, J.N., R.K. JONES & R.F. SEARLE. 1998. Intraepithelial leukocytes in endometriosis and adenomyosis: comparison of eutopic and ectopic endometrium with normal endometrium. Hum. Reprod . **13:** 2910–2915.
24. HILL, J.A. 1992. Cytokines considered critical in pregnancy. Am. J. Reprod. Immunol. **28:** 123–126.
25. HILL, J.A. 1992. Immunology and endometriosis. Fertil. Steril. **58:** 262–264.
26. OOSTERLYNCK, D.J., F.J. CORNILLIE, M. WAER, et al. 1991. Women with endometriosis show a defect in natural killer activity resulting in a decreased cytotoxicity to autologous endometrium. Fertil. Steril **56:** 45–51.
27. OTA, H., S. IGARASHI, J. HATAZAWA, et al. 1997. Distribution of heat shock proteins in eutopic and ectopic endometrium in endometriosis and adenomyosis. Fertil. Steril. **68:** 23–28.
28. NIP, M.M., D. MILLER, P.V. TAYLOR, et al. 1994. Expression of heat shock protein 70 kDa in human endometrium of normal and infertile women. Hum. Reprod. **9:** 1253–1256.
29. BROOKS, P.C., R.L. KLEMKE, S. SCHON, et al. 1997. Insulin-like growth factor receptor cooperates with integrin $\alpha v \beta 5$ to promote tumor cell dissemination in vivo. J. Clin. Invest. **99:** 1390–1398.
30. BROOKS, P.C., S. STROMBLAD, L.C. SANDERS, et al. 1996. Localization of matrix metalloproteinase MMP-2 to the surface of invasive cells by interaction with integrin $\alpha v \beta 3$. Cell **85:** 683–693.
31. OTA, H. & T. TANAKA. 1997. Integrin adhesion molecules in the endometrial glandular epithelium in patients with endometriosis or adenomyosis. J. Obstet. Gynaecol. Res. **23:** 485–491.
32. LESSEY, B.A., L. DAMJANOVICH, C. COUTIFARIS, et al. 1992. Integrin adhesion molecules in the human endometrium. Correlation with the normal and abnormal menstrual cycle. J. Clin. Invest. **90:** 188–195.
33. LESSEY, B.A., A.J. CASTLEBAUM, S.W. SAWIN, et al. 1994. Aberrant integrin expression in the endometrium of women with endometriosis. J. Clin. Endocrinol. Metab. **79:** 643–649.
34. HII L.L.P. & P.A.W. ROGERS. 1998. Endometrial vascular and glandular expression of integrin $\alpha v \beta 3$ in women with and without endometriosis. Hum. Reprod. **13:** 1030–1035.
35. SHARPE-TIMMS, K.L., K.E. COX, B. RAY, et al. 2000. Localization of matrix metalloproteinase (MMP) enzymes, MMP-2 and MMP-3, to luminal endometrial epithelia by interaction with $\alpha v \beta 3$ and $\alpha v \beta 5$ integrins during the window of implantation. Biol. Reprod. **62:** 282.
36. OSTEEN K.G., K.L. BRUNER & K.L. SHARPE-TIMMS. 1996. Steroids and growth factor regulation of matrix metalloproteinases expression and the disease endometriosis. Sem. Reprod. Endocrinol. **14:** 247–255.
37. SHARPE-TIMMS, K.L., L.L PENNEY, R.L. ZIMMER, et al. 1995. Partial purification and amino acid sequence analysis of endometriosis protein-II (ENDO-II) reveals homology with tissue inhibitor of metalloproteinases-1 (TIMP-1). J. Clin. Endocrinol. Metab. **80:** 3784–3787.
38. SHARPE-TIMMS, K.L., L.W. KEISLER, E.W. MCINTUSH, et al. 1998. Tissue inhibitor of metalloproteinase-1 (TIMP-1) concentrations are attenuated in peritoneal fluid and sera of women with endometriosis and restored in sera by gonadotropin-releasing hormone agonist (GnRHa) therapy. Fertil. Steril. **69:** 1128–1134.
39. COX, K.E., M. PIVA & K.L. SHARPE-TIMMS. 2000. Differential expression of matrix metalloproteinase-3 (MMP-3) gene expression in endometriotic lesions as compared to endometrium. Biol. Reprod. In press.

40. RODGERS, W.H., L.M. MATRISIAN, L.C. GIUDICE, *et al.* 1994. Patterns of matrix metal-loproteinase expression in cycling endometrium imply differential functions and regulation by steroid hormones. J. Clin. Invest. **94:** 946–953.
41. MURRAY, M.J. & B.A. LESSEY. 1999. Embryo implantation and tumor metastasis: common pathways of invasion and angiogenesis. Sem. Reprod. Endocrinol. **17:** 275–290.
42. BISCHOF, P., A. MEISSER & A. CAMPANA. 2000. Paracrine and autocrine regulators of trophoblast invasion: a review. Placenta **21:** S55–60.
43. BISCHOF, P., A. MEISSER & A. CAMPANA. 2000. Mechanisms of endometrial control of trophoblast invasion. J. Reprod. Fertil. Suppl. **55:** 65–71.
44. RECHTMAN, M.P., J. ZHANG & L.A. SALAMONSEN. 1999. Effect of inhibition of matrix metalloproteinases on endometrial decidualization and implantation in mated rats. J. Reprod. Fertil. **117:** 169–177.
45. BRUNER, K.L., L.M. MATRISIAN, W.H. RODGERS, *et al.* 1997. Suppression of matrix metalloproteinases inhibits establishment of ectopic lesions by human endometrium in nude mice. J. Clin. Invest. **99:** 2851–2857.
46. NOBLE, L.S., K. TAKAYAMA, K.M. ZEITOUN, *et al.* 1997. Prostaglandin E2 stimulates aromatase expression in endometriosis-derived stromal cells. J. Clin. Endocrinol. Metab. **82:** 600–660.
47. KITAWAKI, J., T. NOGUCHI, T. AMATSU, *et al.* 1997. Expression of aromatase cytochrome P450 protein and messenger ribonucleic acid in human endometriotic and adenomyotic tissues but not in normal endometrium. Biol. Reprod. **57:** 514–519.
48. NISOLLE, M., F. CASANAS-ROUX, C. WYNS, *et al.* 1994. Immunohistochemical analysis of estrogen and progesterone receptors in endometrium and peritoneal endometriosis: a new quantitative method. Fertil. Steril. **62:** 751–759.
49. SUGAWARA, J., T. FUKAYA, T. MURAKAMI, *et al.* 1997. Increased secretion of hepatocyte growth factor by eutopic endometrial stromal cells in women with endometriosis. Fertil. Steril. **68:** 468–472.
50. TSENG, J.F., I.P. RYAN, T.D. MILAM *et al.* 1996. Interleukin-6 secretion *in vitro* is up-regulated in ectopic and eutopic endometrial stromal cells from women with endometriosis. J. Clin. Endocrinol. Metab. **81:** 1118–1122.
51. PIVA, M., R.A. KNITTING, W.T. GRIFFIN, *et al.* 1998. Interleukin-6 (IL-6) up regulates expression of Endometriosis Protein-I (ENDO-I) mRNA, a haptoglobin-like gene that is differentially expressed by pelvic endometriosis [abstr]. Am. Soc. Reprod. Med. O-171. San Francisco, CA.
52. AKOUM, A., A. LEMAY, C. BRUNET, *et al.* 1995. Secretion of monocyte chemotactic protein-1 by cytokine-stimulated endometrial cells of women with endometriosis. Fertil. Steril. **63:** 322–328.
53. JOLICOEUR, C., M. BOUTOUIL, R. DROUIN, *et al.* 1998. Increased expression of monocyte chemotactic protein-1 in the endometrium of women with endometriosis. Am. J. Pathol. **152:** 125–133.
54. MCBEAN, J.H. & J.R. BRUMSTEAD. 1993. In vitro CA-125 secretion by endometrium from women with advanced endometriosis. Fertil. Steril. **59:** 89–92.
55. TAYLOR H.S., C. BAGOT, A. KARDANA, *et al.* 1999. HOX gene expression is altered in the endometrium of women with endometriosis. Hum. Reprod. **14:** 1328–1331.
56. SHARPE, K.L., R.L. ZIMMER, W.T. GRIFFIN, *et al.* 1993. Polypeptides synthesized and released by human endometriosis tissue differ from those of the uterine endometrium in culture. Fertil. Steril. **60:** 839–851.
57. SHARPE-TIMMS, K.L., M. PIVA, E.A. RICKE, *et al.* 1998. Endometriotic lesions synthesize and secrete a haptoglobin-like protein. Biol. Reprod. **58:** 988–994.
58. PIVA, M. & K.L. SHARPE-TIMMS. 1999. Peritoneal endometriotic lesions differentially express a haptoglobin-like gene. Mol. Hum. Reprod. **5:** 71–78.
59. SHARPE-TIMMS, K.L., E.A. RICKE, M. PIVA & G.M. HOROWITZ. 2000. Differential expression and localization of de-novo synthesized endometriotic haptoglobin in endometrium and endometriotic lesions. Hum. Reprod. **5:** 2180–2185.
60. LANGLOIS, M.R. & J.R. DELANGHE. 1996. Biological and clinical significance of haptoglobin polymorphism in humans. Clin. Chem. **42:** 1589–1600.
61. DOBRYSZYCKA, W. 1997. Biological functions of haptoglobin: new pieces to an old puzzle. Eur. J. Clin. Chem. Clin. Biochem. **35:** 647–654.

62. SHARPE-TIMMS, K.L., R.L. ZIMMER, E.A. RICKE, et al. 2000. Aberrant adherence of peritoneal macrophages in endometriosis [abstr]. Am. Soc. Reprod. Med. O–57. San Diego, CA.

63. VIERIKKO, P., A. KAUPPILA, L. RONNBERG & R. VIHKO. 1985. Steroidal regulation of endometriosis tissue: lack of induction of 17β-hydroxysteroid dehydrogenase activity by progesterone, medroxyprogesterone acetate, or danazol. Fertil. Steril. 43: 218-224.

64. LECHNER, J.F., M.A. LAVECK, B.I. GERWIN & E.A. MATIS. 1989. Differential responses to growth factors by normal human mesothelial cultures from individual donors. J. Cell Physiol. 139: 295–300.

65. MEGELA, C., M. BALDUCCI, C. BULLETTI, et al. 1991. Tissue factors influencing growth and maintenance of endometriosis. Ann. N.Y. Acad. Sci. 622: 257-265.

66. BERGQVIST, A., O. LJUNGBERG & L. SKOOG. 1993. Immunohistochemical analysis of oestrogen and progesterone receptors in endometriotic tissue and endometrium. Hum. Reprod. 8: 1915-1922.

67. BERGQVIST, A. & M. FERNO. 1993. Oestrogen and progesterone receptors in endometriotic tissue and endometrium: comparison of different cycle phases and ages. Hum. Reprod. 8: 2211–2217.

68. NISOLLE, M., F. CASANAS-ROUX, C. WYNS, et al. 1994. Immunohistochemical analysis of estrogen and progesterone receptors in endometrium and peritoneal endometriosis: a new quantitative method. Fertil. Steril. 62: 751–759.

69. HOWELL, R.J., M. DOWSETT & D.K. EDMONDS. 1994. Oestrogen and progesterone receptors in endometriosis: heterogeneity of different sites. Hum. Reprod. 9: 1752–1758.

70. JONES, R.K., J.N. BLUMER & R.F. SEARLE. 1995. Immunohistochemical characterization of proliferation, oestrogen receptor and progesterone receptor expression in endometriosis: comparison of eutopic and ectopic endometrium with normal cycling endometrium. Hum. Reprod. 10: 3272–3279.

71. HAINING, R.E.B., I.T. CAMERON, C. VAN PAPENDORP, et al. 1991. Epidermal growth factor in human endometrium: proliferative effects in culture and immunocytochemical localization in normal and endometriotic tissues. Hum. Reprod. 6: 1200–1205.

72. PRENTICE, A., E.J. THOMAS, A. WEDDELL, et al. 1992. Epidermal growth factor receptor expression in normal endometrium and endometriosis: an immunohistochemical study. Br. J. Obstet. Gynecol. 99: 395–398.

73. HUANG, J. & J. YEH. 1994. Quantitative analysis of epidermal growth factor receptor gene expression in endometriosis. J. Clin. Endocrin. Metab. 79: 1097–1101.

74. MELLOR, S.J. & E.J. THOMAS. 1994. The actions of estradiol and epidermal growth factor in endometrial and endometriotic stroma. Fertil. Steril. 62: 507–513.

75. FERRIANI, R.A., D.S. CHARNOCK-JONES, A. PRENTICE, et al. 1993. Immunohistochemical localization of acidic and basic fibroblast growth factors in human endometrium and endometriosis and the detection of their mRNA by polymerase chain reaction. Hum. Reprod. 8: 11–16.

76. SHARPE-TIMMS, K.L., P.L. BRUNO, L.L. PENNEY & J.T. BICKEL. 1994. Immunohistochemical localization of granulocyte-macrophage colony stimulating factor (GM-CSF) in matched endometriosis and endometrial tissues. Am. J. Obstet. Gynecol. 171: 450–455.

77. KLEIN, N.A., G.M. PERGOLA, R.R. TEKMAL, et al. 1994. Cytokine regulation of cellular proliferation in endometriosis. Ann. N.Y. Acad. Sci. 734: 322–332.

78. SAHAKIAN, V., J. ANNERS, S. HASKILL & J. HALME. 1993. Selective localization of interleukin-1 receptor antagonist in eutopic endometrium and endometriotic implants. Fertil. Steril. 60: 276–279.

79. KOBAYASHI, H., W. IDA, T. TERAO & Y. KAWASHIMA. 1993. Quantitative and qualitative assessment of CA-125 production by human endometrial epithelial cells: comparison of eutopic and heterotopic epithelial cells. Int. J. Cancer 54: 426–434.

80. ISAACSON, K.B., C. COUTIFARIS, C. GARCIA & C.R. LYTTLE. 1989. Production and secretion of complement component 3 by endometriotic tissue. J. Clin. Endocrinol. Metab. 69: 1003–1009.

81. ISAACSON, K.B., Q. XU & C.R. LYTTLE. 1991. The effect of estradiol on the production and secretion of complement component 3 by the rat uterus and surgically induced endometriotic tissue. Fertil. Steril. **55:** 395–402.

82. SHARPE, K.L. & M.W. VERNON. 1993. Polypeptides synthesized and released by rat endometriotic tissue differ from those of the uterine endometrium in culture. Biol. Reprod. **48:** 1334–1340.

83. SHARPE, K.L., R.L. ZIMMER, W.T. GRIFFIN & L.L. PENNEY. 1993. Polypeptides synthesized and released by human endometriosis tissue differ from those of the uterine endometrium in culture. Fertil. Steril. **60:** 839–851.

84. SHARPE-TIMMS, K.L., M. PIVA, E.A. RICKE, et al. 1998. Endometriotic lesions synthesize and secrete a haptoglobin-like protein. Biol. Reprod. **58:** 988–994.

85. SHARPE-TIMMS, K.L., E.A. RICKE, M. PIVA & G.M. HOROWITZ. 2000. Differential in vivo expression and localization of endometriosis protein-I (ENDO-I), a haptoglobin homologue, in endometrium and endometriotic lesions. Hum. Reprod. **15:** 101–105.

86. PIVA, M. & K.L. SHARPE-TIMMS. 1999. Peritoneal endometriotic lesions differentially express a haptoglobin-like gene. Mol. Hum. Reprod. **5:** 71–78.

87. BERGQVIST, A., M. FERNO & S. MATTSON. 1996. A comparison of cathepsin D levels in endometriotic tissue and in uterine endometrium. Fertil. Steril. **65:** 1130–1134.

88. OSTEEN, K.G., K.L. BRUNER & K.L. SHARPE-TIMMS. 1996. Steroid and growth factor regulation of matrix metalloproteinase expression and endometriosis. Sem. Reprod. Endocrinol. **14:** 247–255.

89. COX, K.E., M. PIVA & K.L. SHARPE-TIMMS. 2001. Differential expression of matrix metalloproteinase-3 (MMP-3) gene expression in endometriotic lesions as compared to endometrium. Biol. Reprod. In press.

90. SHARPE-TIMMS, K.L., L.L. PENNEY, R.L. ZIMMER, et al. 1995. Partial purification and amino acid sequence analysis of endometriosis protein-II (ENDO-II) reveals homology with tissue inhibitor of metalloproteinases-1 (TIMP-1). J. Clin. Endocrinol. Metab. **80:** 3784–3787.

91. SHARPE-TIMMS, K.L., L.W. KEISLER, E.W. MCINTUSH & D.H. KEISLER. 1998. Tissue inhibitor of metalloproteinase-1 (TIMP-1) concentrations are attenuated in peritoneal fluid and sera of women with endometriosis and restored in sera by gonadotropin-releasing hormone agonist (GnRHa) therapy. Fertil. Steril. **69:** 1128–1134.

92. FERNANDEZ-SHAW, S., D.H. BARLOW, J.M. MARSHALL, et al. 1995. Plasminogen activators in ectopic and uterine endometrium. Fertil. Steril. **63:** 45–51.

93. JONES, R.K., J.N. BULMER & R.F. SEARLE. 1996. Immunohistochemical characterization of stromal leukocytes in ovarian endometriosis: comparison of eutopic and ectopic endometrium with normal endometrium. Fertil. Steril. **66:** 81–89.

94. SUGAWARA, J., T. FUKAYA, T. MURAKAMI, et al. 1997. Increased secretion of hepatocyte growth factor by eutopic endometrial stromal cells in women with endometriosis. Fertil. Steril. **68:** 468–472.

The Mechanisms of Placental Viral Infection

HIDEKI KOI, JIAN ZHANG, AND SAMUEL PARRY

Center for Research on Reproduction and Women's Health, University of Pennsylvania School of Medicine, Philadelphia, Pennsylvania 19104, USA

ABSTRACT: The placenta is a dynamic organ whose structure and function change throughout pregnancy. There is compelling evidence that the placenta plays an integral role in the vertical transmission of viruses, such as cytomegalovirus and human immunodeficiency virus, from the mother to the fetus. Although the sequelae of congenital viral infection (i.e., fetal anomalies, intrauterine fetal death, and persistent postnatal infection) may be devastating, very little is known about the passage of viruses across the placenta and the pathologic consequences of placental viral infection. We postulate that the syncytiotrophoblast, which forms a continuous barrier between the maternal and fetal circulation, is relatively resistant to viral infection. In support of this hypothesis, we observed that the susceptibility of trophoblast cells to infection by adenovirus and herpes simplex virus and the expression of viral receptors were reduced as trophoblast cells terminally differentiated into syncytiotrophoblast. Conversely, we observed that undifferentiated, extravillous trophoblast cells, which are susceptible to adenovirus infection, underwent pathologic changes (i.e., apoptosis) when infected by adenovirus in the presence of decidual lymphocytes (which were used to simulate the maternal immune response to viral infection). Based on these findings, we speculate that viral infection of extravillous trophoblast cells may negatively impact the process of placental invasion and predispose the mother and fetus to adverse reproductive outcomes that result from placental dysfunction.

KEYWORDS: placenta; trophoblast; virus; adenovirus; adeno-associated virus; herpes simplex virus; human immunodeficiency virus; apoptosis

INTRODUCTION

Congenital viral infection is associated with fetal anomalies, postnatal infection, and fetal demise. Although transplacental passage of these viruses is a critical aspect of these infections, few investigators have characterized placental viral infection and the role placental trophoblast cells have in passage of virus from the maternal to the fetal circulation. To define the mechanisms by which trophoblast cells influence viral infection, we studied the interactions of wild-type viruses and replication-deficient viral vectors with choriocarcinoma cell lines, primary trophoblast cells, and placental villous explants. Our findings suggest that the villous trophoblast is relatively resistant to viral infection because of decreased expression of viral receptors,

Address for correspondence: Samuel Parry, M.D., Assistant Professor, Center for Research on Reproduction and Women's Health, University of Pennsylvania School of Medicine, 1352 Biomedical Research Building II/III, 421 Curie Boulevard, Philadelphia, PA 19104-6142. Voice: 215-573-4916; fax: 215-573-5408.

parry@mail.med.upenn.edu

but that viral infection of extravillous trophoblast cells may impair placental invasion of the maternal uterine wall, causing obstetric conditions that result from placental dysfunction.

PLACENTAL DEVELOPMENT

Development of the placenta is largely dependent on the differentiation of trophoblast cells along two pathways.[1,2] In one pathway, a subset of undifferentiated cytotrophoblast cells in anchoring placental villi invades maternal tissues and blood vessels within the decidua and myometrium. These intermediate, or extravillous, trophoblast cells engage in a dialogue with maternal cells and probably mediate suppression of the maternal immune system against the semi-allogeneic conceptus.[3,4] The inflammatory response to infection at the maternal–fetal interface has been postulated to abrogate normal placentation and predispose the mother and fetus to adverse reproductive outcomes, including miscarriage, fetal growth restriction, and preeclampsia.[4–6] In the other pathway of placental development, mononucleated cytotrophoblast cells within the placental villi differentiate into the multinucleated syncytiotrophoblast. As pregnancy progresses, cytotrophoblast cells become more sparse within the placental villi, and the syncytiotrophoblast forms the only continuous layer separating the maternal intervillous space and the fetal capillary endothelium. Importantly, superficial breaks in this barrier do not appear to be significant factors in the vertical transmission of viruses, at least in the case of human immunodeficiency virus (HIV).[7]

THE ROLE OF THE PLACENTA IN CONGENITAL VIRAL INFECTION

A number of clinically relevant viruses are vertically transmitted to the fetus subsequent to maternal infection, including HIV, hepatitis B virus, hepatitis C virus, varicella zoster virus, rubella virus, parvovirus B19, and cytomegalovirus. However, clinical and experimental data suggest that the placenta is a relatively effective barrier to many of these viruses. For example, the maternal–infant transmission rate of HIV is only 25% in mothers who do not receive prophylaxis with zidovudine during pregnancy, and most perinatal transmission likely occurs during childbirth when the fetus is exposed to maternal blood and cervicovaginal secretions.[8] Not surprisingly, primary cytotropblast cells and placental villous explants are relatively resistant to HIV infection.[9,10] Similarly, the rate of vertical transmission of varicella zoster virus is less than 2%, and, in one study, only 3 of 19 placentas from mothers with primary varicella zoster infection during pregnancy demonstrated findings consistent with placental infection.[11] Finally, villous explants from human placentas at term are not susceptible to cytomegalovirus infection.[12]

In our laboratory, we studied the susceptibility of trophoblast cells to adenovirus and herpes simplex virus-1 (HSV-1) infections.[2,13,14] Adenovirus is the most common viral pathogen identified in fetal samples obtained from abnormal pregnancies.[15,16] In one series, adenovirus was detected in the amniotic fluid of only 2% (3/154) of controls.[16] However, nonimmune fetal hydrops was associated with a high incidence of viral infection (50/91 cases), and adenovirus was detected in the amniotic fluid from 60% of these patients.[16] Additionally, adenovirus was detected in the amniotic fluid of 30% (10/33) of women whose pregnancies were complicated by conditions usually attributed to abnormal placental function (i.e., fetal growth restriction, oligohydramnios).[16] Thus, we believe that viral infection, particularly adenovirus infection, is a previously unrecognized factor in adverse obstetric outcomes.

Transplacental transmission of HSV occurs rarely, although congenital infection during the first two trimesters has been associated in isolated reports with fetal anomalies such as microcephaly, intracranial calcifications, and chorioretinitis.[17–19] The infrequency with which congenital HSV infection occurs may be attributed to several factors, including (1) the prevalence in reproductive-aged women of protective antibodies against HSV, (2) the fact that viremia is not a cardinal feature of HSV infections, and (3) the possibility that the placenta functions as a physical barrier preventing vertical transmission of HSV from the maternal to the fetal circulation. However, primary maternal genital infections with HSV are common during pregnancy and increase the risk of miscarriage, presumably as a result of placental infection and dysfunction.[20–22] Additionally, involvement of other visceral organs may complicate primary HSV infections.[23] Thus, these observations indicate that the placenta is exposed to HSV during primary infection in some women, but that the placenta generally prevents vertical transmission of the virus.

ADENOVIRUS

We discovered that the ability of adenovirus to infect placental trophoblast cells is related to the state of trophoblast differentiation.[2,13] A replication-deficient adenovirus-5 vector containing the *lacZ* gene, which codes for intracellular β-galactosidase, was used to transduce primary cytotrophoblast cells and human choriocarcinoma cell lines (BeWo and JEG-3 cells). BeWo cells can be induced to undergo terminal differentiation in response to treatment with cAMP, but JEG-3 cells cannot. Cytotrophoblast cells undergo spontaneous differentiation (syncytialization) over 24–48 hours in culture. Recombinant adenovirus efficiently transduced cytotrophoblast cells as detected by a blue staining reaction involving the β-galactosidase substrate, X-gal.[13] However, there was a marked reduction in the transduction efficiency of primary cytotrophoblast cells that underwent terminal differentiation in culture over 24–48 hours. Similarly, BeWo cells treated with cAMP were not efficiently transduced, but JEG-3 cells were transduced by the adenovirus vector 48 hours after treatment with cAMP. In all of these experiments, terminal differentiation was confirmed by visualization of syncytium formation and by documenting increased production of human chorionic gonadotropin and/or progesterone.

Differentiated trophoblast cells were successfully transfected by an adenovirus-based plasmid, pAdlacZ, complexed with a cationic phospholipid, which demonstrates that syncytialized trophoblast cells retain the transcriptional and translational machinery to express the *lacZ* gene.[13] Additionally, Southern blot analysis of trophoblast cells infected with the adenovirus vector containing the *lacZ* gene revealed the presence of *lacZ* DNA in undifferentiated, but not differentiated, trophoblast cells. These results indicate that recombinant adenovirus vectors efficiently transduce undifferentiated trophoblast cells, but cannot transduce terminally differentiat-

TABLE 1. Summary of findings that describe the presence (+) or absence (–) of CAR RNA transcripts and protein in trophoblast cells at various stages of differentiation; also, the ability of adenovirus to transduce trophoblast cells and to bind to these cells in a fiber-dependent fashion

Cell type	CAR	Transducibility by adenovirus	Specific binding by adenovirus fiber
First trimester			
Extravillous trophoblast	+	+	+
Villous cytotrophoblast	Weak +	Not tested	Not tested
Villous syncytiotrophoblast	Weak +	Not tested	Not tested
Third trimester			
Extravillous trophoblast	+	+	+
Villous cytotrophoblast	–	+	–
Villous syncytiotrophoblast	–	–	–

ed trophoblast secondary to failed viral uptake by these cells.[2] On the basis of these findings, we speculated that receptors mediating adenovirus attachment and entry may be differentially expressed on trophoblast cells.

Adenovirus entry into target cells involves attachment of the knob domain of the viral fiber protein to the coxsackievirus B and adenovirus receptor (CAR), and internalization of the virus is mediated by the binding of its penton base with $\alpha_v\beta_3$ and $\alpha_v\beta_5$ integrins.[24–26] Accordingly, the expression of CAR and $\alpha_v\beta_3$ and $\alpha_v\beta_5$ integrins is strongly correlated with host cell infectivity/resistance to adenovirus.[25,27,28] The integrins $\alpha_v\beta_3$ and $\alpha_v\beta_5$ are known to be expressed in undifferentiated and differentiated trophoblast.[29,30] Therefore, we focused our investigation on the placental expression of CAR.

Northern hybridization, flow cytometry, and immunostaining revealed that placental expression of the recently identified coxsackievirus and adenovirus receptor (CAR) varies with gestational age and trophoblast phenotype.[31] CAR is continuously expressed in invasive, or extravillous, trophoblast cells, but not in villous trophoblast cells (TABLE 1). In first-trimester placentas, CAR was detected on villous cytotrophoblast cells and at lower levels within the syncytiotrophoblast. Extravillous trophoblast cells, which invade the uterine wall and maternal vasculature, expressed CAR. In third-trimester placentas, villous cytotrophoblast cells and syncytiotrophoblasts were negative for CAR. However, extravillous trophoblast cells continued to express CAR.

Binding assays using adenovirus fiber protein were performed to determine whether CAR mediates adenovirus attachment to trophoblast cells on which the receptor is expressed.[31] We observed that adenovirus fiber protein specifically bound to extravillous trophoblast cells and that pretreatment of these cells with fiber protein reduced the transduction efficiency of recombinant adenovirus vectors. Thus, CAR appears to be the primary receptor for adenovirus in extravillous trophoblast cells.

CAR protein and RNA were not present in villous trophoblast cells isolated from third-trimester placentas, although primary villous cytotrophoblast cells from these placentas were efficiently transduced by adenovirus vectors.[13,31] Preincubation with adenovirus fiber protein did not inhibit the transduction of cytotrophoblast cells by adenovirus vectors, and specific binding of adenovirus fiber protein to villous cytotrophoblast cells was not observed. Consequently, we speculate that an alternate, fiber-independent mechanism for adenovirus attachment to villous cytotrophoblast cells exists, or that viral internalization following low-affinity binding is reduced as villous trophoblast cells syncytialize. Regarding the first possibility, alternate receptors for adenovirus, such as the α_2 domain of the heavy chain of human MHC class 1 molecules, have been identified. However, binding to the α_2 domain is a fiber-dependent process, and villous trophoblast cells do not express classic MHC 1 or 2 molecules.[32,33] Instead, trophoblast cells express a novel MHC molecule, HLA-G, the expression of which is downregulated by viral infection.[6] Therefore, attachment of adenovirus to villous cytotrophoblast cells via the α_2 domain is not likely. Other fiber-independent receptors for adenovirus have been proposed but have not been studied in trophoblast cells. Regarding the second possibility, we observed significant levels of nonspecific binding by fiber protein to villous cytotrophoblast and syncytiotrophoblast. This nonspecific binding reflects low-affinity binding to high-capacity sites that are not likely to be viral receptors in the traditional sense. It is possible, however, that internalization of virus subsequent to low-affinity, high-capacity binding of fiber protein is reduced as trophoblast cells syncytialize, accounting for their resistance to infection.

Our findings demonstrate that CAR is expressed at all stages of gestation by extravillous trophoblast cells, to which adenovirus attachment is fiber-mediated.[31] Villous cytotrophoblast cells do not express CAR beyond the first trimester of pregnancy, and adenovirus attachment to these cells is fiber-independent. The villous syncytiotrophoblast also does not express CAR beyond the first trimester of pregnancy, and adenovirus does not efficiently infect these cells. Hence, the terminally differentiated syncytiotrophoblast may function as a barrier to transplacental adenovirus infection.

HERPES SIMPLEX VIRUS

Similar to our findings for adenovirus, we found that transduction of trophoblastic cells by recombinant HSV-1 vectors is affected by cellular differentiation.[14] Isolated cytotrophoblast cells, extravillous trophoblast cells, and BeWo cells were efficiently transduced by recombinant HSV-1 vectors. Treatment of BeWo cells with cyclic-AMP reduced transduction by the HSV vector, but when BeWo cells were transfected with HSV-based plasmids, lacZ expression was not affected by treatment with cyclic-AMP. Southern blot analysis demonstrated 2.75 times less transgene DNA in cyclic-AMP-treated BeWo cells compared to untreated BeWo cells. We conclude that inefficient transduction of differentiated trophoblastic cells with HSV is due to diminished viral entry, which may be an important factor that limits maternal–fetal transmission of HSV.

Attachment of HSV to target cells is mediated by heparan sulfate, and entry is regulated by three recently identified entry mediators (HveA, HveB, HveC).[34–36] Because heparan sulfate is a ubiquitous glycoprotein on cell surfaces, we hypothesized that the villous syncytiotrophoblast is resistant to HSV secondary to decreased expression of the HSV entry mediators. Our preliminary findings using primary trophoblast cells and placental villous explants suggest that the differential expression of the HSV entry mediators in trophoblast cells is related to their susceptibility to HSV infection and that the syncytiotrophoblast may serve as an effective barrier against maternofetal transmission of HSV (unpublished data).

OTHER VIRUSES

In contrast to our findings with adenovirus and HSV, treatment with cAMP augments trophoblast transduction by adeno-associated virus (AAV) vectors containing the *lacZ* transgene.[2,14] Southern blot analysis suggests that the augmentation is due to increased virus uptake by a yet to be determined mechanism. The cAMP effect appears to be selective for trophoblast cells, since it was not observed with other cell types that are permissive to AAV infection. It is interesting that AAV, to which trophoblast cells appear to be uniquely receptive, has recently been reported to infect mouse embryos and induce abortion.[37] Among women with adverse reproductive outcomes, including miscarriage and spontaneous preterm birth, AAV DNA was found more frequently than among healthy controls.[38,39] Given our experimental findings and the clinical observations made by other investigators, we believe that future studies of AAV as a previously unrecognized cause of reproductive failure are warranted.

Currently, we are studying the placental expression of HIV receptors, and we are initiating a comprehensive analysis of transplacental transmission of HIV. Our preliminary results suggest that HIV receptors are not expressed in villous trophoblast cells, which appear to be resistant to HIV infection (unpublished data). Consequently, we believe that the villous syncytiotrophoblast may serve as a relatively effective barrier to the vertical transmission of HIV.

VIRAL-INDUCED PLACENTAL DYSFUNCTION

In addition to investigating the role of the placenta in transmitting viruses from the mother to her fetus, we are also studying the pathologic significance of placental viral infection. We observed that extravillous trophoblast cells, which express CAR at all stages of gestation and are efficiently transduced by adenovirus vectors, underwent apoptosis when infected by wild-type adenovirus in the presence of decidual lymphocytes (which were used to simulate the maternal immune response to viral infection).[31] Briefly, extravillous trophoblast cells were infected with wild-type ad-

TABLE 2. Adenovirus-induced apoptosis of extravillous trophoblast cells

Adenovirus (1,000 vp/cell)[a]	−	−	+	+
Decidual cells	−	+	−	+
Percent of apoptotic cells	0.10%	0.67%	0.50%	3.53%*

[a]vp = viral particles.

* $p < 0.01$, compared to the rate of apoptosis observed in untreated cells.

enovirus (100–1000 particles/cell) and incubated for two hours. The cells were washed with fresh medium, and decidual lymphocytes were added in a 1:10 ratio to the extravillous trophoblast cells. After overnight co-culture, the cells were fixed, and apoptosis was detected in the extravillous trophoblast cells by 3'-end labeling of DNA fragments (Apop-Tag detection kit, Oncor, Gaithersburg, MD). The number of apoptotic trophoblast nuclei were counted blindly in randomly selected high-power fields, and the morphology of all cells that were detected by fluorescent microscopy was reviewed using phase-contrast microscopy. The morphology of the larger extravillous trophoblast cells was easily distinguished from decidual lymphocytes. Infection with wild-type adenovirus alone, or co-culture of trophoblast cells with decidual lymphocytes (in the absence of adenovirus infection), did not induce cytopathic effects. However, we observed that adenovirus infection in the presence of maternal decidual lymphocytes resulted in the detachment of nonviable trophoblast cells from the culture plates. Trophoblast cells were approximately 80% confluent before treatment with adenovirus and/or decidual lymphocytes, but trophoblast cells were only 30–50% confluent after the detached cells were rinsed away. Furthermore, cocultures of extravillous trophoblast cells with decidual lymphocytes after incubation with wild-type adenovirus demonstrated significantly increased numbers of apoptotic nuclei compared to background levels of apoptosis observed in untreated extravillous trophoblast cells (TABLE 2). Thus, adenovirus infection and/or the maternal immune response to adenovirus infection induced the death of placental cell types that expressed CAR. Consequently, we postulate that adenovirus infection of extravillous trophoblast cells may negatively impact the process of placental invasion and predispose the mother and fetus to adverse reproductive outcomes that result from placental dysfunction. A similar hypothesis was recently proposed by another group of investigators, who demonstrated that cytomegalovirus infection limited extravillous trophoblast invasion into a gel matrix in their *in vitro* system.[40]

SUMMARY

We believe that a better understanding of the molecular basis of the interactions between viruses and trophoblast cells may yield novel strategies to prevent vertical transmission of viruses. The observations presented here confirm our initial hypothesis that differential expression of adenovirus and HSV receptors on trophoblast governs, in part, the susceptibility of the placenta to viral infection. Currently, we are studying the transplacental transmission of HIV, which continues to be a vexing clinical problem, particularly in underdeveloped regions where the prevalence of HIV is greatest and anti-retroviral medications may not be available. Simultaneously, we are investigating the pathologic effects of placental viral infection and will determine whether adverse reproductive outcomes that result from placental dysfunction are associated with viral infection of invasive trophoblast cells.

REFERENCES

1. DAMSKY, C.H., M.L. FITZGERALD & S.J. FISHER. 1992. Distribution patterns of extra-cellular matrix components and adhesion receptors are intricately modulated during

first trimester cytotrophoblast differentiation along the invasive pathway, in vivo. J. Clin. Invest. **89:** 210–222.
2. PARRY, S., J. HOLDER & J.F. STRAUSS III. 1997. Mechanisms of trophoblast–virus interaction. J. Reprod. Immunol. **37:** 25–34.
3. PAZMANY, L., O. MANDELBOIM, M. VALÉS-GÓMEZ, *et al.* 1999. Protection from natural killer cell-mediated lysis by HLA-G expression on target cells. Science **274:** 792–795.
4. KING, A. & Y.W. LOKE. 1999. The influence of the maternal immune response on placentation in human subjects. Proc. Nutr. Soc. **58:** 69–73.
5. REDMAN, C.W.G., G.P. SACKS & I.L. SARGENT. 1999. Preeclampsia: an excessive maternal inflammatory response to pregnancy. Am. J. Obstet. Gynecol. **180:** 499–506.
6. SCHUST, D.J., A.B. HILL & H.L. PLOEGH. 1996. Herpes simplex virus blocks intracellular transport of HLA-G in placentally derived cells. J. Immunol. **157:** 3375–3380.
7. BURTON, G.J., S. O'SHEA, T. ROSTRON, *et al.* 1996. Significance of placental damage in vertical transmission of human immunodeficiency virus. J. Med. Virol. **50:** 237–243.
8. CONNOR, E.M., R.S. SPERLING, R. GELBER, *et al.* 1994. Reduction of maternal–infant transmission of human immunodeficiency virus type 1 with zidovudine treatment. N. Engl. J. Med. **331:** 1173–1180.
9. KILANI, R.T., L. CHANG, M.I. GARCIA-LLORET, *et al.* 1997. Placental trophoblasts resist infection by multiple human immunodeficiency virus (HIV) type 1 variants even with cytomegalovirus coinfection but support HIV replication after provirus transfection. J. Virol. **71:** 6359–6372.
10. TSCHERNING-CASPER, C., N. PAPADOGIANNAKIS, M. ANVRET, *et al.* 1999. The trophoblastic epithelial barrier is not infected in full-term placentae of human immunodeficiency virus-seropositive mothers undergoing antiretroviral therapy. J. Virol. **73:** 9673–9678.
11. QURESHI, F. & S.M. JACQUES. 1996. Maternal varicella during pregnancy: correlation of maternal history and fetal outcome with placental histopathology. Hum. Pathol. **27:** 191–195.
12. MUHLEMANN, K., M.A. MENEGUS & R.K. MILLER. 1995. Cytomegalovirus in the perfused human term placenta *in vitro*. Placenta **16:** 367–373.
13. MACCALMAN, C.D., E.E. FURTH, A. OMIGBODUN, *et al.* 1996. Transduction of human trophoblast cells by recombinant adenoviruses is differentiation dependent. Biol. Reprod. **54:** 682–691.
14. PARRY, S., J. HOLDER, M.W. HALTERMAN, *et al.* 1998. Transduction of human trophoblastic cells by replication-deficient recombinant viral vectors. Am. J. Pathol. **152:** 1521–1529.
15. WENSTROM, K.D., W.W. ANDREWS, N.E. BOWLES, *et al.* 1998. Intrauterine viral infection at the time of second trimester genetic amniocentesis. Obstet. Gynecol. **92:** 420–424.
16. VAN DEN VEYVER, I.B., J. NI, N. BOWLES, *et al.* 1998. Detection of intrauterine viral infection using the polymerase chain reaction. Molec. Genet. Metab. **63:** 85–95.
17. CHALHUB, E.G., J. BAENZIGER, R.D. FEIGEN, *et al.* 1977. Congenital herpes simplex type II infection with extensive hepatic calcification bone lesions and cataracts: complete postmortem examination. Dev. Med. Child Neurol. **19:** 527–534.
18. MONIF, G.R., K.R. KELLNER & W.H. DONNELLY, JR. 1985. Congenital herpes simplex type II infection. Am. J. Obstet. Gynecol. **152:** 1000–1002.
19. HUTTO, C., A. ARVIN, R. JACOBS, *et al.* 1987. Intrauterine herpes simplex virus infections. J. Pediatr. **110:** 97–101.
20. BROWN, Z.A., J. BENEDETTI, R. ASHLEY, *et al.* 1991. Neonatal herpes simplex virus infection in relation to asymptomatic maternal infection at the time of labor. N. Engl. J. Med. **324:** 1247–1252.
21. BROWN, Z.A., S. SELKE, J. ZEH, *et al.* 1997. The acquisition of herpes simplex virus during pregnancy. N. Engl. J. Med. **337:** 509–515.
22. GRONROOS, M., E. HONKONEN, P. TERHO, *et al.* 1983. Cervical and serum IgA and serum IgG antibodies to *Chlamydia trachomatis* and herpes simplex virus in threatened abortion: a prospective study. Br. J. Obstet. Gynaecol. **90:** 167–171.

23. DIAMOND, C., K. MOHAN, A. HOBSON, *et al.* 1999. Viremia in neonatal herpes simplex virus infections. Pediatr. Infect. Dis. J. **18:** 487–489.
24. BERGELSON, J.M., J.A. CUNNINGHAM, G. DROGUETT, *et al.* 1997. Isolation of a common receptor for coxsackie B virus and adenoviruses 2 and 5. Science **275:** 1320–1323.
25. TOMKO, R.P., R. XU & L. PHILIPSON. 1997. HCAR and MCAR: the human and mouse cellular receptors for subgroup C adenoviruses and group B coxsackieviruses. Proc. Natl. Acad. Sci. USA **94:** 3352–3356.
26. WICKHAM, T.J., P. MATHIAS, D.A. CHERESH, *et al.* 1993. Integrins $\alpha_v\beta_3$ and $\alpha_v\beta_5$ promote adenovirus internalization but not virus attachment. Cell **73:** 309–319.
27. HUANG, S., R.I. ENDO & G.R. NEMEROW. 1995. Upregulation of integrins $\alpha_v\beta_3$ and $\alpha_v\beta_5$ on human monocytes and T lymphocytes facilitates adenovirus-mediated gene delivery. J. Virol. **69:** 2257–2263.
28. DELPORTE, C., R.S. REDMAN & B.J. BAUM. 1997. Relationship between the cellular distribution of the $a_v\beta_{3/5}$ integrins and adenoviral infection in salivary glands. Lab. Invest. **77:** 167–173.
29. VANDERPUYE, O.A., C.A. LABARRERE & J.A. MCINTYRE. 1991. A vitronectin receptor-related molecule in human placental brush border membranes. Biochem. J. **280:** 9–17.
30. OMIGBODUN, A., C. TESSLER, G. COUKOS, *et al.* 1995. Human trophoblast adhesion to osteopontin is regulated by cell differentiation and divalent cations. J. Soc. Gynecol. Invest. **2:** O126 (Abstract).
31. KOI, H., J. ZHANG, A. MAKRIGIANNAKIS, *et al.* 2001. Differential expression of the coxsackievirus and adenovirus receptor regulates adenovirus infection of the placenta. Biol. Reprod. **64:** 1001–1009.
32. HONG, S.S., L. KARAYAN, J. TOURNIER, *et al.* 1997. Adenovirus type 5 fiber knob binds to MHC class 1 α2 domain at the surface of human epithelial and B lymphoblastoid cells. EMBO J. **16:** 2294–2306.
33. COADY, M.A., D. MANDAPATI, B. ARUNACHALAM, *et al.* 1999. Dominant negative suppression of major histocompatibility complex genes occurs in trophoblasts. Transplantation **67:** 1461–1467.
34. MONTGOMERY, R.I., M.S. WARNER, B.J. LUM, *et al.* 1996. Herpes simplex virus-1 entry into cells mediated by a novel member of the TNF/NGF receptor family. Cell **87:** 427–436.
35. WARNER, M.S., R.J. GERAGHTY, W.M. MARTINEZ, *et al.* 1998. A cell surface protein with herpesvirus entry activity (HveB) confers susceptibility to infection by mutants of herpes simplex virus type 1, herpes simplex virus type 2, and pseudorabies virus. Virology **246:** 179–189.
36. GERAGHTY, R.J., C. KRUMMENACHER, G.H. COHEN, *et al.* 1998. Entry of alphaherpes viruses mediated by poliovirus receptor-related protein 1 and poliovirus receptor. Science **280:** 1618–1620.
37. BOTQUIN, V., A. CID & J.R. SCHLEHOFER. 1993. Induction of differentiation of embryonic cells and interference with development of mouse embryo by adeno-associated virus type 2. J. Cancer Res. Clin. Oncol. **119:** 24–29.
38. TOBIASCH, E., M. RABREAU, K. GELTNEKY, *et al.* 1994. Detection of adeno-associated virus DNA in human genital tract tissue and in material from spontaneous abortion. J. Med. Virol. **44:** 215–222.
39. BURGUETE, T., M. RABREAU, M. FONTANGES-DARRIET, *et al.* 1999. Evidence for infection of the human embryo with adeno-associated virus in pregnancy. Hum. Reprod. **14:** 2396–2401.
40. FISHER, S., O. GENBACEV, E. MAIDJI, *et al.* 2000. Human cytomegalovirus infection of placental cytotrophoblasts in vitro and in utero: implications for transmission and pathogenesis. J. Virol. **74:** 6808–6820.

Biochemistry and Molecular Biology of Trophoblast Invasion

P. BISCHOF, A. MEISSER, AND A. CAMPANA

Department of Obstetrics and Gynaecology, University of Geneva, Maternité, 1211 Geneva 14, Switzerland

ABSTRACT: Cytotrophoblastic cells (CTBs) from first-trimester placenta form columns of invasive CTBs. This invasive behavior is due to the ability of CTBs to secrete matrix metalloproteinases (MMPs), since tissue inhibitor of MMPs (TIMP) inhibits their invasiveness in the extracellular space. Although CTBs behave like metastic cells, *in vivo* they are only transiently invasive (first trimester), and their invasion is normally limited only to the endometrium and to the proximal third of the myometrium. This temporal and spatial regulation of trophoblast invasion is believed to be mediated in an autocrine way by trophoblastic factors and in a paracrine way by uterine factors. Several types of regulators have been investigated: hormones, extracellular matrix glycoproteins, and cytokines or growth factors. This review is not intended to be an exhaustive catalogue of potential regulators of trophoblast invasion but is aimed at summarizing the most important categories of factors affecting trophoblast–endometrium interactions.

KEYWORDS: trophoblast invasion; matrix metalloproteinases; cytotrophoblastic cells

INTRODUCTION

Cytotrophoblastic cells (CTBs) are derived from the trophectodermal cells of the blastocyst and represent a heterogeneous population during early pregnancy. CTBs follow one of two existing differentiation pathways: Villous CTBs (vCTBs) form a monolayer of polarized epithelial stem cells that proliferate and fuse to form syncytiotrophoblasts (STBs) covering the entire surface of the villous CTBs. CTBs can also break through the syncytium at selected sites (anchoring villi) to form multilayered columns of nonpolarized CTBs. These motile and highly invasive extravillous CTBs (evCTBs) are found as cytokeratin-positive cells in the decidua, the intima of the uterine spiral arteries, and the proximal third of the myometrium (FIG. 1).

Trophoblast invasion, like tumor invasion, is due to the active secretion of proteolytic enzymes capable of digesting the different extracellular matrices (ECMs) of the host's tissues. Serine proteases, cathepsins, and metalloproteinases have been implicated in invasive processes.[1] Matrix metalloproteinases (MMPs), also called matrixins, form a family of at least 17 human zinc-dependent endopeptidases collectively capable of degrading essentially all components of the ECM. According to

Address for correspondence: P. Bischof, P.B. Laboratoire d'Hormonologie, Maternité, 1211 Geneva 14, Switzerland. Voice: 41 22 382 43 36; fax 41 22 382 43 10.

paul.bischof@hcuge.ch

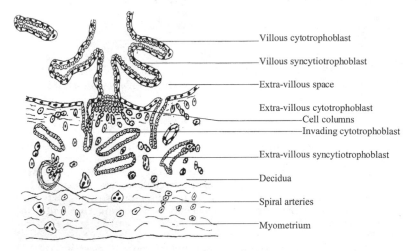

FIGURE 1. The placental bed at about 10 weeks of pregnancy.

TABLE 1. Classification of matrix metalloproteinases

Subfamily	MMP	Other names	Substrates
Gelatinases	MMP-2	Gelatinase A 72-kDa gelatinase	Col IV, V, VII, X, gelatin fibronectin, elastin
	MMP-9	Gelatinase B 92-kDa gelatinase	Col IV, V, Gelatin
Collagenases	MMP-1	Interstitial collagenase Fibroblast collagenase	Col I, II, III, VII, X , MMP-5, Entactin
	MMP-8	Neutrophil collagenase, PMNL collagenase	Col I, III
	MMP-13	Collagenase-3	Col I
Stromelysins	MMP-3	Stromelysin-1 Transin-1	Col III, IV, IX, X, gelatin, laminin, fibronectin, elastin, casein
	MMP-7	PUMP-I, matrilysin	Casein, fibronectin, gelatin
	MMP-10	Stromelysin-2 Transin-2	Col II, IV, V, fibronectin, gelatin
	MMP-11	Stromelysin-3	Col IV
	MMP-12	Metalloelastase	Elastin, fibronectin
Membrane bound	MMP-14	MT1-MMP, MMP-X1	MMP-2
	MMP-15	MT2-MMP	MMP-2
	MMP-16	MT3-MMP	MMP-2
	MMP-17	MT4-MMP	

ABBREVIATIONS: Col: collagen; MW: molecular weight; PMNL: polymorphonuclear leukocytes; PUMP-1: putative metalloprotease-1.

their substrate specificity and structure, members of the MMP gene family can be classified into four subgroups (TABLE 1).[2] Gelatinases (MMP-2 and MMP-9) digest type IV collagen (the major constituent of basement membranes) and denatured collagen (gelatin). Collagenases (MMP-1, -8, -13) digest types I, II, III, VII, and X collagens. They are thus appropriately designed for digesting the collagens of the ECM of the interstitium. Stromelysins (MMP-3, 7, 10, 11, and 12) have relatively broad substrate specificity and digest type IV, V, and VII collagens as well as laminin, fibronectin, elastin, proteoglycans, and gelatin. The substrate of the membrane metalloproteinases (MMP-14, -15, -16) is essentially proMMP-2, and these enzymes allow activation of proMMP-2 at the cell surface on the invasive front. Most MMPs are secreted as inactive proenzymes (proMMPs) that become activated in the extracellular compartments with the exception of MMP-11 and MT-MMPs. Several enzymes are capable of activating the promatrixins, the most well known being plasmin. The activity of MMPs in the extracellular space is specifically inhibited by tissue inhibitor of metalloproteinases (TIMP), which binds to the highly conserved zinc-binding site of active MMPs at molar equivalence. The TIMP gene family consists of four structurally related members—TIMP-1, -2, -3, and -4.

In vitro, CTBs invade an acellular amniotic membrane or a reconstituted basement membrane like Matrigel, thus behave like metastatic cells.[3] This invasive behavior is due to the ability of CTBs to secrete MMPs since TIMP inhibits their invasiveness in the extracellular space.[4] Although CTBs behave like metastatic cells, *in vivo* they are only transiently invasive (first trimester), and their invasion is normally limited only to the endometrium and to the proximal third of the myometrium.[5] This temporal and spatial regulation of trophoblast invasion is believed to be mediated in an autocrine way by trophoblastic factors and in a paracrine way by uterine factors. Several types of regulators have been investigated: hormones, cytokines, growth factors and extracellular matrix components.

REGULATION OF METALLOPROTEINASES

Extracellular matrix components are known to influence adhesion, spreading, migration, and differentiation of cells through specific cell-surface receptors called integrins.[6] Villous and evCTBs express different integrins; and, while CTBs migrate from the villi into the decidua, they modulate their integrin repertoire. These changes in integrin expression are linked with the acquisition of the invasive phenotype and with the expression of MMPs.[7]

Hormones such as progesterone and human chorionic gonadotropin (hCG) are important regulators. It was recently shown[8] that progesterone downregulates the production of MMP-9 in first-trimester CTBs and this effect is mediated through the progesterone receptor because an anti-gestagen opposed this effect. These results are in line with the observation that trophoblastic gelatinase production is much higher in first-trimester CTBs than at term when progesterone production is maximal. This effect of progesterone cannot be direct and must be mediated intracellularly by other factors since there is no progesterone response element in the regulatory region of the *MMP-9* gene to which the progesterone–receptor complex can bind.

hCG significantly increases the collagenolytic activity and the degree of invasion of Jeg-3 cells, a choriocarcinoma cell line.[9] These *in vitro* results fit very well with

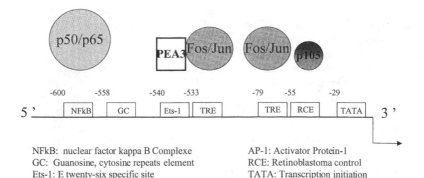

NFkB: nuclear factor kappa B Complexe   AP-1: Activator Protein-1
GC: Guanosine, cytosine repeats element   RCE: Retinoblastoma control
Ets-1: E twenty-six specific site   TATA: Transcription initiation

FIGURE 2. The regulatory region of the human *MMP-9* gene. NFkB: nuclear factor kappa B complex; GC: guanosine, cytosine repeat element; Ets-1: E 26-specific site; AP-1: activator protein-1; RCE: retinoblastoma control; TATA: transcription initiation.

in vivo observations showing that the degree of trophoblast invasion in ectopic pregnancy is significantly more pronounced (reaching the myosalpinx) when hCG levels are high.[10] Nevertheless, an understanding of how hCG affects trophoblast invasion still awaits further studies.

The literature on the effects of cytokines and growth factors on the invasive behavior of CTBs is extensive and has been recently reviewed.[11] Interleukin-1, -6, -15, tumor necrosis factor-α, insulin-like growth factor II, insulin-like growth factor binding protein-1, and epidermal growth factor promote CTB invasion by stimulating MMPs. In contrast, interleukin-10, leukemia inhibitory factor, and transforming growth factor-β inhibit invasion and MMP expression. Cytokines influence secretion and/or activity of MMPs. Although there is a certain degree of cell specificity, pro-inflammatory cytokines exert a stimulatory effect, whereas anti-inflammatory cytokines are generally inhibitors of MMPs. Cytokines exert their effects mainly by inducing the transcription of immediate early-response genes whose products act as transcription factors activating other genes, including those of MMPs.

Despite a large body of data, a complete understanding of the mechanism of regulation of trophoblast invasion is still lacking. Because nuclear transcription factors involved in the activation or repression of the *MMP-9* gene are less abundant than the paracrine or autocrine regulators studied so far, investigations are now focused on *MMP-9* gene regulation, particularly since in *in-vitro* models MMP-9 secretion seems to be a prerequisite for invasion of Matrigel by human CTBs.[4]

TRANSCRIPTION FACTORS INVOLVED IN THE REGULATION OF THE *MMP-9* GENE

The *MMP-9* gene is composed of 13 exons and 12 introns for a total size of 7.7 kb. The regulatory region (5′ flanking) of this gene (FIG. 2) contains multiple *cis*-regulatory elements. These *cis*-regulatory elements are specific DNA sequences that bind *trans*-activators or *trans*-repressors (transcription factors). These transcription factors are nuclear proteins (sometimes also cytoplasmic from which position they translocate into the nucleus), which upon binding activate or repress the gene's transcription machinery. Starting from the transcription initiation site (TATA, FIG. 2) and traveling upstream toward the 5′ end of the *MMP-9* promoter, both a TATA box and a retinoblastoma control element (RCE) will be encountered. RCE binds a protein called p105^{RB1} (the product of oncogene RB1). The next *cis*-regulatory element is a 12-*O*-tetradecanoyl phorbol 13-acetate (TPA)-responsive element (TRE) binding the activator protein-1 (AP-1, a heterodimer of Jun and Fos proteins). Another TRE is coupled to ets-1, to which the PEA3 (polyoma enhancer binding protein) products bind. Farther upstream there is an NFκB site (which binds p50–p65 heterodimers encoded by the *c-REL* oncogene family).

The most widely known transcription factor is the AP-1 complex. All genes inducible by the tumor promoter TPAs have a consensus sequence known as the TRE site, which binds AP-1.[12] The AP-1 complex is a heterodimer of Jun and Fos, the products of the proto-oncogenes *c-jun* and *c-fos*, which belong to the family of immediate early response genes.[12]

TPA not only increases trophoblastic *MMP-9* gene activity but also increases *MMP-9* mRNA. Because the maximal mRNA response appears only after 24 hr of incubation and cycloheximide significantly inhibits the stimulatory effect of TPA or tumor necrosis factor (TNF) on *MMP-9* messages, we hypothesized that TPA and TNF stimulate the synthesis of MMP-9 by inducing the transcription of early response genes. As observed with the band-shift assay, TPA and TNF induce in CTBs an increased binding of nuclear proteins to TRE sequences. These nuclear proteins were identified by monoclonal antibodies to Jun and Fos, and by transfection of CTB with antisense probes to *c-jun* and *c-fos* mRNA, which inhibited the trophoblastic secretion of MMP-9.[13] These results allow us to conclude that indeed TPA and TNF induce transcription of *c-jun* and *c-fos* oncogenes, the products of which bind to a TRE sequence in the promoter region of the *MMP-9* gene. This binding induces transcription of the *MMP-9* gene and increases the secretion of trophoblastic MMP-9.

ACKNOWLEDGMENTS

The authors wish to thank the Swiss National Science Foundation for their continuing support over the last twelve years.

REFERENCES

1. WESTERMARCK, J. & V.M. KÄHÄRI. 1999. Regulation of matrix metalloproteinase expression in tumour invasion. FASEB J. **13:** 781–792.
2. NAGASE, H. 1997. Activation mechanisms of matrix metalloproteinases. Biol. Chem. **378:** 151–160.
3. KLIMAN, H.J. & R.F. FEINBERG. 1990. Human trophoblast-extracellular matrix (ECM) interactions in vitro ECM thickness modulates morphology and proteolytic activity. Proc. Natl. Acad. Sci. USA **87:** 3057–3061.
4. LIBRACH, C.L., Z. WERB, M.L. FITZGERALD, *et al.* 1991. 92-kDa type IV collagenase mediates invasion of human cytotrophoblasts. J. Cell Biol. **113:** 437–449.
5. PIJNENBORG, R., G. DIXON, W.B. ROBERTSON & I. BROSENS. 1980. Trophoblastic invasion of human decidua from 8 to 18 weeks of pregnancy. Placenta **1:** 3–19.

6. HEINO, J. 1993. Integrin-type extracellular matrix receptors in cancer and inflammation. Ann. Med. **25:** 335–342.
7. BISCHOF, P., L. HAENGGELI & A. CAMPANA. 1995. Gelatinase and oncofetal fibronectin secretion are dependent upon integrin expression on human cytotrophoblasts. Hum. Reprod. **10:** 734–742.
8. SHIMONOVITZ, S., A. HURWITZ, D. HOCHNER-CELNIKIER, *et al.* 1998. Expression of gelatinase B by trophoblast cells. Down-regulation by progesterone. Am. J. Obstet. Gynecol. **1788:** 457–461.
9. ZYGMUNT, M., D. HAHN, K. MUNSTEDT, *et al.* 1998. Invasion of cytotrophoblastic JEG-3 cells is stimulated by hCG in vitro. Placenta **19:** 587–593.
10. OKTAY, K., R.G. BRZYSKI, E.B. MILLER & D. KRUGMAN. 1994. Association of serum beta-hCG levels with myosalpingeal invasion and viable trophoblast mass in tubal pregnancy. Obstet. Gynecol. **84:** 803–861.
11. BISCHOF P. & A. CAMPANA. 2000. Molecular mediators of implantation. *In* Implantation and Miscarriages. P. Bischof, Ed. Baillière's Clinical Obstetrics and Gynaecology. Vol. 14. In press.
12. ANGEL, P., M. IMAGAWA, R. CHIU, *et al.* 1987. Phorbol ester-inducible genes contain a common *cis* element recognized by a TPA-modulated *trans*-acting factor. Cell **49:** 729–739.
13. BISCHOF, P., K. TRUONG & A. CAMPANA. 2000. Unpublished results.

Uterine Contractility: Vaginal Administration of the β-Adrenergic Agonist, Terbutaline

Evidence of Direct Vagina-to-Uterus Transport

CARLO BULLETTI, DOMINIQUE DE ZIEGLER,[a,b] BEATRICE DE MOUSTIER,[a] VALERIA POLLI, GIANFRANCO BOLELLI, FRANCA FRANCESCHETTI, AND C. FLAMIGNI

1st Institute of Obstetrics and Gynecology, University of Bologna, 40138 Bologna, Italy

[a]*Columbia Laboratories, Paris, France*

[b]*Nyon Medical Center, Nyon, Switzerland*

ABSTRACT: Spontaneous uterine contractility during the menstrual cycle is required for menstruation, gamete transport, and, most likely, embryo nidation. Abnormal uterine contractility has been linked to dysmenorrhea, a condition associated with painful uterine cramping. Based on previous studies with progesterone, we have postulated the existence of a portal system that is responsible for some degree of direct vagina-to-uterus transport of administered compounds (i.e., the "first uterine pass effect"). It is possible that treatment with uterorelaxing substances, particularly β-adrenergic agonists, may alleviate the uterine discomfort that accompanies dysmenorrhea. However, side effects encountered with oral administration of β-agonists limit their utility. Alternatively, vaginal delivery of β-agonists could solve this dilemma by enhancing their efficacy and reducing side effects. Therefore, in the current study we used hysterectomy specimens and an *in vitro* uterine perfusion system to test the vagina-to-uterus transport of [³H]terbutaline, a well-known β-agonist. With the use of autoradiographic and scintillation counting techniques, our results clearly show progressive diffusion of labeled terbutaline from the rim of vaginal tissue through the uterus during the first 12 hours of perfusion. This indicates that uterine targeting of terbutaline can be accomplished through vaginal administration, suggesting a new therapeutic modality in women's health care.

KEYWORDS: dysmenorrhea; endometriosis; endometrium; first uterine pass; myometrium; terbutaline; transvaginal drug delivery; uterine contractility

INTRODUCTION

Human uterus exhibits spontaneous contractility during the menstrual cycle, facilitating gamete transportation, menstruation, and possibly embryo nidation. However, abnormal uterine contractility may cause dysmenorrhea. Recently, accu-

Address for correspondence: Carlo Bulletti, M.D., 1st Institute of Obstetrics and Gynecology, University of Bologna, Via Massarenti, 13, 40138 Bologna, Italy. Voice: 39.541.393844 or 39.541.705741; fax: 39.541.705741.

Bull@infotel.it

mulated evidence indicates that progesterone administered vaginally induces endometrial effects that largely surpass expectations according to the relatively low circulatory levels achieved.[1] This enhanced uterine action is believed to result from some degree of direct vagina-to-uterus transport of progesterone administered vaginally, the "first uterine pass effect."[2] Ultimately, direct diffusion of progesterone to the uterus results in higher uterine tissue-to-blood ratios[3,4] in the case of vaginal administration compared to intramuscular injection.

The existence of direct vagina-to-uterus transport occurring through a local functional "portal" system makes the vaginal route an ideal option for administering all uterotropic drugs. Preferential delivery associated with vaginal administration permits maximization of the desired effects on the uterus, while minimizing circulatory levels and, consequently, side effects. Evidence of the clinical advantage of this phenomenon already exists with progesterone. Experience with a sustained release gel of progesterone shows that direct delivery to the uterus and low systemic levels significantly limit side effects.[5] This is clinically important because it may improve treatment compliance in hormone replacement therapy (HRT).

First among uterotropic drugs, other than progesterone, that could benefit from vaginal administration are uterorelaxing substances, particularly β-adrenergic agonists. These compounds, including terbutaline, are effective in treating the painful uterine cramping of dysmenorrhea.[6] Yet, the magnitude of side effects encountered when β-agonists are administered orally[7] or systemically has precluded their use in treating a condition as benign as dysmenorrhea. Vaginal delivery of β-agonists, however, can solve the dilemna of efficacy versus side effects. By targeting drug delivery to the uterus, vaginal terbutaline offers the potential of efficiently treating dysmenorrhea, while not raising blood levels above the side effects threshold. Local therapy could therefore correct the underlying disorder responsible for dysmenorrhea, the dyskinetic uterine contractions (cramping), instead of merely treating its symptom, pain.

It remains to be determined, however, whether nonsteroidal hydrophilic substances such as terbutaline can benefit from the direct transport phenomenon linking the vagina to the uterus identified with progesterone. To clarify this issue, we studied the fate of [^{3}H]terbutaline deposited on the rim of vaginal tissue remaining attached to the hysterectomy specimen using the *ex vivo* human uterus perfusion system we described.

MATERIALS AND METHODS

Surgical Specimens

Thirty-four uteri were obtained surgically with a rim of 1.5–2 cm of vaginal tissue from women 31–44 years of age undergoing abdominal hysterectomy for early stage cervical carcinoma (CIN) or uterine prolapse. All patients consented freely to participate in the study and to have their uteri used until completion of the experiment. The study was approved by our Institutional Review Board. All uteri were sent to pathology for definitive analysis on completion of the functional study. The subjects were carefully selected preoperatively as previously described.[8–11] The hysterectomies were programmed to obtain specimens during the proliferative ($n = 8$) and secretory ($n = 16$) phases of the menstrual cycle. Histologic examination of the endometrium confirmed the menstrual cycle phase. Six uteri established the nonspecific uptake by uterine tissues of membrane-impermeable dextran at different intervals (3, 6, 9, 12, 18, 24, and 48 hours). Twenty-four experiments were used to determine the accumulation of terbutaline in the endometrium and myometrium 3 ($n = 2$), 6 ($n = 4$), 9 ($n = 4$), 12 ($n = 4$), 18 ($n = 4$), 24 ($n = 3$), and 48 ($n = 3$) hours after the application of terbutaline on the cuff of vaginal tissue removed on hysterectomy. Finally, four uteri used for autoradiography studies were exposed to a single tracer, [³H]terbutaline.

Perfusion Procedure

Uterine perfusions were performed using a technique that has been reported extensively elsewhere.[8–11] Briefly, this method allows good preservation of the organ for up to 52 hours, as reflected by oxygenation and responsiveness of tissue samples.

Vaginal Administration of Test and Reference Substances: Calculation of Tissue Extractions

[³H]Terbutaline was custom prepared by NEN Research Products, Dupont (Boston, MA, USA) with the following characteristics. D,L-Terbutaline, (Ring-³H(N)) (C12H19NO3), lot #3246-109 and assay #3246-113, radioactivity 1×10.4 mCi, and weight 1×0.098 mg, was received in a Pyrex ampule sealed under nitrogen in solution in 0.05M KH_2PO_4, pH 3-EtOH (1:2) at 1.84 mCi/ml with specific activity 23.Ci/mmol. Aliquots containing 27.2 ml (50 mCi) of D,L-terbutaline, (Ring-³H(N)), were applied on the vaginal rim remaining attached to each uterus after surgical removal and before extracorporeal perfusion 1 hour after placing the uterus in the *invitro* perfusion device. For this, a mixture of [³H]terbutaline and cold terbutaline was dissolved in mineral oil. Transport to the uterus (calculated as whole organ) and vaginal and endometrial or myometrial extraction were measured 3, 6, 9, 12, 18, 24, and 48 hours after application of oil mixed with either the radioactive test terbutaline or radioactive dextran. Furthermore, radioactive water and butanol were used as freely diffusible reference substances. Venous perfusate was collected from the open circulatory system at preset time intervals for measurement of radioactivity. The solution applied vaginally consisted of either a mixture of [³H]terbutaline (test substance) and [¹⁴C]butanol (reference substance), for assessment of specific terbutaline extraction, or [¹⁴C]dextran (test) and [³H]water (reference), for assessment of nonspecific tissue extraction. [³H]Terbutaline was the sole radioactive product used in the autoradiography experiments. All experiments were interrupted at predetermined time intervals after vaginal application of the mixture of ³H and cold terbutaline. Samples of vagina, myometrium, and endometrium were taken with a through-cut biopsy needle (Travenol Laboratories, Deerfield, IL) or a Novak curette, respectively. These samples (approximatively 100 mg) were used for histologic study and determination of ³H and ¹⁴C concentrations. For this the samples were dissolved in 1 ml of Soluene (Packard Instruments, Chicago, IL) and mixed with 15 ml of scintillation fluid (Dimilume 30, Packard Instruments). Aliquots of the original oil solution used to administer the radioactive tracers and of the venous effluent were prepared similarly for double-isotope liquid scintillation counting using an LKB 1215 Rackbeta 2 scintillation spectrometer (LKB-Produkter AB, Bromma, Sweden). Radioactivity in the original preparations used was adjusted to maintain a ratio of at least 3:1 of ^{3}H-labeled test to ^{14}C-labeled reference radioactivity, which was used to minimize errors resulting from ^{14}C radioactivity overlapping into the ^{3}H channel. Isotope counts per minute were converted to disintegrations per minute (dpm), making standard quench corrections.

The vaginal, endometrial, and myometrial influx indices of [^{14}C]dextran relative to ^{3}H-labeled water were calculated as previously reported by Pardridge et al.[12-16] Following this paradigm, the dextran index was calculated as (^{14}C/^{3}H) in endometrium (vagina or myometrium)/(^{14}C/^{3}H) in the mixture applied on the vaginal cuff. Similarly, when [^{3}H]terbutaline and [^{14}C]butanol were used, the terbutaline index (test) was calculated as (^{3}H/^{14}C) in endometrium (vagina or myometrium)/(^{3}H/^{14}C) in the mixture used on the vaginal tissue. The oil solution applied on the vagina contained approximately 27.2 μCi [^{3}H]terbutaline and 4.5 μCi of [^{14}C]butanol. Finally, a mixture containing about 2 μCi [^{14}C]dextran and 5 μCi [^{3}H]H$_2$O was applied to the vaginal cuff to determine true extraction of terbutaline from uterine tissues and transit time of this mixture through the organ when a constant flow rate of 25 ml/min was maintained in the arterial perfusion. Because of its membrane impermeability, [^{14}C]dextran was used as a reflector of nonspecific transport from the vaginal collar to the uterine tissues.

Uterine extraction of isotopes applied on vaginal tissue was taken as evidence of direct vagina-to-uterus transport or the first uterine pass effect of these substances.[17] Because the experimental uterine perfusion model avoided recirculation of the perfusate, contamination of arterial flow by residual vascular radioactivity during second passage through the organ was not possible. [^{14}C]Butanol served as reference isotope because of its freely diffusible characteristics. The net vaginal, endometrial, and myometrial extractions of [^{3}H]terbutaline and [^{14}C]butanol were determined for each experiment concluded at set time intervals after application of the test substance on the vaginal cuff. Following the method described,[12-16] extraction of test terbutaline was calculated with the following formula: Et = TII × Eb, where Et and Eb represent the percent extraction of terbutaline and butanol, respectively, at time intervals after vaginal application of the test substance and TII the tissue influx index. Statistical analysis was performed by the two-tailed Student's t test with two independent means as determined for each individual experiment

Autoradiography

Autoradiography was performed from thin transverse and longitudinal sections (about 5 mm) of perfused uteri obtained 3, 6, 9, and 12 hours after vaginal application of a standard dose of [^{3}H]terbutaline. Transverse uterine sections of the organ featuring the endometrial tissue in its center were obtained at different distances from the internal os of the cervix. This served to assess with autoradiography data the time dependency of the uterine invasion by vaginally administered terbutaline. Tissue sections were positioned on Hyperfilm ^{3}H 18 × 24 cm (code RPN 535), obtained from Amersham Italia s.r.l. (Milan, Italy), for 28 days at −80°C and Kodak Scientific Imaging Film X-OMAT AR 8 × 10 in, 20.3 × 25.4 cm obtained from Eastman Kodak Company (Rochester, New York).

TABLE 1. Efflux of terbutaline (mean ± SD) from uterine vein and its tissue extraction (mean ± SD) after vaginal application of [^{3}H]terbutaline

Time intervals (hr)	Outflow vein recovery (% of total dose)	$(n)^a$	Extractions (% of total dose) Endometrial	Myometrial	Vaginal
3	3.3 + 1.4	(24)	1 + 0.1 (2)	0.9 + 0.4	0.5 + 0.1
6	22.1 + 9	(24)	3.1 + 1.1 (4)	9.5 + 0.3	0.8 + 0.2
9	26.6 + 6.3	(24)	9.9 + 3.6 (4)	13.8 + 1.8	1.4 + 0.4
12	21.3 + 9.2	(24)	18.9 + 1.7 (4)	18.4 + 3.4	2.1 + 0.6
18	17.4 + 7.2	(24)	6 + 3.3 (4)	7.7 + 2.8	1.9 + 1
24	7 + 5	(24)	6.1 + 1.5 (3)	16 + 13.2	0.9 + 0.7
48	5.9 + 5.5	(24)	5.3 + 1.3 (3)	2.8 + 0.8	0.9 + 0.3

^{a}Number of samples (n) in parentheses.

RESULTS

Background dextran (nonspecific) accumulations in the endometrium and myometrium were 9% and 6% of the labeled terbutaline extracted by these tissues. Hence, this value needed to be subtracted from the amounts of [^{3}H]terbutaline counted in all tissue samples. FIGURE 1 shows the endometrial extraction of terbutaline and the correspondent venous outflow of this compound during the 48 hours of uterine perfusion that followed vaginal application of labeled terbutaline. TABLE 1 reports terbutaline efflux (mean + SD) as well as extraction in vagina, myometrium, and endometrium (100 mg of tissue) from the organ (venous effluent) 3–48 hours after vaginal application of [^{3}H]terbutaline.

[^{3}H]Terbutaline appeared in uterine effluent during the third hour of perfusion (3.3% ± 1.4% of total dose). Efflux from the uterus increased during the first 9 hours of perfusion (26.8% ± 6.3% of total dose) and decreased thereafter from the twelfth (21.3% ± 9.2%) to the forty-eighth hour of perfusion (7% ± 5%). Uterine extraction of [^{3}H]terbutaline and [^{14}C]butanol increased from the third to the twelfth hour of perfusion. It decreased at the eighteenth hour and tended to remain constant for up to 48 hours of uterine perfusion.

After 12 hours of perfusion, autoradiography of uterine sections showed uniform accumulation of radioactivity by the endometrium in all sections obtained from the cervical to the fundal area, as illustrated in FIGURE 1A and B. Progression of the front of migration of terbutaline and butanol into the uterine organ was established from all the experiments reported here (extraction data and autoradiography).[17]

DISCUSSION

We showed that progressive diffusion of [^{3}H]terbutaline through the uterus occurred 1–12 hours after placing the radioactive preparation on the rim of vaginal tis-

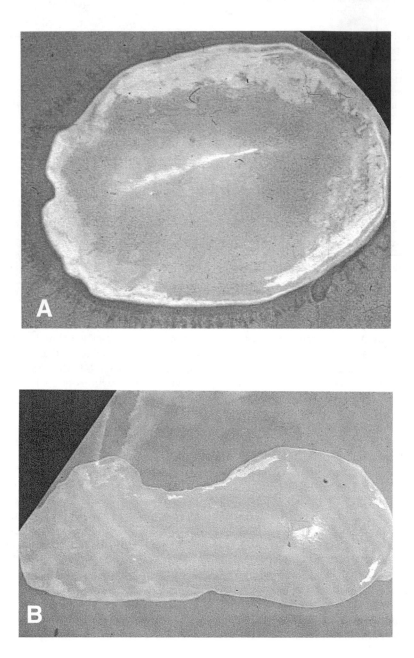

FIGURE 1. (A,B) Autoradiography of layers of human uterus obtained 12 hours after vaginal application of radioactive terbutaline and uterine perfusion *in vitro*. Terbutaline accumulates in the endometrium (middle of the radiograph), around the organ, in the external third of the muscle, and, apparently, around the vessels.

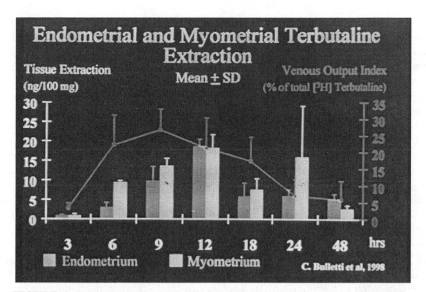

FIGURE 2. Terbutaline efflux (mean ± SD) from uterine vein and its endometrial, myometrial, and vaginal extractions (mean ± SD) after vaginal application of tritiated terbutaline. Terbutaline outflow decreased from the 12 to 48 hours of perfusion The zenith of both myometrial and endometrial accumulations was reached after 12 hours of the vaginal application of terbutaline.

sue that remained attached to the hysterectomy specimen. Because of the nature of the experimental model (open circulatory system), our results confirmed and extended our prior demonstration of direct vagina-to-uterus transport of vaginally administered substances. In prior work, we demonstrated that this direct transport, or first uterine pass effect, occurs with readily diffusible substances such as progesterone.[17] Our present data confirm that the local vagina-to-uterus transport phenomenon first identified with progesterone is also seen with hydrophilic substances, such as terbutaline, that are not as readily diffusible as progesterone. Hence, these results support our contention that a true "functional portal" system links the vagina to the uterus with a capacity to transport substances as different as liposoluble progesterone and hydrosoluble products such as terbutaline.

The difference in tissue diffusibility between progesterone (liposoluble) and terbutaline (hydrosoluble) is likely to account for the different kinetics observed for the uterine diffusion of these two substances. Readily diffusible progesterone reached the fundal end of the uterus approximately 5–6 hours after placement of [3H]progesterone on the rim of vaginal tissue.[17] In the case of terbutaline, comparable diffusion to the entire uterus occurred markedly later after [3H]terbutaline placement on the remaining fragments of vaginal tissue. Although differences in tissue diffusibility translate in different kinetics of direct vagina-to-uterus diffusion, our results indicate, however, that the "portal" system linking vagina to uterus is not product specific.

The relatively minimal differences in diffusion kinetics between [3H]progesterone[17] and [3H]terbutaline support the hypothesis of vascular involvement with countercurrent exchange as the primary underlying mechanism for this phenomenon.[4] Alternatively, if the vagina-to-uterus transport were solely dependent on passive "through tissue" diffusion, it would be reasonable to expect more profound differences between the findings obtained with substances whose tissue diffusion characteristics are as different as those of progesterone and terbutaline.

Identification of a functional portal system connecting the vagina to the uterus, capable of transporting substances as different as progesterone and terbutaline, raises questions about the functional role of such system. Stated differently, why would nature design a local transport system if not for a specific function? With this problematic in mind, it is reasonable to postulate that prostaglandins contained in sperm may be the primary product destined to benefit from direct vagina-to-uterus transport. By this mechanism, prostaglandins could activate uterine contractions without raising the circulating levels of prostaglandins. Ultimately, activation of uterine contractility by direct transport of sperm prostaglandins to the uterus will facilitate sperm transport towards the fallopian tubes.

The slower kinetics of vagina-to-uterus diffusion of [³H]terbutaline as compared to that of [³H]progesterone is a favorable characteristic for the possible use of vaginal terbutaline in the treatment of dysmenorrhea. In dysmenorrhea, slow vagina-to-uterus transfer of terbutaline offers a good prospect that treatment applied just before the onset of menses will remain effective for up to 48 hours and therefore cover the acme of painful uterine cramping.

Targeting terbutaline action to the uterus by its vaginal administration may provide exceptional practical advantages. Indeed, the major limitations to the clinical use of terbutaline in gynecology are its serious side effects (tachycardia and tremor) encountered at therapeutic concentrations. In pilot trials, Kullander and Svanberg[18] and Åkerlund et al.[7] showed that terbutaline can effectively treat dysmenorrhea. In this trial, however, side effects (tachycardia and tremor) were unacceptably high for a condition as benign as dysmenorrhea, precluding the use of terbutaline for this condition. Because of the high incidence of dysmenorrhea and the absence of treatment other than symptomatic alleviation of cramping by nonsteroidal anti-inflammatory drugs, the emerging possibility of directly antagonizing the primary dyskinetic process at its origin is clinically important. It potentially offers a significant therapeutic leap in women's health care. This study also confirms the advantages offered by the vaginal route for substances mainly targeted to the uterus because of the well-established vagina–uterus transportation.[19–22]

REFERENCES

1. FANCHIN, R., D. DE ZIEGLER, C. BERGERON, et al. 1997. Transvaginal administration of progesterone: dose-response data support a first uterine pass effect. Obstet. Gynecol. **90:** 396–401.
2. DE ZIEGLER, D. 1995. Hormonal control of endometrial receptivity. Hum. Reprod. **10:** 4–7.
3. MILES, R.A., R.J. PAULSON, R.A. LOBO, et al. 1994. Pharmacokinetics and endometrial tissue levels of progesterone after administration by intramuscular and vaginal routes: a comparative study. Fertil. Steril. **62:** 485–490.
4. CICINELLI, E., D. DE ZIEGLER, C. BULLETTI, et al. 2000. Direct transport of progesterone from vagina to uterus. Obstet. Gynecol. **95:** 403–406.

5. WARREN, M.P., B.M.K. BILLER & M.M. SHANGOLD. 1999. A new clinical option for hormone replacement therapy in women with secondary amenorrhea: effects of cyclic administration of progesterone from the sustained release vaginal gel Crinone (4% and 8%) on endometrial morphologic features and withdrawal bleeding. Am. J. Obstet. Gynecol. **180:** 42–48.

6. ANDERSSON, K.-E., I. INGERMARSSON & C.G.A. PERSSON. 1973. Relaxing effects of β-receptor stimulators in isolated, gravid human myometrium. Life Sci. **13:** 335–344.

7. ÅKERLUND, M. & K.-E. ANDERSSON. 1976. Effects of terbutaline on human myometrial activity and endometrial blood flow. Obstet. Gynecol. **47:** 529–535.

8. BULLETTI, C., V.M. JASONNI, S. LUBICZ, *et al.* 1986. Extracorporeal perfusion of the human uterus. Am. J. Obstet. Gynecol. **154:** 683–638.

9. BULLETTI, C., V.M. JASONNI, G. MARTINELLI, *et al.* 1987. A 48-hour preservation of an isolated human uterus: endometrial responses to sex steroids. Fertil. Steril. **47:** 122–129.

10. BULLETTI, C., V.M. JASONNI, P. CIOTTI, *et al.* 1988. Extraction of estrogens by human perfused uterus. Effects of membrane permeability and binding by serum proteins on differential influx into the endometrium and myometrium. Am. J. Obstet. Gynecol. **159:** 509–515.

11. BULLETTI, C., V.M. JASONNI, S. TABANELLI, *et al.* 1988. Early human pregnancy *in vitro* utilizing an artificially perfused uterus. Fertil. Steril. **49:** 991–996.

12. PARDRIDGE, W.M. & L.J. MIETUS. 1979. Transport of steroid hormones through the rat blood–brain barrier: primary role of albumin-bound hormone. J. Clin. Invest. **64:** 145–154.

13. PARDRIDGE, W.M. 1981. Transport of protein-bound hormones into tissues *in vivo*. Endocrine Rev. **2:** 103–123.

14. LAUFER, L.R., J.C. GAMBONE, G. CHAUDHURI, *et al.* 1983. The effect of membrane permeability and binding by human serum proteins on sex steroid influx into the uterus. J. Clin. Endocrinol. Metab. **56:** 1282–1287.

15. VERHEUGEN, C., W.M. PARDRIDGE, H. JUDD & G. CHAUDHURI. 1984. Differential permeability of uterine and liver vascular beds to estrogens and estrogen conjugates. J. Clin. Endocrinol. Metab. **59:** 1128–1132.

16. STEINGOLD, K.A., W. CEFALU, W.M. PARDRIDGE, *et al.* 1986. Enhanced hepatic extraction of estrogens used for replacement therapy. J. Clin. Endocrinol. Metab. **62:** 761–766.

17. BULLETTI, C., D. DE ZIEGLER, F. FLAMIGNI, *et al.* 1997. Targeted drug delivery in gynecology: the first uterine pass effect. Hum. Reprod. **12:** 1073–1079.

18. KULLANDER, S. & L. SVANBERG. 1985. On resorption and the effects of vaginally administered terbutaline in women with premature labor. Acta Obstet. Gynecol. Scand. **64:** 613–616.

19. MIZUTANI, T., S. NISHIYAMA, I. AMAKAWA, *et al.* 1995. Danazol concentrations in ovary, uterus, and serum and their effect on the hypothalamic-pituitary-ovarian axis during vaginal administration of danazol suppository. Fertil. Steril. **63:** 1184–1189.

20. HAUSKNECHT, P.R. 1995. Methotrexate and misoprostol to terminate early pregnancy. N. Engl. J. Med. **333:** 537–540.

21. EL-REFAEY, H., D. RAJASEKAR, M. ABDALLA, *et al.* 1995. Induction of abortion with mifepristone (RU 486) and oral or vaginal misoprostol. N. Engl. J. Med. **332:** 983–987.

22. DE ZIEGLER, D., E. SHAERER, L. SEIDLER, *et al.* 1995. Transvaginal administration of progesterone: the vaginal paradox and the first uterine pass effect hypothesis. Gynecol. Obstet. **3:** 267–272.

Contractility of the Nonpregnant Uterus

The Follicular Phase

D. DE ZIEGLER,[a,d] C. BULLETTI,[b] R. FANCHIN,[c] M. EPINEY,[a] AND
P.-A. BRIOSCHI[a]

[a]Department of Obstetrics and Gynecology, Hôpital de Nyon, Nyon, Switzerland

[b]1st Institute of Obstetrics and Gynecology, University of Bologna, 40138 Bologna, Italy

[c]Department of Obstetrics and Gynecology and Reproductive Medicine, Hôpital Antoine
Béckère, 92141 Clamart, France

[d]Columbia Laboratories, Paris, France

ABSTRACT: Recent renewed interest in uterine contractility stems from the possibility of directly visualizing uterine contractility on images generated by
high-resolution ultrasound probes. During the menstrual cycle, three typical
patterns of uterine contractility have been recognized. During the luteofollicular transition and early follicular phase (menses), the contractile event involves
all layers of the myometrium and exerts antegrade (from fundus to cervix) expulsive forces. Characteristically, uterine contractions are often perceived by
women at the time of menses, sometimes reaching the level of painful cramps
(dysmenorrhea). In the late follicular phase, uterine contractility involves only
the subendometrial layers of the myometrium and is never perceived by wom-
en. The primary function of uterine contractility in the late follicular phase is
to facilitate the retrograde (cervix to fundus) transport of sperm towards the
distal end of the fallopian tubes where fertilization normally takes place. Finally, the uterus reaches a stage of quiescence after ovulation (under the influence
of progesterone) that characterizes the major part of the luteal phase. The
present review summarizes our understanding of the physiological role of uterine contractility during the follicular phase and the possible implications in
pathological circumstances such as endometriosis and dysmenorrhea.

KEYWORDS: uterine contractility; sperm transport; endometriosis; dysmenorrhea

INTRODUCTION

There is currently ample evidence that the nonpregnant uterus contracts throughout the menstrual cycle. Interest in studying uterine contractility was recently re-
vived with the availability of high-resolution vaginal ultrasound probes that allow
direct visualization of the contractile process. Typically, three distinct patterns are
recognized during the menstrual cycle:

Address for correspondence: Dr. D. de Ziegler, Department of Ob Gyn, Hôpital de Nyon,
Nyon, Switzerland. Voice: 00331 53423007; fax: 00331 53423001.
ddeziegler@compuserve.com

Luteofollicular transition (menses): After circulating levels of progesterone decrease following the demise of the corpus luteum, contractility increases with, as primary features, an increase in uterine contraction (UC) amplitude, frequency, and resting tone. During the luteofollicular transition (menses), UC participates in the forward emptying of the uterine contents.

Late follicular phase: During the late follicular phase of the menstrual cycle, a progressive increase in uterine contractility parallels the rise in E_2 levels. Ultimately, UC frequency increases to a mean value of 3.5–5 UC/min just prior to ovulation. The primary function of uterine contractility in the late follicular phase is to transport sperm from the vagina to the distal end of the fallopian tube where fertilization normally occurs.

Luteal phase: After ovulation, the uterus undergoes a characteristic period of quiescence.

This article reviews the physiological characteristics of uterine contractility that prevail during the luteofollicular transition and late follicular phases. We also outline the pathophysiological consequences of the dyskinetic alterations in uterine contractility that sometimes occur during these phases of the menstrual cycle. Because our understanding of uterine contractility hinges primarily on human investigations, we also review advances in the investigative methods currently available for clinical trials. We underscore the specific advantages and limitations of each of these methods.

UTERINE CONTRACTILITY DURING THE LUTEOFOLLICULAR TRANSITION AND EARLY FOLLICULAR PHASES

Physiology

During the luteofollicular transition and early follicular phases (at the time of menses), UC is predominantly antegrade, that is, propagating from the fundus to the cervical end of the uterus.[1,2] This pattern of contractility is instrumental in the forward emptying of uterine contents (menstrual blood). At this stage in the menstrual cycle, UC is also a primary factor in hemostasis. Characteristically, the prevailing pattern of contractility during menses represents a miniature replica of the expulsive contractions of labor. During this phase of the menstrual cycle, UCs are often perceived by patients. On occasion, UCs can even become frankly painful (a condition known as dysmenorrhea) to the point where the patient may require specific medication and/or time off from work. Studies based on intrauterine pressure (IUP) recordings (FIG. 1) and UTZ findings typically show a rather low (by reference to the late follicular phase) UC frequency of approximately 2–3/min (range, 0.5–6), but a characteristically high mean UC amplitude of up to 60 mm Hg. Mean resting tone is also elevated during menses, when it commonly averages 40 mm Hg, the highest value observed during the menstrual cycle. The elevated resting tone and high UC amplitude during menses reflect the active involvement of all layers of the myometrium during the contractile process. Notably, this has been documented in studies assessing uterine contractility by electrophysiology, and evidence of transparietal involvement of all layers of the myometrium hase been reported. By contrast, solely the subendometrial layers of the myometrium participate in the contactile process at other times in the menstrual cycle.[2] Recently, ultrasound-based studies have abounded.

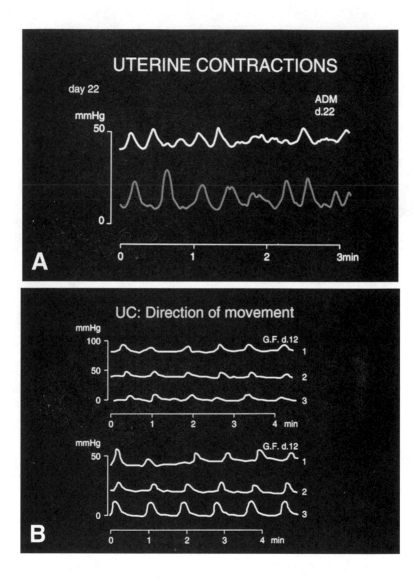

FIGURE 1. Uterine contractility assessed by recording intrauterine pressure (IUP). *Early follicular phase*: this phase of the menstrual cycle is characterized by high uterine contraction (UC) amplitude and resting tone. *Late follicular phase*: UCs were recorded from triple-ended uterine catheters. The direction of contraction was assessed by computing the time lag between the high points of each contraction recorded in different segments of the uterine cavity. *Upper* and *lower parts* of FIGURE 1B illustrate the abrupt reversal of direction sometimes observed in the same patient within a short time interval (10 min). *Luteal phase*: this phase is characterized by a prompt decrease in UC frequency and amplitude. From Martinez-Gaudio et al.[1]

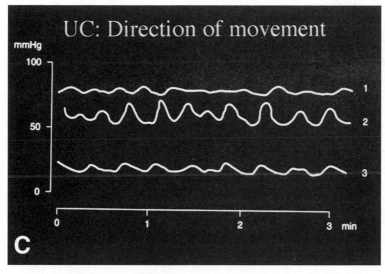

FIGURE 1. *Continued.*

By and large, these all concurred to confirm the early IUP data with reports of similar UC frequencies at the time of menses.[3, 4]

Today, no one questions the obvious advantage of the noninvasiveness of ultrasound-based assessments of uterine contractility. Yet, we must also admit that ultrasound has so far failed to recognize the characteristics of contractility that are specific to each pattern in the menstrual cycle and, notably, at the time of menses. The shortcomings of ultrasound-based measurements of uterine contractility have long been identified and include the lack of information on resting pressure, which clearly hampers the value of assessments made during menses. Now, it has become evident that ultrasound also has other limitations. Notably, ultrasound-based studies have not lived up to the early hopes brought by the foreseen possibility of directly visualizing the respective involvement of each myometrial layer. Specifically, ultrasounds have not yet been able to distinguish the physiologic (normal) pattern(s) of uterine contractility during menses from the dyskinetic ones (abnormal) associated with dysmenorrhea. Hence, the primary clinical question on uterine contractility at the time of menses remains: Are there differences in the relative involvement of the various layers of the myometrium identifiable clinically that permit is to single out physiological UCs (antegrade expulsion of uterine contents) from disrupted ones susceptible to pathological consequences (retrograde bleeding, dysmenorrhea, etc.)? Unfortunately to this date, this query remains beyond the reach of ultrasound studies.

As stated, during the early follicular phase, most UCs feature antegrade displacement (from fundus to cervix) of the contractile process (FIG. 1). This information was first provided by early studies in which IUP was recorded from multiple-tip pressure probes.[1] In these studies, UC displacement was analyzed by computing the time lag between the UC high points, detected by the different pressure tips located in the fundal, middle, and lower uterine areas of the uterus, respectively, with multiple-barrel pressure catheters. Later, most ultrasound-based studies of the apparent displacement of the contractile event on accelerated image sequences have concurred to confirm the predominance of antegrade contractions over all other forms of UC during the early follicular phase (menses).[2–4] Yet, as discussed later in more detail, the weakness of ultrasound data on UC direction resides in the inherent subjectivity of assessments made from looking at fast plays of ultrasound sequences or any other method used to date to interpret UC displacement from ultrasound scans. Too hastily we think, extrapolations have been drawn from these readings and used to conclude on true direction of transport of uterine contents. When discussing uterine contractility during the late follicular phase, the conclusions drawn from ultrasound data are often far-fetched and/or possibly erroneous. Certainly, these ultrasound-based measurements of the direction of UC displacement have not been validated.

Alternative methods have currently been proposed for assessing UC direction. Among them, interesting data have been generated from studying the displacement of uterine contents identified by various contrast media and/or makers, notably, Tc-99–labeled macroalbumin aggregates (MAA) or X-ray contrast medium. Because all these approaches looking at the displacement of uterine contents have primarily been used to assess sperm transport during the preovulatory phase, they will all be discussed and their results compared when analyzing uterine contractility in the late follicular phase.

The specific characteristics of UCs experienced during the early follicular phase (menses) and their association with the subjective perception of painful cramps (potentially leading to frank dysmenorrhea) have not yet been fully clarified. By inference from studies of uterine contractility during other phases of the menstrual cycle (when UCs are never perceived, let alone painful), we can formulate the following hypothesis: During the luteofollicular transition (menses), the "transmural" involvement of UCs (i.e., the implication of all the myometrial layers rather than just the subendometrial ones) is likely the primary factor linked to their painful perception. Probably, this latter characteristic is also crucial to another function of uterine contractility at the time of menses, hemostasis. We are still in need of investigative tools capable of providing precise, reliable, and clinically usable markers that reflect the painful characteristics of UC during the early follicular phase. We must recognize however, that to this day, the results of UTZ studies have not provided the awaited help originally hoped.

Pathophysiology

Two medical entities appear to result and/or be associated with alterations in early follicular phase contractility, dysmenorrhea, and endometriosis.

Dysmenorrhea

Primary dysmenorrhea is a clinical condition characterized by painful, possibly invalidating uterine cramps just prior to or at the time of menses. A common disorder that mainly affects young women, dysmenorrhea can become invalidating for many women from one to several days each month and can be the cause of numerous missed workdays. In women with dysmenorrhea, early follicular phase uterine contractility is characterized by an increase in resting IUP (resting tone) and UC amplitude, duration, and frequency.[5] These characteristics of dysmenorrhea can all be assessed by IUP recording; unfortunately, it is an invasive method. Yet to this day, despite high expectation placed on ultrasound evaluations, only one of the characteristics of dysmenorrhea, UC frequency, can reliably be assessed. Unfortunately, this parameter of dysmenorrhea, the increase in UC frequency measurable by UTZ, is the weakest of all UC characteristics for reflecting the extent of menstrual cramps and dysmenorrhea.[6] Hence, despite the advent of ultrasound, we still need a reliable marker(s) of UC alterations responsible for dysmenorrhea that could easily and non-invasively serve in large-scale clinical trials.

Furthermore, because the endometrium is inherently thin at the time of menses, ultrasound imaging can never reach the quality that we are accustomed to during the end-follicular phase and early to midluteal phase studies. Ultrasound is therefore of little help in studying dysmenorrhea and comparing the efficacy of different treatments. The inherent characteristics of early follicular phase uterine contractility and its disruption in dysmenorrhea still evade all forms of noninvasive scrutiny.

Endometriosis

Endometriosis, a serious and potentially devastating disease of unknown origin, mainly affects gynecological and other lower pelvic organs. One of the two hypotheses put forth to explain the growth and development of endometrial implants in various areas of the pelvic cavity proposes a culprit role for retrograde bleeding. This is also known as "Sampson's retrograde menstruation theory." According to this classical hypothesis, retrograde bleeding recurring month after month will keep disseminating endometrial fragments into the pelvic cavity, where they will, in turn, implant and develop.[7] Sampson's theory of retrograde menstruation has long been opposed to the alternate hypothesis of "coelomic metaplasia." Until now, however, no compelling evidence has led to the overwhelming supremacy of either one of these two theories. Furthermore, breaking from a lingering opposition between these two concepts, the views that now prevail favor complementary rather than antagonizing roles for these two mechanisms. Hence, in this multimechanism view of endometriosis, retrograde bleeding is seen as one of the phenomena (rather than the sole mechanism) that fuels pelvic endometriosis. In an ultrasound-based study, unfortunately not confirmed by further work or even reproduced by others, Salamanca *et al.*[8] observed predominantly retrograde UC at the time of menses in women with documented endometriosis. On the contrary, in the experience of these investigators, antegrade contractions predominated during menses in unaffected controls. These findings were quick to gather adepts to the concept that endometriosis is intimately linked to some not yet identified form of dyskinetic alterations in uterine contractility during the early follicular phase. A limiting factor in this study, however, is the lack of validation of ultrasound studies for assessing the direction of contractility.

Inferences from studies of other forms of smooth muscle dyskinesia, notably, the irritable bowel syndrome,[9] have led some to postulate that the alterations in uterine contractility found at the heart of endometriosis are probably of the hyperkinetic type.[10] During the early follicular phase, the net result of these dyskinetic changes is likely to be variable degrees of impediment to proper antegrade emptying of menstrual blood. This, because of the high-pressure environment prevailing in the uterine cavity, will in turn lead to a disorganized evacuation of menstrual blood that will tend

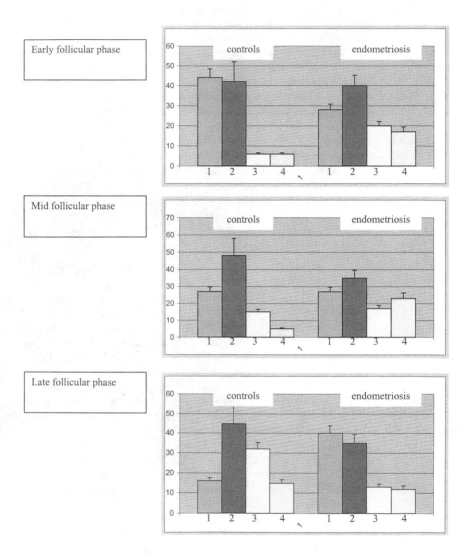

FIGURE 2. Direction of contractility assessed by studying the displacement of uterine contents. The displacement of Tc-99–labeled macroalbumin aggregates (MMA) was studied with a technique called hysterosalpingoscintigraphy (HSS). MMAs were placed in the vaginal fornix during the early (*upper diagram*), mid (*middle diagram*), and late follicular phase (*lower diagram*) in women with endometriosis (*right 4 columns*) and unaffected controls (*left 4 columns*). Sets of 4 columns (1–4) represent Tc activity detected by gamma camera in the lower and mid-portion of the uterus (*columns 1 and 2*) and in the ipsi- and contralateral tubes (by reference to the developing follicle), *columns 3 and 4*. Results show an increase in retrograde transport towards the tubes in the early follicular phase in women with endometriosis and disruption of the targeted transport towards the ipsilateral tube seen in the late follicular phase in nonaffected controls. Adapted from Leyendecker *et al.*[13]

to exit the uterine cavity through all possible openings (including retrograde bleeding through the tubes). Hence, according to this hypothesis, it is the loss of the proper antegrade pattern of UC at the time of menses (rather than its outright reversal) that ultimately leads through various patterns of chaotic uterine contractility to an increase in retrograde bleeding. Ultimately, retrograde bleeding will be one of the factors fueling the development of endometriotic implants through direct seeding of endometrial tissue in the pelvic cavity and activation of chronic inflammation.

Reports of women undergoing peritoneal dialysis at the time of menses provided the first hard-line evidence underscoring that most, if not all, women encounter some degree of retrograde bleeding, at least some of the time.[11] Other reports assessed the amount of endometrial debris present in the pelvic cavity just after menses.[12] The latter studies showed that women with endometriosis had more endometrial debris recovered in the pelvis that displayed stronger disposition to grow in culture than did that obtained from controls unaffected by endometriosis.[12] Studies discussed in further detail in later sections of this article looked at the vagina-to-uterus transport of macroalbumin aggregates (MAA) labeled with Tc-99 placed in the vaginal fornix.[13,14] In the early follicular phase, Leyendecker's team (FIG. 2) found more extensive retrograde transport towards the uterus and tubes of Tc-99 MAA placed in the vaginal fornix in women with documented endometriosis than did unaffected controls.[13]

CONTRACTILITY DURING THE LATE FOLLICULAR PHASE

Physiology

Irrespective of the method used, investigators in the field nearly unanimously described an increase in UC frequency at or near the time of ovulation.[1,3,15–17] A consensus also exists for identifying E_2 as the primary utero-stimulant in the menstrual cycle. Hence, logically, it is the increase in E_2 levels occurring in the late follicular phase that has been seen as the primary triggering stimulus for the preovulatory increase in UC frequency. Just prior to ovulation, mean UC frequency peaks at approximately 4–5 UC/min.

Characteristically, however, despite the relatively high UC frequency (up to 5 UC/min), these are notoriously painless during the late follicular phase. By and large, ultrasound-based data have all tended to confirm older electrophysiologic studies suggesting that the subendometrial layers of the myometrium are solely involved in late follicular phase contractility.[15] Hence, late follicular UCs have sometimes been dubbed "subendometrial contractions" by investigators using UTZ-based approaches. The impression of intense displacement given by viewing UTZ scans has also led other investigators to describe late follicular phase UCs as "wavelike contractions."

As stated earlier, most investigators using either IUP- or UTZ-based approaches have concurred in describing the predominance of retrograde contractions during the late follicular phase. Because sperm has been found in the pelvic cavity within minutes of intercourse (well before it could have traveled there on "its own steam"), retrograde uterine contractility that predominates in the late follicular phase has been instrumental in the rapid transport of sperm.[14] Hence, contractility of the female tract (uterus and tubes) stands out as the primary motor that assures the rapid transport of sperm from the cervical area to the distal end of the fallopian tubes where fertilization normally takes place.

IUP-based studies have attempted to document UC direction by computing the time lag between the high points of contractions recorded in different sections of the uterus. Using triple-ended catheters, Martinez-Gaudio et al.[1] showed that retrograde displacement of IUP waves predominated during the late follicular phase. Yet, these investigators observed that the opposite (antegrade displacement towards the cervical end) also occurred occasionally. Sometimes, complete reversal of UC displacement with a switch from retrograde to antegrade propagation of the contractile wave was described in the same patient less than 10 minutes after a typical retrograde pattern had been observed.[1]

UTZ-based studies have also concurred in describing the predominance of retrograde displacement based on the subjective assessment of the direction of contractility on fast plays of UTZ images.[3,16,17] But, as stated before, interpretations of the direction of UC based on UTZ visualization have never been validated and are possibly misleading. To more precisely study the actual displacement of uterine contents under the influence of uterine contractility, Leyendecker's team adapted an existing Tc-99-based hysterosalpingo-scintigraphy (HSS) technique.[13,14] Until then, HSS had been developed to replace hysterosalpingograms (HSG). This had failed because HSS images are less reliable than conventional HSGs in anatomical studies of the fallopian tubes. Leyendecker's team should be credited, however, for expending HSSs' indications for studying the functionality of the uterotubal contractile unit rather than solely assessing its anatomical characteristics, as done with HSGs. Hence, while we think that HSSs will not replace HSGs for studying tubal patency, they definitely can play a role in studying retrograde contractility and its disorders. In their studies, Leyendecker's team showed that Tc-99-labeled MAA placed in the vaginal fornix rapidly traveled towards the uterus and the fallopian tubes (FIG. 2). According to these investogatprs, retrograde transport towards the fallopian tubes only occurred if a developing follicle >16 mm was present in the ovary. And then, retrograde transport exclusively occurred towards the tube on the side of the developing follicle.[14]

Deviating from the HSS approach, we used an x-ray–based procedure (de Ziegler et al. 2000. ASRM) for studying retrograde transport of uterine contents in the late follicular phase in cycling women and oligoanovulators primed with exogenous E_2. For this, we duplicated the clinical conditions that commonly prevail in intrauterine insemination (IUI) protocols, the basis for most treatment offered to patients diagnosed with "unexplained" infertility in whom uterine dyskinesia is most likely to occur. For this, we used an embryo transfer catheter (Frydman's catheter) and gently deposited approximately 0.5 ml of an iodine-based contrast medium (Isteropack) in the middle portion of the uterine cavity and followed its displacement either retrogradely into the tubes or antegradely back in the vagina with successive spot x-rays (1–3 images). Studying a population of infertile women whose tubes were proved patent, we observed prompt emptying of uterine contents towards the fallopian tube and the pelvic cavity in approximately 60% of women (FIG. 3). By contrast, all the x-ray medium was rapidly expelled from the uterus back into the vagina in the remaining 40% of women (FIG. 4). In 100% of women showing positive retrograde

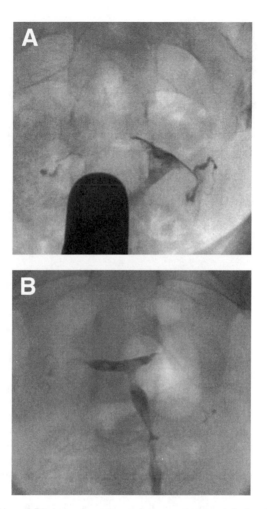

FIGURE 3. (A and B) Assessing retrograde sperm transport during the late follicular phase using a mock intrauterine insemination (IUI) technique. In the late follicular phase, intrauterine deposition of 0.5 cc of X-ray contrast medium (Isteropack) was followed by prompt expulsion of the contrast medium towards both tubes and the pelvic cavity (positive retrograde transport).

transport, this took place towards both tubes (the one facing the developing follicle and the opposite one). Hence, in sharp distinction from data reported by Leyendecker's team,[13,14] our x-ray–based studies did not show the characteristic lateralization of retrograde transport reported by these investigators when using a Tc-99 HSS approach (de Ziegler *et al.* 2000. ASRM). We postulate that the observed discrepancy with Leyendecker's data reflects differences in sensitivity between of the two investigative methods used.

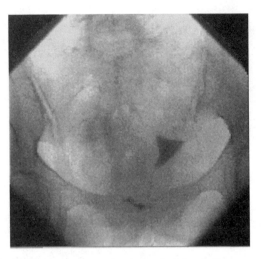

FIGURE 4. Lack of sperm transport in uterine dyskinesia. In some women, mock IUIs were not followed by expulsion of the medium towards the tubes. On the contrary, after a short retention time, the contrast medium was rapidly expelled back towards the vagina.

Pathophysiology

Using HSS, Leyendecker's group reported a characteristic disruption of the retrograde transport of Tc-99 MAA normally seen in the late follicular phase, in women with endometriosis.[13] Based on their findings, these investigators claimed that endometriosis is associated with a state of hyperkinetic dyskinesia. Furthermore, the disordered contractility that prevails in women affected by endometriosis has been postulated to also alter the proper retrograde transport of sperm that normally takes place in the late follicular phase of the menstrual cycle. Interestingly, we made concordant observations in our x-ray–based study of late follicular phase contractility. Using our mock IUI paradigm, we also found that most women with proven endometriosis failed to show proper retrograde transport of the uterine contents towards the fallopian tubes on the day of the luteinizing hormone surge. The latter finding provides a plausible explanation for the poor success of IUI treatment in endometriosis.

The proposition that endometriosis is associated with uterine dyskinesia led to the hypothesis that functional alterations of uterine contractility associated with this disease affect all the UC patterns seen during the menstrual cycle. Hence, following this line of thought, alterations in the early follicular phase pattern of contraction will affect the proper emptying of uterine contents at the time of menses with the net result being increasing retrograde bleeding. Similarly, during the late follicular phase, alterations in normal retrograde contractions will affect the rapid transport of sperm and alter fertility.[14] This hypothesis, therefore, offers new interesting views for explaining both the genesis of endometriosis (retrograde bleeding) and the infertility that accompanies even the most benign forms of this disease (mild to moderate endometriosis). To date, however, retrograde contractility has not been tested in conditions that normally accompany intercourse, that is, exposure of the uterus to the stimulating influences of prostaglandins present in semen and delivered to the vagina.

Different approaches have been contemplated for correcting uterine dyskinesia. Leyendecker's team studied the administration of the uterocontractant oxytocin in women who lacked retrograde contractility in the late follicular phase. In a small series of patients who failed to show retrograde transport of uterine contents after mock IUI, we followed a slightly different approach. In these women, we studied the effect of a beta-mimetic with uterorelaxant properties[18] on the dyskinetic alterations of late follicular phase contractility. In an uncontrolled proof-of-principle trial, five of seven women reverted to a retrograde contractile pattern after 2 months of treatment with vaginally administered beta-mimetics (from cycle day 5 to day 20). While promising, these early findings need confirmation. They suggest that uterorelaxants such as beta-mimetics may restore the physiological pattern of uterine contractility (notably during the late follicular phase) and consequently improve fecundity in women with uterine dyskinesia.

CONCLUSION

Two drastically distinct patterns characterize uterine contractility during the early and late follicular phases. In the early follicular phase, that is, menses, contractions involving all the layers of the myometrium are typically felt by women and sometimes even become frankly painful. Disruption of the physiological process is seen in conditions such as dysmenorrhea and endometriosis, when hyperkinetic alterations of uterine contractions (dyskinesia) induce painful uterine cramps and/or enhance retrograde bleeding. In the late follicular phase, subendometrial peristaltic waves that are never perceived by women are instrumental in the retrograde transport of sperm towards the fallopian tubes, where fertilization takes place. Dyskinetic alteration of this latter process with or without clinical evidence of endometriosis is likely to play a role in at least a fraction of cases of so-called "unexplained" infertility. Improvements in our understanding of the dyskinetic alterations encountered in endometriosis, dysmenorrhea, and infertility may lead to the development of specific therapies, notably, the use of local (intravaginal) application of uterorelaxants in restoring normal contractility.

REFERENCES

1. MARTINEZ-GAUDIO, M., T. YOSHIDA & L.P. BENGTSSON. 1973. Propagated and nonpropagated myometrial contractions in menstrual cycles. Am. J. Obstet. Gynecol. **115:** 107–111.
2. DE VRIES, K., E.A. LYONS, G. BALLARD, *et al.* 1990. Contractions of the inner third of the myometrium. Am. J. Obstet. Gynecol. **162:** 679–682.
3. ABRAMOWICZ, J.S. & D.F. ARCHER. 1990. Uterine endometrial peristalsis: a transvaginal ultrasound study. Fertil. Steril. **54:** 451–454.
4. IJLAND, M.M., J.L.H. EVERS, G.A.J. DUNSELMAN, *et al.* 1997. Relation between endometrial wavelike activity and fecundability in spontaneous cycles. Fertil. Steril. **67:** 492–496.

5. WOODBURY, R.A., R. TORPIN, G.P. CHILD, et al. 1947. Myometrial physiology and its relation to pelvic pain. JAMA **134:** 1081–1085.
6. STRÖMBERG, P., M. ÅKERLUND, M.I. FORSLING, et al. 1984. Vasopressin and prostaglandins in premenstrual pain and primary dysmenorrhea. Acta Obstet. Gynecol. Scand. **63:** 533–538.
7. SAMPSON, J.A. & N.Y. ALBANY. 1927. Peritoneal endometriosis due to menstrual dissemination of endometrial tissue into the peritoneal cavity. Am. J. Obstet. Gynecol. **14:** 422–469.
8. SALAMANCA, A. & E. BELTRAN. 1995. Subendometrial contractility in menstrual phase visualized by transvaginal sonography in patients with endometriosis. Fertil. Steril. **64:** 193–195.
9. JAMIESON, D.J. & J.F. STEEGE. 1996. The prevalence of dysmenorrhea, dyspareunia, pelvic pain, and irritable bowel syndrome in promary care practices. Obstet. Gynecol. **87:** 55–58.
10. SANFILIPPO, J.S., N.G. WAKIM, K.N. SCHIKLER & M.A. YUSSMAN. 1986. Endometriosis in association with uterine anomaly. Am. J. Obstet. Gynecol. **154:** 39–43.
11. HALME, J., M.G. HAMMOND, J.F. HULKA, et al. 1984. Retrograde menstruation in healthy women and in patients with endometriosis. J. Am. Coll. Obstet. Gynecol. **64:** 151–154.
12. BULLETTI, C., S. ROSSI, A. ALBONETTI, et al. 1996. Uterine contractility in patients with endometriosis. J. Am. Assoc. Gynecol. Laparoscopists **3:** S5.
13. LEYENDECKER, G., G. KUNZ, L. WILDT, et al. 1996. Uterine hyperperistalsis and dysperistalsis as dysfunctions of the mechanism of rapid sperm transport in patients with endometriosis and infertility. Hum. Reprod. **11:** 1542–1551.
14. KUNZ, G., D. BEIL, H. DEININGER, et al. 1996. The dynamics of rapid sperm transport through the female genital tract: evidence from vaginal sonography of uterine peristaltis and hysterosalpingoscintigraphy. Hum. Reprod. **11:** 627–632.
15. LYONS, E.A., P.J. TAYLOR, X.H. ZHENG, et al. 1991. Characterization of subendometrial myometrial contractions throughout the menstrual cycle in normal fertile women. Fertil. Steril. **55:** 771–774.
16. IJLAND, M.M., J.L.H. EVERS, G.A.J. DUNSELMAN, et al. 1996. Endometrial wavelike movements during the menstrual cycle. Fertil. Steril. **65:** 746–749.
17. CHALUBINSKI, K., J. DEUTINGER & G. BERNASCHEK. 1993. Vaginosonography for recording of cycle–related myometrial contractions. Fertil. Steril. **59:** 225–228.
18. ÅKERLUND, M. & K.-E. ANDERSSON. 1976. Effects of terbutaline on human myometrial activity and endometrial blood flow. Obstet. Gynecol. **47:** 529–535.

Assessing Uterine Receptivity in 2001

Ultrasonographic Glances at the New Millennium

RENATO FANCHIN

Department of Obstetrics and Gynecology and Reproductive Medicine, Hôpital Antoine Béclère, 92141, Clamart, France

ABSTRACT: The understanding and control of embryo implantation represents the major challenge for assisted reproductive technologies. Along with developments in basic research and efforts to optimize embryo quality, the improvement of noninvasive and reliable methods to assess uterine receptivity constitutes an important step toward meeting such a challenge. Today, ultrasound-based approaches to evaluate endometrial echogenicity and uterine perfusion and contractility are available for practical use. Increasing evidence indicates that echogenic patterns of the endometrium reflect histologic processes that are involved in the establishment of receptivity. This constitutes a possible explanation for the reported association between premature hyperechogenic patterns of the endometrium and poor implantation rates. Nevertheless, additional studies aiming at correlating further morpho-biochemical events in the endometrium with its echogenicity patterns are needed. Further, developments in vascular assessment by Doppler, Doppler-related, and vascular detection technologies will also be instrumental in monitoring and improving vascular changes that lead to uterine receptivity. Finally, data supporting the hypothesis that uterine contractility, as visualized by ultrasound, influences *in vitro* fertilization–embryo transfer (IVF-ET) pregnancy rates encourage further investigation on both the regulation and control of uterine contractions. This article discusses some of the advantages and limitations of ultrasonographic assessments of uterine receptivity in the perspective of the new millennium.

KEYWORDS: uterine receptivity; ultrasound; endometrium; uterine contractions; Doppler; *in vitro* fertilization

INTRODUCTION

Unfortunately, the feeling of surprise and disappointment caused in the early 1980s by the observation that 80–85% of noncavitating embryos transferred fail to implant still perseveres in the new millennium. In 2001, the main barrier limiting *in vitro* fertilization and embryo transfer (IVF-ET) results still is embryo implantation. Both the understanding of mechanisms involved in this process and the possibility of anticipating and treating its disorders represent fundamental steps in the improvement of IVF-ET outcome.

Address for correspondence: Renato Fanchin, Department of Obstetrics and Gynecology and Reproductive Endocrinology, Hôpital Antoine Béclère, 157, rue de la Porte de Trivaux, 92141, Clamart, France. Voice: (0033 1) 45374053; fax: (0033 1) 45374980.
renato.fanchin@abc.ap-hop-paris.fr

Governed by multiple interactive events, embryo implantation depends schematically on the quality of embryos and the status of uterine receptivity. During the last two decades, several developments in controlled ovarian hyperstimulation (COH), fertilization, and embryo culture techniques have led to an optimization in the number and quality of embryos available for ET. In contrast, uterine receptivity has failed to benefit from parallel improvements, and its disarrangement is likely to represent an important cause of the suboptimal embryo implantation rates observed in IVF-ET.

UTERINE RECEPTIVITY: WHEN AND HOW

Extensive and often successful research efforts have been made to determine when the uterus becomes receptive to the embryo and what are the decisive factors that are involved in this intricate process. The early concept that the endometrium is optimally receptive to implantation only during a defined period[1,2] seems also to be valid in humans.[3,4] Although the exact time frame of the so-called "implantation window" still is fuzzy, it is well accepted that it encompasses the fifth to the seventh days after ovulation and is surrounded by a refractory endometrial status.[3-6] The period of maximal endometrial receptivity is marked by a wealth of coordinated morphological and biochemical events. Morphological changes include characteristic histologic transformations, such as reduced mitotic activity, glandular secretion, and stromal edema,[7] that are often accompanied by the presence of globular protrusions in the surface membrane of epithelial cells, named pinopodes.[1,2,8] In addition, other modifications on the surface membrane of epithelial cells may occur, possibly including thinning of the glycocalix layer as demonstrated in several animal species.[9,10] Concurrent changes occur in cell-to-cell and cell-to-extracellular matrix binding that are orchestrated by cyclic variations in the expression of adhesion molecules such as cadherins[11] and integrins.[12] Similarly, cytokines[13] such as the leukemia inhibitory factor (LIF),[14] some interleukins, tumor necrosis factor (TNF)-α, growth factors, and interferon seem to play specific autocrine, paracrine, and juxtacrine roles in the establishment of the receptive status of the endometrium. Further, part of these morphologic and biochemical mechanisms may be significantly influenced by the presence of the implanting embryo in the uterine cavity.[15]

UTERINE RECEPTIVITY: PRACTICAL DILEMMAS

The relatively minimal clinical translation of the bulk of this basic scientific knowledge may be explained by several factors. First, despite the physiologic importance of the events cited above, in humans, control of endometrial receptivity seems not to be as stringent as in some other species, and implantation can occur under a wide range of morphological and biochemical conditions.[16] The implication of this is that no factor considered independently plays a determining role in the establishment of endometrial receptivity. Therefore, in an effort to assess the receptivity status of the endometrium, all of these factors should be investigated simultaneously, which is impractical for clinical purposes. Also, the embryo–uterus dialogue that takes part in the implantation process may further encumber the practical value of preimplantation endometrial measurements.[15]

Second, tissue sampling, which is often required for the direct assessment of markers of uterine receptivity, is inherently impossible in actual ET cycles. Given that the complex morphological, endocrine, and paracrine–autocrine interactions may undergo intercycle and interindividual variations, it is difficult to extrapolate information obtained from experimental cycles.

Finally, it is noteworthy that nearly all the morphologic and biochemical mechanisms that the uterus undergoes during its acquisition of receptivity are directly or indirectly regulated by ovarian hormones.[17] Indeed, in IVF-ET with egg donation, sequential administration of physiologic doses of E_2 and progesterone to women deprived of ovarian function has been shown to successfully restore endometrial receptivity and authorize the establishment of viable pregnancies.[3,4,18,19] In a recent series, blastocysts being transferred to egg donation candidates led to embryo implantation and pregnancy rates as high as 66% and 88%, respectively.[19] This indicates that the endometrium can be highly receptive as the exclusive result of physiologic hormonal replacement. Further, the outstanding pregnancy rates reported,[19] which may be explained by optimum embryo and endometrial conditions, clearly surpass those commonly observed in conventional IVF-ET. A plausible explanation for the poorer outcome of conventional IVF-ET compared to egg donation is the possible adverse effect of COH used for conventional IVF-ET on the endometrium.[18,20] In COH, administration of exogenous gonadotropins may exert, directly[21] or through its supraphysiologic effects in ovarian hormones,[18,20–24] unsuitable consequences on the endometrium, probably in proportion to the doses administered and the magnitude of the ovarian response.[22,23,25]

UTERINE RECEPTIVITY: ASSESSING IT TODAY (AND NONINVASIVELY)

These dilemmas have led numerous investigators to focus on noninvasive prognostic factors of uterine receptivity in actual ET cycles. Indeed, classical morphologic assessment of endometrial maturation provided by histologic dating,[7] which has long been regarded the "gold standard" in the evaluation of uterine receptivity, as well as the research of subtler morphobiochemical markers of the receptive uterine status,[26] are impractical in real IVF-ET cycles, owing to the reasons listed above. Hence, as an alternative to endometrial biopsies, high-resolution transvaginal ultrasonography makes it possible to monitor, noninvasively and in the definitive treatment cycle, some of the important events involved in the endometrial preparation to embryo implantation.

Along with the identification of morphologic abnormalities of the endometrium and myometrium, transvaginal ultrasonography provides information on at least three distinct levels that have been recognized as influencing uterine receptivity: endometrial echogenicity, uterine vascular network, and uterine contractility.

A New Look at Endometrial Echogenicity

Many publications have indicated that high-resolution transvaginal ultrasonography makes it possible to monitor, noninvasively, histologic changes in the endometrium through the analysis of endometrial echogenicity.[27–32] Endometrial echogenicity displays cyclic changes during the menstrual cycle. During the follicular phase, the endometrium is hypoechogenic as compared with the surrounding myometrium. After ovulation, endometrial echogenicity increases progressively, with hyperechogenic changes developing from the base toward the surface of the endometrium,[32] probably as a result of rising progesterone levels.[33]

Measurements of endometrial echogenicity performed during the late follicular phase of COH have long been tested as potential prognostic indicators of embryo implantation. However, reports have drawn disparate conclusions. Some investigators have ascertained that endometrial echogenic patterns in the late follicular phase predict IVF-ET outcome.[34–39] Others, on the contrary, have failed to find a relationship between endometrial echogenicity and implantation rates.[40,41] This controversy may be explained by operator-dependent variability, the use of arbitrary and heterogeneous classifications, and the lack of control for confounding factors, such as poor embryo quality and uterine cavity abnormalities, that influence the analysis of results.

Recently, this led us to examine a selected subset of IVF-ET patients to clarify whether endometrial echogenicity on the day of hCG administration might reflect endometrial receptivity.[42] In that study, to overcome possible subjectivity of ultrasound measurements, endometrial echogenicity was assessed objectively using a computer-assisted module for the analysis of ultrasound images. Briefly, 228 consecutive COH cycles undertaken in 221 IVF-ET candidates using similar COH protocols were studied. To limit the possibility of confounding factors in the analysis of our results, we selected only women aged <38 years, whose uteri were morphologically normal, as confirmed by hysteroscopy and ultrasound, and who had at least two good-quality embryos available for ET. Women whose uterine position did not allow adequate visualization of endometrial texture in transvaginal ultrasonography were not included.

Controlled ovarian hyperstimulation was performed by using time-release gonadotropin releasing-hormone (GnRH) agonist and recombinant follicle-stimulating hormone (FSH). On the day of hCG administration, women underwent ultrasound scans of a sagittal plane of the uterus using a 7.5-MHz transvaginal probe (Siemens Elegra, Siemens, Paris, France) at approximately 11:00 A.M. by the same operator. Ultrasound settings (in particular, gain and scan depth) were adjusted for optimal results. By design, the endometrium could be visualized in all scans. To improve consistency, our measurements were performed during the rest interval between two uterine contractions. Images were digitized and analyzed online with the use of a computer-assisted module specifically developed for the assessment of endometrial echogenicity and thickness (IôTEC 3.1; IôDP, Paris, France).

As shown in FIGURE 1, after digitation of uterine images, our expert system performed multiple transverse cuts across representative sections of the endometrial surface. Gray-level analysis was then performed automatically in all cuts, and means of results were displayed graphically. The magnitude of the base-to-surface expansion of endometrial hyperechogenicity was calculated as the ratio of the extent of the submyometrial hyperechogenic transformation over the whole thickness of the endometrium. Endometrial borders were set arbitrarily as the outer limits of the hyperechogenic myometrium–endometrium interfaces. Endometrial thickness (truly double endometrial thickness) was calculated as the greatest distance between the outer limits of the proximal and distal endometrial interfaces. Sensitivity of endome-

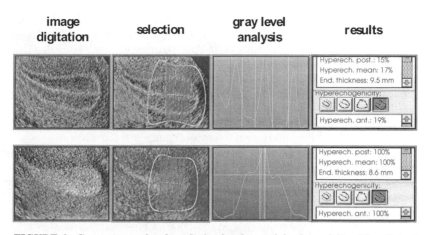

FIGURE 1. Computer-assisted analysis of endometrial echogenicity. After digitation of uterine images, multiple transverse cuts across representative sections of the endometrial surface were performed, and gray level analysis was displayed graphically. Endometrial echogenicity was calculated as the ratio of the extent of the hyperechogenic transformation over the whole thickness of the endometrium. The upper and the bottom lines of pictures represent the analysis of a hypoechogenic and hyperechogenic endometrium, respectively.

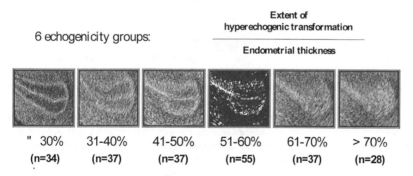

FIGURE 2. Relationship between the degreee of endometrial echogenicity and IVF-ET outcome. Cycles were sorted into six groups according to the extent of the upward hyperechogenic transformation of the endometrium.

trial echogenicity and thickness calculations was 0.01 (1%) and 0.1 mm, respectively. Intraanalysis coefficients of variation of our measurements were <5%.

As depicted in FIGURE 2, to simplify the interpretation of a possible relationship between the degree of endometrial echogenicity and IVF-ET outcome and on the basis of our previous experience, we determined six arbitrary groups according to the extent of hyperechogenic transformations of the endometrium, which over the whole endometrial thickness was <30% ($n = 34$), 31–40% ($n = 37$), 41–50% ($n = 37$), 51–60% ($n = 55$), 61–70% ($n = 37$), or >70% ($n = 28$).

The results of this investigation showed that all echogenicity groups were similar in regard to age of patients, indications for IVF-ET, ovarian reserve assessment (cycle day 3 FSH and E_2 levels), number of 75 IU-FSH ampules administered, duration of COH, plasma E_2 and P levels on the day of hCG administration, number of mature oocytes retrieved, and number of available and transferred embryos. Endometrial thickness was comparable in all six echogenicity groups at 10.2 ± 0.3 mm (range: 6.2 to 15.2 mm), 10.4 ± 0.4 mm (range: 5.1 to 15.2 mm), 9.9 ± 0.3 mm (range: 6.9 to 15.3 mm), 10.0 ± 0.3 mm (range: 5.4 to 15.7 mm), 9.4 ± 0.3 mm (range: 6.0 to 14.6 mm), and 10.2 ± 0.4 mm (range: 6.6 to 14.2 mm), respectively.

In contrast to the similarity in individual, COH, and embryology data among groups, we observed a dramatic decrease in clinical and ongoing pregnancy as well as in implantation rates from the lowest to the highest endometrial echogenicity groups (59%, 50%, 35%; 57%, 46%, 23%; 35%, 22%, 17%; 20%, 15%, 6%; 16%, 8%, 7%, and 11%, 7%, 3% respectively, in the ≤30%, 31–40%, 41–50%, 51–60%, 61–70%, and >70% echogenicity groups; $p < 0.001$). Conversely, no relationship between endometrial thickness on the day of hCG administration and IVF-ET outcome was observed.

Several characteristics concurred to single out that investigation[42] from others previously published on the same topic.[34–41] Participants have been controlled for age (<38 years), absence of uterine abnormalities, and the number and quality of embryos transferred (≥2). Women whose uterine position impaired adequate visualization of endometrial texture were excluded. The assessment of endometrial echogenicity has been performed objectively with a computer-assisted image analysis system. This has enabled us to avoid the use of arbitrary and subjective classifications and sort data accumulated from 228 IVF-ET cycles into multiple groups according to a precise degree of upward extension of hyperechogenic transformation.

These strict methodological attributes and the similarity of all echogenicity groups in regard to population, COH, and embryology characteristics allowed us to conclude that there is a relationship between the degree of endometrial hyperechogenicity on the day of hCG administration and pregnancy rates. Hence, the results of that investigation[42] confirmed and extended earlier observations that the echogenic status of the endometrium assessed in the late follicular phase predict endometrial receptivity status.[30,31,34–41]

The histologic bases for the upward extension of endometrial echogenicity remain, however, unknown. Some reports have shown that echogenicity status reflects the degree of histologic development of the endometrium.[27–29,32] Therefore, the degree of extension of hyperechogenic transformations of the endometrium observed on the day of hCG administration may denote an acceleration of secretory changes and a proportional forward slide of the period of endometrial receptivity. In the menstrual cycle, hyperechogenic endometrial features during the follicular phase are infrequent.[43] During this phase, endometrium-to-myometrium interfaces and uterine cavity appear hyperechogenic, whereas the remaining part of the endometrial thickness displays a hypoechogenic or isoechogenic signal in relation to the surrounding myometrium.[27–32] This ultrasonographic aspect may be a reflection of glandular straightness, reduced glandular secretion, and/or reduced stromal edema that characterize the proliferative endometrium, with a decreased number of interfaces to ultrasound.

During the luteal phase, a progressive base-toward-surface extension of endometrial hyperechogenicity is seen in natural cycles,[27–29] E_2–progesterone replacement cycles,[32] and COH[30,31] cycles. This probably is a result of the endometrial exposure to progesterone, although it is conceivable that additional endocrine or paracrine-autocrine mechanisms also partake in this process. We recently reported that premature exposure of the endometrium to progesterone during the follicular phase leads to a faster progression of endometrial echogenicity during the early luteal phase in COH cycles.[33] These data further support the effects of progesterone on endometrial echogenicity.

From a histologic standpoint, stromal edema has been retained as the key event responsible for hyperechogenic signals.[32] Indeed, the contact of interstitial fluid with glands and vessels walls is likely to generate echoes in the endometrium and, therefore, increase endometrial echogenicity.[32] Some arguments, however, challenge this hypothesis. In the menstrual cycle, stromal edema occurs on approximately days 21–22.[7] It is, therefore, a relatively late feature in the timed cascade of the histologic transformations of the endometrium. Even the unbalanced hormonal milieu induced by COH and its putative consequences on the endometrium are probably insufficient to boost endometrial secretory transformations to such a degree. Indeed, the study reported above[42] indicated a remarkable advance of hyperechogenic transformation in a large fraction of women, often surpassing 50% of the endometrium on the day of hCG administration. Therefore, other histologic events, such as glandular coiling (day 16 onward) and/or secretion (day 17 onward), may contribute to increasing endometrial echogenicity. As a result of endometrial exposure to supraphysiologic progesterone levels during the follicular phase of COH,[23,25,33] these early postovulatory histologic features may theoretically occur prematurely, on the day of hCG administration. However, the lack of correlation between circulating progesterone levels and endometrial echogenicity values, observed in previous investigations[36,43] and confirmed by our own results,[42] is inconsistent with this hypothesis. Direct effects on the endometrium of other hormones, such as androgens[22,24] or exogenous gonadotropins,[21] constitute alternative mechanisms to explain the premature increase in endometrial echogenicity during the late follicular phase of COH. This latter point requires, however, further examination.

We observed a progressive decrease in pregnancy and implantation rates with the extension of endometrial echogenicity on the day of hCG administration. The perception of this gradual phenomenon was possible because of the optimal sensitivity and precision of our measurements. Indeed, the strength of the correlation between endometrial texture patterns, histologic findings, and IVF-ET outcome is susceptible to variance according to subjective evaluation of scans[25] and the use of arbitrary classifications.[31,34,35,39] The computer-assisted image analysis module employed in this study was developed specifically for the assessment of the degree of hyperechogenic transformation of the endometrium and improved both the reliability and objectivity of our calculations.

Another computer-assisted analysis of the endometrium was reported by Leibovitz et al.[44] Their system was based on the calculation of the intensity of echogenic signals relative to the surrounding myometrium. These authors have reported a progressive and significant increase of endometrium-to-myometrium relative echogenicity coefficients during the luteal phase of spontaneous and COH cycles.[44]

The progressive fall in pregnancy rates observed[42] leads us to speculate that the greater the submyometrial hyperechogenicity, the more advanced the histologic transformations of the endometrium and, probably, the lower the endometrial receptivity. Our observation that pregnancy rates remained over 10% even in the >70% echogenicity group suggests that other factors, possibly linked to embryo quality, may compensate for the reduction in the endometrial receptivity[23] and allow ongoing pregnancies. Hence, additional investigation of unselected patients with poor-quality embryos will clarify the possibility of a more drastic decrease in implantation rates in hyperechogenic groups.

It is also noteworthy that endometrial thickness was not correlated with plasma E_2 levels on the day of hCG administration in the present analysis. Indeed, time-dependent (rather than concentration-dependent)[43] thickening of the endometrium occurs throughout the follicular phase of the menstrual cycle[43,45] as a probable consequence of the proliferative action of estrogens. The present data confirm the hypothesis that supraphysiological E_2 levels induced by COH do not accelerate either the pace or the magnitude of endometrial development[43] beyond values triggered by physiological concentrations of estrogens. Futher, tissue and/or vascular mechanisms may concur to modulate the action of estrogens on the endometrium. Indeed, the present and previously published series[27,30,31,33,34,37,38–41,43,46] showed conspicuous inter-subject variability in endometrial thickness during the late follicular phase. Incidentally, the present study failed to identify any relationship between endometrial thickness on the day of hCG administration and IVF-ET outcome.

In conclusion, the present data indicate that the more advanced the hyperechogenic transformation of the endometrium at the time of hCG administration, the lower the pregnancy and implantation rates in IVF-ET. The mechanism put forth to explain this inverse relation is an alteration of the endometrial receptivity, which presumably results from hastened secretory transformations of the endometrium. It is possible that the low pregnancy rates observed in the hyperechogenic groups in this selected series may decrease even further in older women with poor-quality embryos. In these cases, cycle cancellation or delaying ET by cryopreserving embryos may be judicious alternatives. Antiprogestin administration[47] in the late follicular phase of COH to reduce the possible progesterone-induced acceleration of endometrial hyperechogenicity may constitute an attractive measure to restore endometrial receptivity. These issues deserve further investigation.

Assessing Uterine Perfusion

During the past 10 years, increasing evidence has supported the hypothesis that a relationship exists between uterine perfusion and receptivity to embryo implantation.[48,49] Developments in color Doppler imaging[50,51] and high-frequency transvaginal ultrasound probes have made it possible to both visualize and assess[53] uterine blood vessels. These novel techniques allowed the monitoring of physiologic modifications in the uterine perfusion occurring during the menstrual cycle.[54–60] Indeed, most of the vascular adaptations of the uterus are modulated by ovarian hormones. In the proliferative phase of spontaneous[54,56] and E_2–progesterone replacement cycles,[61,62] E_2 affects uterine perfusion with a reduction in vascular resistance of uterine arteries; incidentally, this reduction seems to be larger in the artery ipsilateral to the dominant follicle.[54,58] After ovulation, presumably in response to progesterone, a further decrease in vascular impedance is observed that is maximal at the midluteal phase, during the periimplantation phase.[55,56,59] These vascular changes are likely to participate in the embryo implantation process. It is noteworthy that the uterus seems to be a privileged target for these cyclic vascular adaptations,[60] which also involve possible additional vasoactive processes including neuronal factors, prostaglandins,[60] and L-arginine–nitric oxide pathways.[63]

Spurred not only by these ovarian-driven periodic changes in uterine perfusion, but also by the improvement in technologies for vascular assessment and the putative noninvasive characteristics of ultrasound, numerous investigators became interested in studying uterine vascularization in search of predictors of uterine receptivity. Most of them have focused preferentially on uterine artery blood flow measurements,[64–71] since these vessels could be easily recognized and studied. For quantitative purposes, the pulsatility index (PI) became widely used because of its accurate reflection of blood flow impedance and because it may be used when the end diastolic frequency shift is absent or reversed.[72] More recently, smaller uterine vessels situated, in particular, in the myometrium and the endometrium have been studied by using color Doppler[73] or power Doppler[74,75] technologies in both two-dimensional and three-dimensional[76] analyses.

Most of uterine artery Doppler studies,[49,64–67,70,71] but not all,[68,75] have associated increased uterine impedance with lower pregnancy rates in IVF-ET. In these trials, Doppler measurements were usually performed on the day of hCG administration,[65,70] oocyte retrieval,[49] or ET,[64,67,71] with comparable predictive values.[76] Pulsatility index cut-off values for prognosticating poor endometrial receptivity ranged from 2.5[67] to 3.3.[65,71] In search of physiopathologic bases for the relation between PIs and IVF-ET outcome, some investigators have assessed morphological and immunocytochemical markers of endometrial receptivity. Significant correlation between uterine artery PI values and PP14,[78] E_2 receptors, and endometrial histology[69] was observed.

Both the accurate mapping of smaller blood vessels directly supplying the endometrium and the study of their possible influence on endometrial receptivity have been greatly improved by the development of power-Doppler technology.[79] In contrast to color Doppler, power Doppler can detect slow and opposite blood flows in tiny vessels with reduced dependency on the beam–vessel angle. Three recent studies have addressed the possible relation between endometrial vascularization assessed by power Doppler and IVF-ET outcome[74–76] with different methods. With the use of power Doppler, Yuval et al.[74] quantified intra- and subendometrial blood flow using three different blood flow indexes. These authors failed to find any relation between index values and the outcome of IVF-ET. In contrast, Yang et al.,[75] undertaking a qualitative assessment of intra-endometrial vascularization, identified a critical endometrial surface (5 mm^2) under which endometrial receptivity might be hampered. To overcome some limitations of previous studies, particularly those due to the arbitrary selection of a single uterine plane to perform the analysis of endometrial vascularization, Schild et al.[76] used three-dimensional power Doppler assessment. These investigators concluded that spiral artery blood flow is a useful predictor of IVF-ET results.

In conclusion, the measurement of uterine perfusion status by Doppler remains an instrumental approach in the assessment of uterine receptivity. Unfortunately, its accuracy depends on a number of factors such as subjectivity, ultrasound apparatus, and tissue impedance. Future improvements of noninvasive vascular assessment technologies will possibly refine the predictive value of uterine perfusion on uterine receptivity and extend our comprehension of the vascular processes implicated in the uterine preparation for embryo implantation. Also, in an effort to optimize uterine receptivity, measures to improve uterine vascularization have been proposed, such as L-arginine administration[63] or sildenafil (Viagra®).[80] Nevertheless, larger studies remain necessary to confirm their effectiveness.

"uterine-contractility.com":
BEFORE CONTACTING THE IMPLANTATION SITE

The nonpregnant uterus shows constant contractile activity that is, in part, regulated by ovarian hormones and that undergoes periodic changes throughout the menstrual cycle. Uterine contraction frequency progressively increases during the follicular phase, to peak at nearly four to five contractions per minute in the late follicular phase, probably in response to the utero-stimulating effects of estradiol. During the luteal phase, however, uterine contraction frequency decreases sharply to reach a nearly quiescent status, presumably as a result of the utero-relaxing effects of progesterone. All indicate that the high uterine contraction frequency observed in the late follicular phase assists the sperm ascension toward the distal end of the Fallopian tubes where fertilization takes place. Conversely, the utero-quiescence observed in the mid-luteal phase may assist the proper positioning of the embryo[81] in the middle section of the uterine cavity and help embryo implantation.

Assessment of Uterine Contractility

Traditionally, uterine contractility has been assessed by measuring changes in intrauterine pressure,[82–84] an approach that has remained the reference for detecting uterine contractions. For this, pressure probes introduced into the uterine cavity provide information on uterine contraction duration, amplitude, and frequency. The invasiveness of intrauterine pressure measurements has, however, greatly limited the possibility of conducting clinical studies, notably in assisted reproduction. Recently, an alternative method for assessing uterine contractions in nonpregnant women has emerged from studying the uterus with ultrasound. The development of high-resolution, vaginal ultrasound probes has enabled the direct visualization of the contractile activity of the uterus, which can be recorded and studied in real-time motion.[85,86] Today, the ultrasound method has been proven to offer reliable information on uterine contraction frequency and benefits from being totally noninvasive. The "fast play" method, using VHS tapes or digitized sequences, improves visualization of uterine contractions, allowing the quantification of uterine contraction frequency. In an attempt to improve the reliability of uterine contraction measurements, we developed an original approach based on using 3D reconstruction software.[87,88]

As represented in FIGURE 3, we used commercially available 3D reconstruction software for generating time-mode (TM) graphs. For this, instead of swapping the ultrasound probe, as for volume acquisition and 3D reconstruction, the probe was kept steady, and 2D images acquired over time at the rate of two per second, for 2

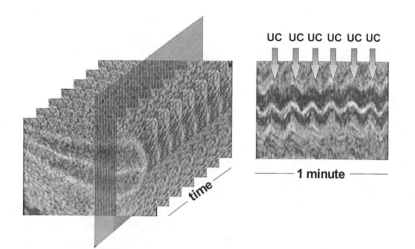

FIGURE 3. Computerized assessment of uterine contraction frequency. After images of a sagittal plane of the uterus were acquired over time at a rate of two images/sec (*left panel*), time-dependent changes in myometrial–endometrial interfaces that correspond to uterine contractions (UC) were assessed (*right panel*). Each vertical arrow indicates one UC.

minutes. Hence, in the electronic matrix acquired, the "z" axis, instead of being the third dimension of volume, became time. This method allowed us to generate time mode or TM graphs anywhere from the fundus to the cervical end of the uterus. On TM graphs, uterine contractions are identified as vertical displacements of the myometrial–endometrial interface and of the uterine cavity line and appear like waves. Using the 3D-derived method, we investigated the possible relationship between uterine contractions at the time of ETs and IVF-ET outcome and the influence on uterine contractility of supraphysiological ovarian hormone levels resulting from controlled ovarian hyperstimulation.

Uterine Contractility and IVF-ET Outcome

In a first study[87] we looked at the uterine contraction frequency at the time of ET and its possible detrimental effect on IVF-ET outcome. We studied 209 women undergoing 220 IVF-ET cycles with controlled ovarian hyperstimulation. To limit the interference of confounding variables affecting embryo quality and/or uterine receptivity, we only selected patients who were under 39 years of age, whose uterus was normal, and who had at least three good-quality embryos available for transfer. For uterine contraction assessment, just before ET all patients underwent transvaginal ultrasound scans and measurement of uterine contraction frequency with the 3D-derived system. In this early study, women who displayed >5.0 contractions per minute had markedly lower implantation and pregnancy rates per ET (4% and 14%, respectively) than those who had ≤3.0 contractions per minute (21% and 53%, respectively), probably by reason of the mechanical expulsion of embryos from the uterine cavity. In addition, the overall mean uterine contraction frequency observed during the early luteal phase of controlled ovarian hyperstimulation (4.3 contractions/min on the day of ET) appeared higher than that measured during the corresponding phase of the menstrual cycle (2.5–3.0 contractions/min).[85,86]

Hormone Regulation of Uterine Contractility

On the basis of these results, we questioned whether IVF-ET patients might have an overall increase in uterine contraction frequency as a result of the high estradiol levels brought about by controlled ovarian hyperstimulation or whether the hormonal changes induced a resistance to the relaxing effects of progesterone. To answer this question, we designed another study[88] on hormonal influence on uterine contractility during COH cycles. Uterine contractility was studied in 59 women undergoing 59 IVF-ET cycles with measurements conducted both on the days of hCG administration and ET. Serum estradiol and progesterone levels were also measured on these two days. We observed that, despite the very high estradiol levels achieved at the end of controlled ovarian hyperstimulation, overall uterine contraction frequency remained at menstrual cycle levels (4.6 uterine contractions/min) on the day of hCG administration. Hence, the supraphysiological levels of estradiol characteristic of IVF-ET do not further stimulate uterine contraction frequency beyond menstrual cycle values. But, uterine contraction frequency remained nearly unchanged on the day of ET, not showing the prompt decrease seen in the menstrual cycle after ovulation.

We also investigated a possible correlation between uterine contraction frequency at the time of ET and ovarian hormones. There was no correlation between ovarian hormones on the day of hCG and uterine contraction frequency. On the day of ET, estradiol levels did not correlate with uterine contraction frequency, but a strong negative correlation existed with progesterone levels. Because of the negative relationship between progesterone and uterine contraction frequency, we divided data into two groups according to whether progesterone levels on the day of ET exceeded 100 ng/ml or not. In the low-progesterone group, uterine contraction frequency remained unchanged from findings made on the day of hCG administration. On the contrary, women whose progesterone was high experienced a sharp decrease in uterine contraction frequency on the day of ET. We believe this is a direct consequence of the high estradiol levels encountered in IVF-ET. We formulated the hypothesis that further increasing the exposure of the uterus to progesterone will overcome the resistance and produce the needed utero-relaxation. Hence, we investigated the effects of vaginal progesterone administration to relax the uterus at the time of ET.

Effects of Vaginal Progesterone Administration on
Uterine Contractility

It has now been amply documented that vaginal progesterone administration provides direct access for progesterone to the uterus, which leads to a high uterine tissue concentration of progesterone. Therefore, vaginal progesterone administration started before ET could be effective in restoring utero-relaxation at the time of ET and may improve embryo implantation. To address this issue, we studied 84 IVF-ET candidates undergoing 84 controlled ovarian hyperstimulation cycles.[89] Luteal support with a vaginal progesterone gel was randomly started either just before oocyte retrieval or at the evening of ET in the control group. Uterine contractility was studied on the day of hCG administration and just before ET, using the ultrasound 3D-derived system. Serum estradiol and progesterone levels were also measured. Similar patient characteristics were observed in women who started progesterone supplementation on the day of oocyte retrieval or ET, with regard to age, indication for IVF-ET, and ovarian reserve data. Data on controlled ovarian hyperstimulation and embryology were also similar for both groups. As expected, serum estradiol levels fell from the day of hCG administration until ET in both groups. After hCG administration, progesterone levels increased progressively in both groups but reached levels slightly higher in women who started progesterone supplementation on the day of oocyte retrieval. Uterine contraction frequency declined significantly at the time of ET in the group receiving luteal support with early vaginal progesterone, starting on the day of oocyte retrieval. On the contrary, uterine contraction frequency remained practically unchanged in the untreated group who started luteal support only after the ET. In support of our prior observation of the negative effect of uterine contractility on IVF outcome, we observed a trend for higher pregnancy and implantation rates in women who started luteal support with early vaginal progesterone.

Uterine Contractility on the Day of Blastocyst Transfers

Another issue remaining to be investigated was the possible reduction in uterine contractility on the day of blastocyst transfers, 7 days after hCG administration in controlled ovarian hyperstimulation for IVF-ET.[90] This could provide an additional explanation for the high implantation rates reported with blastocysts.[91] For this, we studied 43 infertile women undergoing 43 GnRH-a and FSH/hCG cycles for IVF-ET. On the day of hCG administration, on the day of noncavitating ET (hCG + 4), and on the day of blastocyst transfers (hCG + 7), 2-min sagittal uterine scans were obtained with a 7.5-MHz vaginal ultrasound probe; and uterine contraction frequency was assessed according to a method similar to that previously described. The results of that investigation showed a slight, yet significant decrease in UC frequency from the day of hCG (4.4 ± 0.2 contractions/min) to hCG + 4 (3.5 ± 0.2 contractions/min). A remarkable additional decrease occurred on hCG + 7 (1.5 ± 0.2 contractions/min). We concluded that, on the day of blastocyst transfers, UC frequency is reduced to a nearly quiescent status, and these favorable conditions might assist blastocyst implantation.

IN CONCLUSION

The improvement of noninvasive and reliable methods to assess endometrial receptivity constitutes an important challenge for the new millennium. Today, ultrasound-based approaches that evaluate endometrial echogenicity, uterine perfusion, and contractility are available for practical use. Increasing evidence indicates that echogenic patterns of the endometrium reflect histologic features that are involved in establishing receptivity. This constitutes a possible explanation for the reported association between premature hyperechogenic patterns and poor implantation rates. Other studies aiming at correlating additional morpho-biochemical events in the endometrium with its echogenicity patterns remain needed, however. Further, developments in vascular assessment by Doppler or related technologies will also be instrumental in monitoring and improving vascular changes that lead to endometrial receptivity. Finally, data supporting the hypothesis that uterine contractility, as visualized by ultrasound, influences IVF-ET pregnancy rates should encourage further investigation on regulation and control of uterine contractions. Undoubtedly, the improvement of existing tools and the development of new noninvasive techniques are fundamental steps toward the adequate assessment and control of human uterine receptivity.

REFERENCES

1. PSYCHOYOS, A. 1973. Hormonal control of ovoimplantation. Vitam. Horm. **31:** 201–256.
2. PSYCHOYOS, A. 1976. Hormonal control of uterine receptivity for nidation. J. Reprod. Fertil. Suppl. **25:** 17–28.
3. ROSENWAKS, Z. 1987. Donor eggs: their application in modern reproductive technologies. Fertil. Steril. **47:** 895–909.
4. NAVOT, D., N. LAUFER, J. KOPOLOVIC, et al. 1986. Artificially induced endometrial cycles and establishment of pregnancies in the absence of ovaries. N. Engl. J. Med. **314:** 806–811.
5. PSYCHOYOS, A. 1993. Uterine receptivity for egg-implantation and scanning electron microscopy. Acta Eur. Fertil. **24:** 41–42.
6. TABIBZADEH, S. & A. BABAKNIA. 1995. The signals and molecular pathways involved in implantation, a symbiotic interaction between blastocyst and endometrium involving adhesion and tissue invasion. Hum. Reprod. **10:** 1579–1602.
7. NOYES, R.W., A.T. HERTIG & J. ROCK. 1950. Dating the endometrial biopsy. Fertil. Steril. **1:** 3–25.
8. NIKAS, G., A. MAKRIGIANNAKIS, O. HOVATTA, et al. 2000. Surface morphology of the human endometrium. Basic and clinical aspects. Ann. N.Y. Acad. Sci. **900:** 316–324.
9. CHAVEZ, D.J. & T.L. ANDERSON. 1985. The glycocalyx of the mouse uterine luminal epithelium during estrus, early pregnancy, the peri-implantation period, and delayed implantation. I. Acquisition of Ricinus communis I binding sites during pregnancy. Biol. Reprod. **32:** 1135–1142.
10. ANDERSON, T.L., G.E. OLSON & L.H. HOFFMAN. 1986. Stage-specific alterations in the apical membrane glycoproteins of endometrial epithelial cells related to implantation in rabbits. Biol. Reprod. **34:** 701–720.
11. MACCALMAN, C.D., S. GETSIOS & G.T. CHEN. 1998. Type 2 cadherins in the human endometrium and placenta: their putative roles in human implantation and placentation. Am. J. Reprod. Immunol. **39:** 96–107.
12. LESSEY, B.A. & J.T. ARNOLD. 1998. Paracrine signaling in the endometrium: integrins and the establishment of uterine receptivity. J. Reprod. Immunol. **39:** 105–116.
13. SIMON, C., C. MORENO, C. REMOHI, et al. 1998. Cytokines and embryo implantation. J. Reprod. Immunol. **39:** 117–131.
14. STEWART, C.L., P. KASPAR, L.J. BRUNET, et al. 1992. Blastocyst implantation depends on maternal expression of leukaemia inhibitory factor. Nature **359:** 76–79.
15. SIMON, C., C. MORENO, J. REMOHI, et al. 1998. Molecular interactions between embryo and uterus in the adhesion phase of human implantation. Hum. Reprod. **13(Suppl. 3):** 219–232.
16. ROGERS, P.A. 1995. Current studies on human implantation: a brief overview. Reprod. Fertil. Dev. **7:** 1395–1399.
17. DE ZIEGLER, D., R. FANCHIN, B. DE MOUSTIER, et al. 1998. The hormonal control of endometrial receptivity: estrogen (E_2) and progesterone. J. Reprod. Immunol. **39:** 149–166.
18. PAULSON, R.J., M.V. SAUER & R.A. LOBO. 1990. Embryo implantation after human in vitro fertilization: importance of endometrial receptivity. Fertil. Steril. **53:** 870–874.

19. SCHOOLCRAFT, W.B. & D.K. GARDNER. 2000. Blastocyst culture and transfer increases the efficiency of oocyte donation. Fertil. Steril. **74:** 482–486.
20. CHECK, J.H., A. O'SHAUGHNESSY, D. LURIE, *et al.* 1995. Evaluation of the mechanism for higher pregnancy rates in donor oocyte recipients by comparison of fresh with frozen embryo transfer pregnancy rates in a shared oocyte programme. Hum. Reprod. **10:** 3022–3027.
21. FANCHIN, R., E. PELTIER, R. FRYDMAN & D. DE ZIEGLER. 2001. Human chorionic gonadotropin: does it affect human endometrial morphology in vivo? Semin. Reprod. Med. **19:** 31–35.
22. FANCHIN, R., C. RIGHINI, F. OLIVENNES, *et al.* 1997. Premature plasma progesterone and androgen elevation are not prevented by adrenal suppression in in vitro fertilization. Fertil. Steril. **67:** 115–119.
23. FANCHIN, R., C. RIGHINI, F. OLIVENNES, *et al.* 1997. Consequences of premature progesterone elevation on the outcome of in vitro fertilization: insights into a controversy. Fertil. Steril. **68:** 799–805.
24. FANCHIN, R., D. DE ZIEGLER, J. TAIEB, *et al.* 2000. Human chorionic gonadotropin administration does not increase plasma androgen levels in patients undergoing controlled ovarian hyperstimulation. Fertil. Steril. **73:** 275–279.
25. FANCHIN, R., D. DE ZIEGLER, V.D. CASTRACANE, *et al.* 1995. Physiopathology of premature progesterone elevation. Fertil. Steril. **64:** 796–801.
26. LESSEY, B.A., A.J. CASTELBAUM, L. WOLF, *et al.* 2000. Use of integrins to date the endometrium. Fertil. Steril. **73:** 779–787.
27. FLEISCHER, A.C., G. KALEMERIS, J.E. MACHIN, *et al.* 1986. Sonographic depiction of normal and abnormal endometrium with histopathologic correlation. J. Ultrasound Med. **5:** 445–452.
28. YOSHIMITSU, K., G. NAKAMURA & H. NAKANO. 1989. Dating sonographic endometrial images in the normal ovulatory cycle. Int. J. Gynaecol. Obstet. **28:** 33–39.
29. FORREST, T.S., M.K. ELYADERANI, M.I. MUILENBURG, *et al.* 1988. Cyclic endometrial changes: US assessment with histologic correlation. Radiology **167:** 233–237.
30. WELKER, B.G., U. GEMBRUCH, K. DIEDRICH, *et al.* 1989. Transvaginal sonography of the endometrium during ovum pickup in stimulated cycles for in vitro fertilization. J. Ultrasound Med. **8:** 549–553.
31. GONEN, Y. & R.F. CASPER. 1990. Prediction of implantation by the sonographic appearance of the endometrium during controlled ovarian stimulation for in vitro fertilization. J. In Vitro Fert. Embryo Transf. **7:** 146–152.
32. GRUNFELD, L., B. WALKER, P.A. BERGH, *et al.* 1991. High-resolution endovaginal ultrasonography of the endometrium: a noninvasive test for endometrial adequacy. Obstet. Gynecol. **78:** 200–204.
33. FANCHIN, R., C. RIGHINI, F. OLIVENNES, *et al.* 1999. Computerized assessment of endometrial echogenicity: clues to the endometrial effects of premature progesterone elevation. Fertil. Steril. **71:** 174–181.
34. UENO, J., S. OEHNINGER, R.G. BRZYSKI, *et al.* 1991. Ultrasonographic appearance of the endometrium in natural and stimulated in-vitro fertilization cycles and its correlation with outcome. Hum. Reprod. **6:** 901–904.
35. SHER, G., C. HERBERT, G. MAASSARANI, *et al.* 1991. Assessment of the late proliferative phase endometrium by ultrasonography in patients undergoing in-vitro fertilization and embryo transfer (IVF/ET). Hum. Reprod. **6:** 232–237.
36. KHALIFA, E., R.G. BRZYSKI, S. OEHNINGER, *et al.* 1992. Sonographic appearance of the endometrium: the predictive value for the outcome of in-vitro fertilization in stimulated cycles. Hum. Reprod. **7:** 677–680.
37. COHEN, B.M., L. BERRY, V. ROETHEMEYER, *et al.* 1992. Sonographic assessment of late proliferative phase during ovulation induction. J. Reprod. Med. **37:** 685–690.
38. DICKEY, R.P., T.T. OLAR, S.N. TAYLOR, *et al.* 1993. Relationship of biochemical pregnancy to pre-ovulatory endometrial thickness and pattern in patients undergoing ovulation induction. Hum. Reprod. **8:** 327–330.
39. COULAM, C.B., M. BUSTILLO, D.M. SOENKSEN, *et al.* 1994. Ultrasonographic predictors of implantation after assisted reproduction. Fertil. Steril. **62:** 1004–1010.

40. OLIVEIRA, J.B., R.L. BARUFFI, A.L. MAURI, *et al.* 1993. Endometrial ultrasonography as predictor of pregnancy in an in-vitro fertilizaton programme. Hum. Reprod. **8:** 1312–1315.

41. CHECK, J.H., K. NOWROOZI, J. CHOE, *et al.* 1993. The effect of endometrial thickness and echo pattern on in vitro fertilization outcome in donor oocyte–embryo transfer cycle. Fertil. Steril. **59:** 72–75.

42. FANCHIN, R., C. RIGHINI, J.M. AYOUBI, *et al.* 2000. New look at endometrial echogenicity: objective computer-assisted measurements predict endometrial receptivity in in vitro fertilization-embryo transfer. Fertil. Steril. **74:** 274–281.

43. BAKOS, O., O. LUNDKVIST & T. BERGH. 1993. Transvaginal sonographic evaluation of endometrial growth and texture in spontaneous ovulatory cycles—a descriptive study. Hum. Reprod. **8:** 799–806.

44. LEIBOVITZ, Z., S. DEGANI, R. RABIA, *et al.* 1998. Endometrium-to-myometrium relative echogenicity coefficient. A new sonographic approach for the quantitative assessment of endometrial echogenicity. Gynecol. Obstet. Invest. **45:** 121–125.

45. RANDALL, J.M., N.M. FISK, A. MCTAVISH, *et al.* 1989. Transvaginal ultrasonic assessment of endometrial growth in spontaneous and hyperstimulated menstrual cycles. Br. J. Obstet. Gynaecol. **96:** 954–959.

46. LI, T.C., L. NUTTALL, L. KLENTZERIS, *et al.* 1992. How well does ultrasonographic measurement of endometrial thickness predict the results of histological dating? Hum. Reprod. **7:** 1–5.

47. PAULSON, R.J., M.V. SAUER & R.A. LOBO. 1997. Potential enhancement of endometrial receptivity in cycles using controlled ovarian hyperstimulation with antiprogestins: a hypothesis. Fertil. Steril. **67:** 321–518.

48. GOSWAMY, R.K., G. WILLIAMS & P.C. STEPTOE. 1988. Decreased uterine perfusion—a cause of infertility. Hum. Reprod. **3:** 955–959.

49. STERZIK, K., D. GRAB, V. SASSE, *et al.* 1989. Doppler sonographic findings and their correlation with implantation in an in vitro fertilization program. Fertil. Steril. **52:** 825–828.

50. HATA, T., K. HATA, D. SENOH, *et al.* 1989. Transvaginal Doppler color flow mapping. Gynecol. Obstet. Invest. **27:** 217–218.

51. KURJAK, A., I. ZALUD, D. JURKOVIC, *et al.* 1989. Transvaginal color Doppler for the assessment of pelvic circulation. Acta Obstet. Gynecol. Scand. **68:** 131–135.

52. STEER, C.V., J. WILLIAMS, J. ZAIDI, *et al.* 1995. Intra-observer, interobserver, interultrasound transducer and intercycle variation in colour Doppler assessment of uterine artery impedance. Hum. Reprod. **10:** 479–481.

53. TAYLOR, K.J., P.N. BURNS, P.N. WELLS, *et al.* 1985. Ultrasound Doppler flow studies of the ovarian and uterine arteries. Br. J. Obstet. Gynaecol. **92:** 240–246.

54. GOSWAMY, R.K. & P.C. STEPTOE. 1988. Doppler ultrasound studies of the uterine artery in spontaneous ovarian cycles. Hum. Reprod. **3:** 721–726.

55. SCHOLTES, M.C., J.W. WLADIMIROFF, H.J. VAN RIJEN, *et al.* 1989. Uterine and ovarian flow velocity waveforms in the normal menstrual cycle: a transvaginal Doppler study. Fertil. Steril. **52:** 981–985.

56. STEER, C.V., S. CAMPBELL, J.S. PAMPIGLIONE, *et al.* 1990. Transvaginal colour flow imaging of the uterine arteries during the ovarian and menstrual cycles. Hum. Reprod. **5:** 391–395.

57. SANTOLAYA-FORGAS, J. 1992. Physiology of the menstrual cycle by ultrasonography. J. Ultrasound Med. **11:** 139–142.

58. TINKANEN, H., E. KUJANSUU & P. LAIPPALA. 1995. The association between hormone levels and vascular resistance in uterine and ovarian arteries in spontaneous menstrual cycles—a Doppler ultrasound study. Acta Obstet. Gynecol. Scand. **74:** 297–301.

59. TAN, S.L., J. ZAIDI, S. CAMPBELL, *et al.* 1996. Blood flow changes in the ovarian and uterine arteries during the normal menstrual cycle. Am. J. Obstet. Gynecol. **175:** 625–631.

60. ZIEGLER, W.F., I. BERNSTEIN, G. BADGER, *et al.* 1999. Regional hemodynamic adaptation during the menstrual cycle. Obstet. Gynecol. **94:** 695–699.

61. DE ZIEGLER, D., R. BESSIS & R. FRYDMAN. 1991. Vascular resistance of uterine arteries: physiological effects of estradiol and progesterone. Fertil. Steril. **55:** 775–779.

62. ACHIRON, R., D. LEVRAN, E. SIVAN, et al. 1995. Endometrial blood flow response to hormone replacement therapy in women with premature ovarian failure: a transvaginal Doppler study. Fertil. Steril. **63:** 550–554.
63. BATTAGLIA, C., M. SALVATORI, N. MAXIA, et al. 1999. Adjuvant L-arginine treatment for in-vitro fertilization in poor responder patients. Hum. Reprod. **14:** 1690–1697.
64. STEER, C.V., S. CAMPBELL, S.L. TAN, et al. 1992. The use of transvaginal color flow imaging after in vitro fertilization to identify optimum uterine conditions before embryo transfer. Fertil. Steril. **57:** 372–376.
65. COULAM, C.B., M. BUSTILLO & D.M. SOENKSEN. 1994. Ultrasonographic predictors of implantation after assisted reproduction. Fertil. Steril. **62:** 1004–1010.
66. SERAFINI, P., J. BATZOFIN, J. NELSON, et al. 1994. Sonographic uterine predictors of pregnancy in women undergoing ovulation induction for assisted reproductive treatments. Fertil. Steril. **62:** 815–822.
67. CHIEN, L.W., C.R. TZENG, S.R. CHANG, et al. 1995. The correlation of the embryo implantation rate with uterine arterial impedance in in vitro fertilization and embryo transfer. Early Pregnancy **1:** 27–32.
68. TEKAY, A., H. MARTIKAINEN & P. JOUPPILA. 1995. Blood flow changes in uterine and ovarian vasculature, and predictive value of transvaginal pulsed colour Doppler ultrasonography in an in-vitro fertilization programme. Hum. Reprod. **10:** 688–693.
69. STEER, C.V., S.L. TAN, D. DILLON, et al. 1995. Vaginal color Doppler assessment of uterine artery impedance correlates with immunohistochemical markers of endometrial receptivity required for the implantation of an embryo. Fertil. Steril. **63:** 101–108.
70. ZAIDI, J., R. PITTROF, A. SHAKER, et al. 1996. Assessment of uterine artery blood flow on the day of human chorionic gonadotropin administration by transvaginal color Doppler ultrasound in an in vitro fertilization program. Fertil. Steril. **65:** 377–381.
71. CACCIATORE, B., N. SIMBERG, P. FUSARO, et al. 1996. Transvaginal Doppler study of uterine artery blood flow in in vitro fertilization–embryo transfer cycles. Fertil. Steril. **66:** 130–134.
72. MILES, R.D., J.A. MENKE, M. BASHIRU, et al. 1987. Relationships of five Doppler measures with flow in an in vitro model and clinical findings in newborn infants. J. Ultrasound Med. **6:** 597–599.
73. ZAIDI, J., S. CAMPBELL, R. PITTROF, et al. 1995. Endometrial thickness, morphology, vascular penetration and velocimetry in predicting implantation in an in vitro fertilization program. Ultrasound Obstet. Gynecol. **6:** 191–198.
74. YUVAL, Y., S. LIPITZ, J. DOR, et al. 1999. The relationships between endometrial thickness, and blood flow and pregnancy rates in in-vitro fertilization. Hum. Reprod. **14:** 1067–1071.
75. YANG, J.H., M.Y. WU, C.D. CHEN, et al. 1999. Association of endometrial blood flow as determined by a modified colour Doppler technique with subsequent outcome of in-vitro fertilization. Hum. Reprod. **14:** 1606–1610.
76. SCHILD, R.L., S. HOLTHAUS, J. D'ALQUEN, et al. 2000. Quantitative assessment of sub-endometrial blood flow by three-dimensional ultrasound is an important predictive factor of implantation in an in-vitro fertilization programme. Hum. Reprod. **15:** 89–94.
77. COULAM, C.B., J.J. STERN, D.M. SOENKSEN, et al. 1995. Comparison of pulsatility indices on the day of oocyte retrieval and embryo transfer. Hum. Reprod. **10:** 82–84.
78. FAY, T.N., I.J. JACOBS, B. TEISNER, et al. 1990. A biochemical test for the direct assessment of endometrial function: measurement of the major secretory endometrial protein PP14 in serum during menstruation in relation to ovulation and luteal function. Hum. Reprod. **5:** 382–386.
79. WINSBERG, F. 1995. Power Doppler US. Radiology **195:** 873.
80. SHER, G. & J.D. FISCH. 2000. Vaginal sildenafil (Viagra): a preliminary report of a novel method to improve uterine artery blood flow and endometrial development in patients undergoing IVF. Hum. Reprod. **15:** 806–809.
81. PUSEY, J., W.A. KELLY, J.M. BRADSHAW, et al. 1980. Myometrial activity and the distribution of blastocysts in the uterus of the rat: interference by relaxin. Biol. Reprod. **23:** 394–397.

82. HENRY, J.S. & J.S.L. BROWNE. 1943. The contractions of the human uterus during the menstrual cycle. Am. J. Obstet. Gynecol. **45:** 927.
83. HENDRICKS, C.H. 1966. Inherent motility patterns and response characteristics of nonpregnant human uterus. Am. J. Obstet. Gynecol. **96:** 824–843.
84. MARTINEZ-GAUDIO, M., T. YOSHIDA & L.P. BENGTSSON. 1973. Propagated and nonpropagated myometrial contractions in normal menstrual cycles. Am. J. Obstet. Gynecol. **115:** 107–111.
85. ABRAMOWICZ, J.S. & D.F. ARCHER. 1990. Uterine endometrial peristalsis-a transvaginal ultrasound study. Fertil. Steril. **54:** 451–454.
86. LYONS, E.A., P.J. TAYLOR, X.H. ZHENG, et al. 1991. Characterization of subendometrial myometrial contractions throughout the menstrual cycle in normal fertile women. Fertil. Steril. **55:** 771–774.
87. FANCHIN, R., C. RIGHINI, F. OLIVENNES, et al. 1998. Uterine contractions at the time of embryo transfer alter pregnancy rates after in-vitro fertilization. Hum. Reprod. **13:** 1968–1974.
88. FANCHIN, R., J.M. AYOUBI, F. OLIVENNES, et al. 2000. Hormonal influence on the uterine contractility during controlled ovarian hyperstimulation. Hum. Reprod. **15**(Suppl. 1): 90–100.
89. FANCHIN, R., C. RIGHINI, D. DE ZIEGLER, et al. 2001. Effects of vaginal progesterone administraton on uterine contractility at the time of embryo transfer. Fertil. Steril. **75:** 1136–1140.
90. FANCHIN, R., C. RIGHINI, F. OLIVENNES, et al. 2001. Uterine contractility decreases at the time of blastocyst transfers. Hum. Reprod. **16:** 1115–1119.
91. GARDNER, D.K., P. VELLA, M. LANE, et al. 1998. Culture and transfer of human blastocysts increases implantation rates and reduces the need for multiple embryo transfers. Fertil. Steril. **69:** 84–88.

Methods and Devices for the Management of Term and Preterm Labor

R.E. GARFIELD, H. MAUL, L. SHI, W. MANER, C. FITTKOW,
G. OLSEN, AND G.R. SAADE

Reproductive Sciences, Department of Obstetrics & Gynecology, University of Texas Medical Branch, Galveston, Texas 77555-1062, USA

ABSTRACT: In this review, we outline studies showing that the uterus (myometrium) and cervix pass through a conditioning step in preparation for labor. This step is not easily identifiable with present methods designed to assess the uterus or cervix. In the uterus, this seemingly irreversible step consists of changes in the electrical properties that make muscle more excitable and responsive and produce forceful contractions. In the cervix, the step consists of softening of the connective tissue components. Progesterone and nitric oxide appear to have important roles in these processes. The progress of labor can be assessed noninvasively using electromyographic (EMG) signals from the uterus (the driving force for contractility) recorded from the abdominal surface. Uterine EMG bursts detected in this manner characterize uterine contractile events during human and animal pregnancy. A low uterine EMG activity, measured transabdominally throughout most of pregnancy, rises dramatically during labor. EMG activity also increases substantially during preterm labor in humans and rats and may be predictive of preterm labor. A quantitative method for assessing the cervix is also described. A collascope estimates cervical collagen content from a fluorescent signal generated when collagen crosslinks are illuminated with an excitation light of about 340 nm. The system has proved useful in rats and humans at various stages of pregnancy and indicates that cervical softening occurs progressively in the last one-third of pregnancy. In rats, collascope readings correlate with resistance measurements made in the isolated cervix, which may help to assess cervical function during pregnancy and indicate controls and treatments.

KEYWORDS: myometrium; cervix; electromyographic signals; labor; preterm labor; progesterone; nitric oxide; collagen

INTRODUCTION

Preterm labor and subsequent preterm birth are the most common pregnancy complications, with 20% of all pregnant women at high risk. In the United States alone, 10% of the four million babies born each year are premature.[1,2] At $1500 a day for neonatal intensive care, this constitutes national health-care expenditures well over $5 billion.[3] In addition, preterm labor accounts for 85% of infant mortality

Address for correspondence: R.E. Garfield, Reproductive Sciences, Department of Obstetrics & Gynecology, University of Texas Medical Branch, 301 University Blvd., Galveston, TX 77555-1062. Voice: 409-772-7590; fax: 409-772-2261.
 rgarfiel@utmb.edu

and 50% of infant neurological disorders. One of the keys to treating preterm labor is the early detection of labor. If preterm labor is diagnosed early, medical specialists can attempt to stop the labor process or use a number of interventions to improve the outcome for premature infants if prevention of preterm delivery fails.

We recently developed two noninvasive methods for the objective evaluation of the status of the uterus and cervix. One method consists of recording uterine electromyographic (EMG) signals from the abdominal surface. Because action potentials are responsible for the contractility of the uterus, recordings of EMG activity can be used to assess the contractile function of the uterus. The other method detects changes in collagen content of the cervix using an optical system and light-induced autofluorescence (LIF). This system measures the collagen fluorescence in the cervix as an indirect estimate of collagen concentration. These two procedures have been used in animals to determine changes in the uterus and cervix during pregnancy. Preliminary studies of human subjects support the use of these techniques. Our studies provide convincing evidence that recording EMG activity from the abdominal surface and measurement of cervical fluorescence can be clinically useful in evaluating the state of the uterus and cervix.

DIAGNOSIS OF LABOR

Although several methods (described below) have been adopted to monitor labor, they are subjective and do not provide an accurate diagnosis or prediction of when labor will occur. To date, the most important key to preventing preterm labor has been constant contact and care from health-care practitioners.[4] The current state of the art in labor monitoring can be summarized as follows: (1) Current methods are subjective; (2) intrauterine pressure catheters provide the best information, but their use is limited by their invasiveness and the need for ruptured membranes; (3) present uterine monitors are uncomfortable, inaccurate, and depend on the examiner; (4) no method has been successful at predicting preterm labor; and (5) no method has led to effective treatment of preterm labor.

While some methods can identify signals of ongoing labor, none of the methods offer objective data that accurately predict labor over a broad range of patients. The methods range in complexity from simple patient self-awareness to complex electronic pressure sensors. TABLE 1 lists the current methods and their characteristics.

Of the current methods, intrauterine pressure catheters perhaps provide the best information concerning the state of the pregnancy, but the invasive instrument used can increase the risk of infection and requires rupture of the membranes. Tocodynamometers are external pressure measurement devices that are used to detect changes in abdominal contour as an indirect indication of uterine contraction.

The primary advantage of a tocodynamometer is that it does not require an invasive probe. This allows the device to be used for most pregnancies without risk to the fetus or the mother. External toco-monitoring devices are used in over 90% of all hospital births. Physicians have been quick to adopt these devices because they supply uterine contraction data with little risk. Nevertheless, most agree the success of these devices depends on the skill of the examiner. Also, these instruments have not changed treatments for preterm labor. Toco devices have one major drawback: poor accuracy. Many different variables affect the pressure measurement, such as instru-

TABLE 1. Current methods used in uterine monitoring or screening of labor

	Accuracy	Invasive
Monitoring of contractions by exsaminer and correlating with intravaginal monitoring	Moderate	Yes
Monitoring the state of the cervix	Moderate	No
Symptomatic self monitoring	Low	No
Intrauterine pressure monitor	High	Yes
External uterine monitor (tocodynamometer)	Erratic	No
Ultrasound, remote sensing, temperature monitoring, blood flow monitors	Mixed	No
Endovaginal ultrasonography	Low	Yes
Fetal fibronectin screening test ⎫ Salivatory estriol test ⎭	High negative predictive values	No

ment placement, amount of subcutaneous fat, and uterine wall pressure. Also, body movements, gastric activity, and other nonlabor-induced stresses on the device can be mistaken for labor contractions. Therefore, the use of external tocodynamometry is limited to obtaining the frequency of contractions and does not include any direct or indirect measure of functional interest, such as force or efficiency of contraction. Still, the advantages of a noninvasive method in providing uterine contraction data have led to their widespread adoption despite these drawbacks.

Home uterine activity monitoring (HUAM), which is based on external tocodynamometer recordings, has been used to predict preterm labor.[5,6] In a recent study, however, HUAM was no better in lowering the frequency of preterm birth than weekly contact with a nurse.[7]

The state of the cervix on the basis of digital examination is clinically used as a predictor of labor. However, the relationship between softening, effacement, and dilation of the cervix and changes in uterine contractility is variable. Indeed, uterine activity and changes in the cervix occur independently. Measuring the length of the cervix via endovaginal ultrasonography has been used to detect premature labor,[8–13] but the positive predictive value (PPV) is only 25% (75% of patients with a shortened cervix based on ultrasound will deliver at term).

Assay of cervical or vaginal fetal fibronectin (fFN), has been recently suggested as a screening method for patients at risk for premature labor. Results from several studies[14–18] show that fFN may be useful in predicting actual premature labor. Other studies indicate that fFN has limited value.[17] The value of the fFN assay lies in its high negative predictive value (NPV); it has the ability to identify patients that are *not* at risk of premature labor. Similarly, salivary estriol has been shown to have some use because of the high NPV.[19]

Despite all the limitations summarized above, the presence of uterine contractions and cervical softening at 28 weeks' gestation were the best predictors of spontaneous preterm birth in a group of nulliparous women at risk for preterm delivery.[20] We believe that the issue is not whether changes in uterine activity and cervical structure precede labor, but rather finding the appropriate method for detecting these changes.

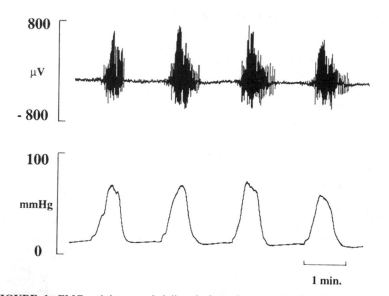

FIGURE 1. EMG activity recorded directly from the uterus (*top*) and intrauterine pressure (*bottom*) obtained from pregnant rat during labor (Garfield, unpublished).

ELECTRICAL PROPERTIES OF THE MYOMETRIUM

The sequence of contraction and relaxation of the myometrium results from the cyclic depolarization and repolarization of the membranes of the muscle cells. The spontaneous electrical discharges in the muscle from the uterus consist of intermittent bursts of spike action potentials.[21–27] Uterine volume (chronic stretch) and ovarian hormones (principally estrogen) contribute to the change in action potential shape through their effect on the resting membrane potential.[28–30] A single spike can initiate a contraction but multiple, coordinated spikes are needed for forceful and maintained contractions.[23] As in other excitable tissues, the action potential in uterine smooth muscle cells results from voltage- and time-dependent changes in membrane ionic permeability.[31]

Studies of isolated myometrial tissues using microelectrodes or extracellular electrodes demonstrate the temporal association between electrical events and contractions.[32–45] In all species, each contraction is accompanied by a burst of action potentials (FIG. 1), which starts slightly earlier than the contraction. The frequency, amplitude, and duration of contractions are determined, respectively, by the frequency of the action potentials within a burst, the duration of a burst, and the total number of cells that are simultaneously active.[23] The frequency of the action potentials within a burst first increases and then decreases. The burst stops before the uterus has relaxed.[23] The electrical and mechanical activity of the myometrium have been recorded in whole animals by many investigators in various species[33–41,46] including humans.[42–45,47]

Our studies to date, as well as those of others,[48–52] provide convincing data that uterine EMG activity can be assessed from abdominal surface measurements (see below).

CHANGES IN ELECTRICAL PROPERTIES OF THE MYOMETRIUM DURING PREGNANCY AND LABOR

We and others have shown that myometrial cells are coupled together electrically by gap junctions composed of connexin proteins.[53,54] The grouping of connexins provides channels of low electrical resistance between cells and thereby furnish pathways for the efficient conduction of action potentials. Throughout most of pregnancy, and in all species studied, these cell-to-cell channels or contacts are low, indicating poor coupling and decreased electrical conductance. This condition favors quiescence of the muscle and the maintenance of pregnancy. At term, however, the cell junctions increase and form an electrical syncytium required for effective contractions. The presence of the contacts seems to be controlled by changing estrogen and progesterone levels in the uterus.[53] As action potentials propagate over the surface of a myometrial cell, the depolarization causes voltage-dependent Ca^{2+} channels (VDCC) to open. When this occurs, Ca^{2+} enters the muscle cell down its chemical gradient to activate the myofilaments and provoke a contraction. We have recently demonstrated by RT-PCR that the expression of VDCC subunits in the rat myometrium increases during term and preterm labor.[55] The increased expression, which appears to be controlled by progesterone withdrawal, may facilitate uterine contractility during labor by increasing portals for Ca^{2+} entry.

A MODEL OF LABOR—A PREPARATORY STAGE

Progesterone seems to exert an overall control of uterine quiescence by (1) suppressing a number of genes in the myometrium that are essential for uterine contractility (connexin 43, calcium channels, receptors, etc.); (2) upregulating the relaxation mechanisms, including the nitric oxide system[56,57]; and finally (3) suppressing the release of proinflammatory cytokines and reducing the availability of prostaglandins.[58,59] The results of experimental and clinical studies with progesterone and its antagonists indicate that parturition is composed of two major steps: a relatively long conditioning (preparatory) phase, followed by a short secondary phase (active labor)[52,54,56,60] (FIG. 2). Similar models have been proposed by others.[61,62] The conditioning step leading to the softening of the cervix takes place during a different time frame from that of the uterus and myometrium, indicating that the myometrium and cervix are regulated in part by independent mechanisms. In the myometrium, this preparatory process involves changes in transduction mechanisms and the synthesis of several new proteins including connexins, ion channels, and receptors for uterotonins. At the same time, there is a downregulation of the nitric oxide system, which leads to withdrawal of uterine relaxation. In the cervix the transition involves a change in the composition of the connective tissue and the invasion by inflammatory cells. It is likely that preparatory changes similar to those occurring in the cervix also take place in fetal membranes. We view the initiation of the conditioning step as the start of parturition. The conditioning phase can be induced with antiprogestins in all species studied thus far, including primates.[60] However, our recent studies show that cervical ripening starts before the drop in circulating progesterone levels, indicating the existence of an additional, progesterone-independent mechanism controlling cervical ripening. At some point during the conditioning step, the process

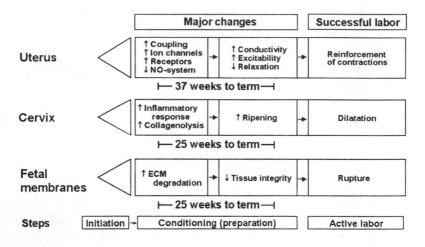

FIGURE 2. Model of the initiation of labor showing changes in the uterus (myometrium), cervix, and fetal membranes. Major alterations occur in these tissues during a conditioning or preparatory step.

becomes irreversible and leads to active labor and delivery. Once active labor has started, delivery cannot be delayed for more than five days in humans because the changes that have occurred in the preparatory phase are by this time well established and thus not reversible, especially not with currently available tocolytics. Active labor, leading eventually to the delivery of the fetus and placenta, starts with the onset of coordinated uterine contractions. In our opinion, the key to understanding parturition and developing suitable treatment methods is the understanding of the processes by which the myometrium and cervix undergo these conditioning or conversion stages (FIG. 2). Unfortunately, the currently available methods, which are based solely on monitoring contractions and manual cervical examination, do not detect whether a patient has entered the conditioning step because changes in these parameters may be independent of this preparatory stage.

EVIDENCE THAT RECORDINGS OF UTERINE EMG ACTIVITY ARE REPRESENTATIVE OF UTERINE CONTRACTILE ACTIVITY

Studies in Rats

We have recently recorded uterine EMG activity directly from the uterine surface and simultaneously from the abdominal surface of pregnant rats, while also monitoring intrauterine pressure.[48,49] Early in pregnancy and until about day 18 of gestation, electromyographic bursts were irregular and of low amplitude. There was also little or no correspondence between activity recorded from the uterus and the abdominal surface. Intrauterine pressure activity was frequent but still irregular and generally of low amplitude (FIG. 3). Later in gestation (day 21 to delivery), the electromyographic activity became more regular, and the signals directly recorded from the

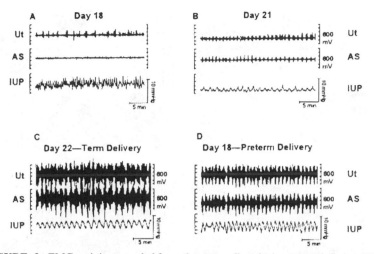

FIGURE 3. EMG activity recorded from the uterus directly (*top* on each figure, Ut) and the abdominal surface (AS) simultaneously with intrauterine pressure (IUP) from pregnant rats. Records were obtained at days 18 (**A**) and 21 (**B**) of gestation and during term (**C**) and preterm (induced with onapristone) delivery (**D**). Note the large and frequent bursts of EMG events from both sites and their correspondence to IUP.[48]

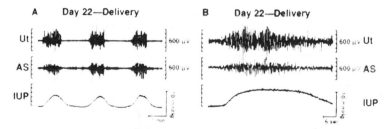

FIGURE 4. Expanded views of EMG bursts from rats recorded simultaneously from uterine (Ut) and abdominal (AS) surface, along with IUP, during term delivery.[48]

uterus (FIG. 3) coincided well with those recorded from the abdominal surface (FIGS. 3 and 4). There was also a tendency for low-amplitude intrauterine pressure to correspond in time with the electromyographic activity recorded from the uterus as well as the abdominal surface. During term and preterm labor in rats, electromyographic activity recorded from both the uterus and abdominal surface occurred concurrently with changes in intrauterine pressure (FIGS. 3 and 4). The electromyographic signals and the intrauterine pressure were frequent (about one contraction per minute) and of high amplitude.

Our study demonstrated that abdominal surface recordings of uterine electrical events are representative of the electrical activity of the uterus, at least just before and during labor. This conclusion is based on the following observations: (1) Action potential bursts obtained from the abdominal surface almost perfectly mirror bursts occurring in the uterus; (2) increases and decreases in electrical bursts at both sites

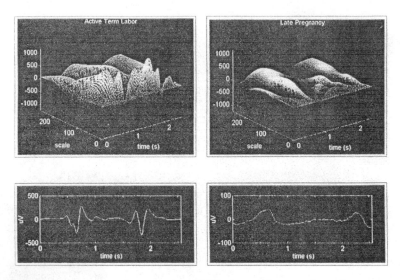

FIGURE 5. Analysis of rat uterine EMG data with use of continuous wavelet transformation.[50]

accompany changes in pressure; (3) changes in activity during term and preterm labor are detected simultaneously at the uterus and the abdominal surface; (4) either pharmacologic stimulation or inhibition results in similar changes in recordings from both sites; (5) cardiac action potentials do not interfere with uterine or abdominal recording; (6) action potentials from the uterus are also propagated to the vaginal surface. This study suggests that this technique can be used to determine when the uterus enters a state required for labor.

We also evaluated the EMG signals from the uterine and abdominal surface by power density spectral and wavelet analysis.[49] These studies indicated that several types of algorithms are useful in evaluating the EMG activity recorded from the abdominal surface. We have also demonstrated increases in all the following parameters during the gestational period leading to labor: amplitude and power of bursts (FIG. 3), high-frequency content of action potential waveforms (FIG. 5), and rate of burst production and duration of bursts.[49] The magnitude of the power spectrum depends not only on the amplitude of the activity but also on the increase in the intensity of the activity during term and preterm labor. The increase in energy of the electrical activity and the increased high-frequency content of the action potentials are favored by the changes that occur in the electrical properties of the myometrium during labor to increase current flow (and contractile force) in the myometrial smooth muscle. These increases do not occur abruptly, but seem to take place gradually during late gestation with the maximum increases occurring during delivery. These data provide convincing evidence that EMG activity can be accurately recorded from the abdominal surface of pregnant rats. In addition, analysis of transabdominally recorded uterine electrical activity allows for the monitoring of a number of important parameters and is not limited, as is the case with external tocodynamometry, to frequency of contractions.

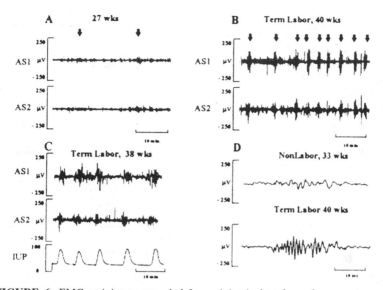

FIGURE 6. EMG activity as recorded from abdominal surface of pregnant women at 27 weeks (**nonlabor, A**) and during term labor (**B and C**). Note the correspondence between EMG bursts and pain (*arrows*, **B**) and intrauterine pressure (IUP, C) during labor. (**D**) shows an expanded and enlarged view of a single burst obtained from a nonlabor patient (*top*) and a patient in labor (*bottom*).[49]

Studies in Humans

We have also recently evaluated the possibility that human uterine electrical events (EMG signals) could be recorded and characterized from the abdominal surface during pregnancy.[49] We studied several hundred patients. The estimated gestational ages ranged from 20 to 42 weeks. Patients included those at term but not in labor, patients in active labor (at term and preterm), postpartum patients, and patients followed longitudinally during pregnancy. Uterine electrical activity was recorded using two sets of bipolar electrodes placed on the abdominal surface. In some patients the intrauterine pressure was also measured with a saline-filled catheter inserted into the uterine cavity. The uterine EMG signals were analyzed in the 0.3–50 Hz frequency range and digitized at 200 samples/sec. Power spectral analysis was performed using fast Fourier transformation (FFT) of the electrical activity in order to assess and characterize the evolution of uterine electrical activity during pregnancy.

The results of this study showed that there was minimal uterine electrical activity, consisting of infrequent and low-amplitude EMG bursts, throughout most of pregnancy (FIG. 6). When bursts occurred before the onset of labor, they often corresponded to periods of perception of contractility by the patient. During term and preterm labor, bursts of EMG activity were frequent, of large amplitude, and correlated with the large changes in the intrauterine pressure and pain sensation. Frequency analysis of the electrical events within bursts recorded during active labor demonstrated a peak frequency of 0.71 ± 0.05 Hz compared with 0.48 ± 0.03 Hz before labor (FIG. 7). Spectral analysis of electrical activity at different periods of ges-

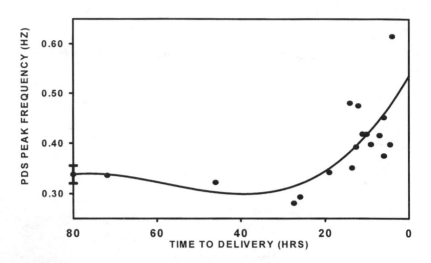

FIGURE 7. The figure shows how the average frequency of the peak in the power spectrum of uterine EMG bursts increases as the time interval from recording to delivery decreases. A measurement-to-delivery time of $t = 0$ would correspond to a recording of EMG activity during actual labor. The mean and standard error of the PDS peak frequency for all patients having a measurement-to-delivery time >80 hours is depicted on the left-hand axis of the figure.[98]

tation showed a dramatic increase in the peaks of energy levels within the bursts (about three- to fourfold) during term (60.2 ± 13.87 µVs) and preterm labor (62.3 ± 22.93 µVs) compared with the energy level of electrical activity recorded early in gestation (11.36 ± 4.03 µVs at 27–36 weeks).

We concluded that the recording of uterine EMG signals from the abdominal surface is a reliable method to follow the evolution of uterine contractility during pregnancy. Analysis of EMG activity might be used to characterize and evaluate uterine contractions during term and preterm labor. This noninvasive technology could be extremely useful in the management of labor and its complications.

Although a prospective study designed to monitor amplitude, burst intensity, and frequency characteristics will be needed to prove that the onset of preterm and term labor can be predicted, our results suggest that parameters such as the percent time active and power density analysis will indicate how close a patient is to term or preterm labor. In humans, this method of analysis may detect whether the stage of uterine preparedness for labor has or has not yet been achieved. With the aid of EMG recordings, monitoring of labor induction or augmentation may become more objective and accurate. Oxytocin may be started or increased earlier if needed or the adequacy of uterine contractions may be ascertained and cesarean section performed sooner than if the health-care providers were relying on external tocodynamometry or had to wait for intrauterine pressure recordings. Our studies offer a possible algorithm that could bring an improvement in clinical diagnosis and treatment. This approach may provide attending obstetricians with a very powerful tool in following the evolution of uterine contractility in the future. It is obvious that more studies are needed before this technology is ready for clinical use in human subjects, but these initial data suggest that it has great promise.

CERVICAL FUNCTION AND ASSESSMENT

The cervix is composed of smooth muscle (ca. 10%) and a large component of connective tissue (90%) consisting of collagen, elastin, and macromolecular components that make up the extracellular matrix.[63–65] Many biochemical and functional changes occur in cervical connective tissue at the end of pregnancy.[66–82] This process, often called cervical ripening, results in softening, dilatation, and effacement of the cervix. Ripening is required for appropriate progress of labor and delivery of the fetus. The exact mechanisms controlling the cervical ripening process are largely unknown.

Presently, there is no objective method to evaluate changes associated with dilation and effacement of the cervix during pregnancy. During pregnancy the cervix is normally firm and closed. At the end of pregnancy, the cervix becomes softer and dilates as the uterine contractions increase during labor. Often, however, the cervix fails to soften and dilate with advancing labor or dilates prematurely before labor. The attending physician currently monitors progress of the cervix by visual inspection or by manual examination. These subjective tests are often inadequate and vary from physician to physician. A more accurate method would be invaluable for the diagnosis of cervical problems such as premature dilation or prolonged labor due to delayed cervical dilation, as well as to determine cervical status before induction of labor. In addition, such a method could lead to appropriate treatments to either dilate or prevent dilation of the cervix. Treatment to increase softening in women at term has been accomplished by treatment with prostaglandins or various mechanical methods.[83–85] However, no treatment to ripen the cervix has reduced the high cesarean section rate associated with dystocia.[86] Cervical cerclage is used for early softening or dilation of the cervix (cervical incompetence). However, this method is associated with many problems, and pharmacological methods to prevent softening are nonexistent.

Fluorescence Spectroscopy of Collagen

Fluorescence spectroscopy is a widely used research tool in the biosciences, primarily because of the amount of information that it can reveal in terms of molecular and physical states.[87–93] Fluorescent spectra offer important details on the structure and dynamics of macromolecules and their locations at microscopic levels. Fluorescence spectroscopy has been used to examine collagen content of a variety of tissues including cancers.[87,91] We used this method recently to evaluate the cervix.

The Collascope and Measurement of Cervical Ripening

We were the first to introduce the use of light-induced autofluorescence (LIF) for the measurement of changes in the cervical tissue during gestation and labor.[94] Collagen gives characteristic fluorescence whose maximum is around 390 nm (FIG. 8). The intrinsic fluorophor is believed to be pyridinoline, which is considered one of the

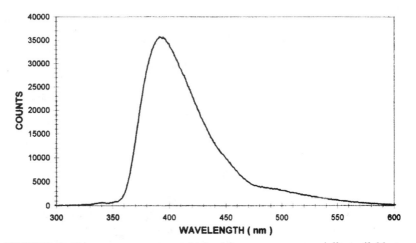

FIGURE 8. Fluorescence spectrum obtained from pure, commercially available type I collagen.

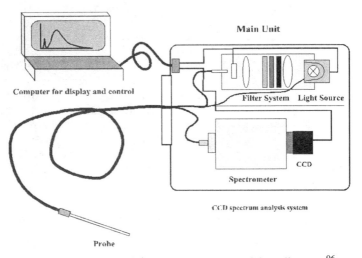

FIGURE 9. Diagram of various components of the collascope.[96]

major crosslinks within the primary structure of collagen fibrils.[9,89,95] In our initial investigations, measurements were obtained from the serosal surface of the medium band of the cervix of rats *in vivo*. The results showed a decrease in fluorescence intensity in the later gestational days and at parturition that corresponded to the decrease in collagen. We also found a drop in collagen fluorescence intensity in rats that were treated with the antiprogesterone compound RU38.486 and that delivered prematurely.

We later assembled a prototype instrument, termed the collascope (FIG. 9), with the help of ISA instruments (ISA Jobin Yvon-Spex, Edison, NJ), specifically to assess the function of the cervix.

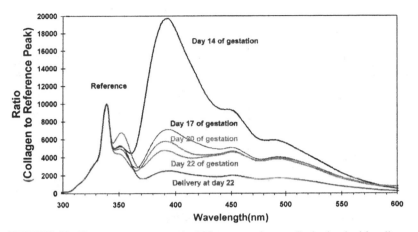

FIGURE 10. Fluorescence spectra (at 390 nm, superimposed) obtained with collascope from rat cervices at various days of gestation and during delivery. Note the decline in fluorescence as pregnancy progresses and the low spectrum observed during delivery. Note also the reference signal at 340 nm, used to normalize the intensity of the excitation signals.[96]

The collascope probe, which is in contact with the measuring site, has two parts: fiber-optical probe and sheath. The fiber-optical probe is a stainless steel rod with optical fiber bundles in the center (1 large fiber for excitation surrounded by 6 small fibers for pickup of fluorescence). Once the probe is in position, the operation of the data collection process is operated by a notebook computer terminal with software that controls the collascope function and analysis. All the data are normalized to a peak of reference light (see FIGS. 10 and 11). The ratio between fluorescence signal from the cervix and reference signal is calculated.

Studies in Rats

With the collascope we were able to measure the fluorescence signal from the cervix in anesthetized rats.[96] The advantage to this technique is that one can follow cervical changes longitudinally in the same animal under a variety of conditions and treatments (FIG. 10).

In the postpartum period, the fluorescence gradually increased from the low value observed during delivery (FIG. 11). FIGURE 12 illustrates the average spectral values in rats that were nonpregnant, pregnant day 13 to day 22, undergoing delivery, and postpartum. These results demonstrate the progressive decline in fluorescence during pregnancy, which reached low values during delivery.

We also measured cervical resistance in rats at various times of gestation to compare these data to those obtained with the collascope. We measured resistance as the slope of the stress–strain curve in cervices removed from rats at various times (FIG. 13). The results of resistance measurements parallel the fluorescence measurements obtained with the collascope (compare FIG. 12 to FIG. 13). We also noted the decline in cervical collagen content in electron micrographs of ripened versus unripe cervix (FIG. 14). In addition, we examined rats at various times before and during preterm labor induced with the antiprogesterone onapristone. This study showed that

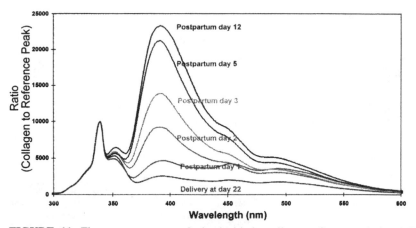

FIGURE 11. Fluorescence spectra obtained with the collascope from rats during delivery and various times postpartum. Note the low values of the spectrum during delivery and the progressive increase in the spectra postpartum.[96]

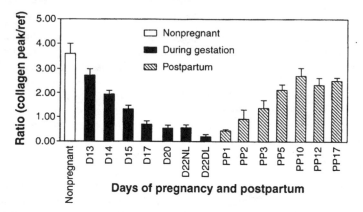

FIGURE 12. Average values of ratio of collagen peak to reference peak obtained in rats that were nonpregnant, at various times during pregnancy, during delivery, and at various times postpartum. Note the progressive decline in fluorescence with lowest values obtained on day 22 (NL = nonlabor, DL = during labor).[96]

ripening occurred with antiprogesterone treatment and that R5020, a progestin agonist, prevented ripening and preterm birth.

We conclude from these studies that the collascope can be used as a noninvasive tool to measure changes in cervical collagen content under a variety of conditions. Results of these measurements correspond with known physiological changes in the cervix during pregnancy.

Studies in Humans

We have also initiated human studies with the collascope.[96] Nonpregnant, pregnant, and postpartum human volunteers were recruited for the study. The first step

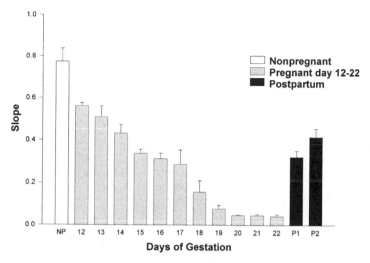

FIGURE 13. Cervical resistance values obtained from isolated cervices in nonpregnant rats, at various times during pregnancy, and postpartum. Resistance was measured as the slope of the stress/strain curve.

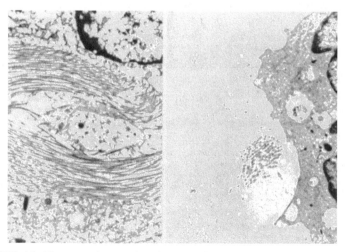

FIGURE 14. Electron micrographs of cervix of pregnant guinea pigs obtained in control animals before term (*left*) and following ripening at term (*right*). Note the large number of collagen fibers present during early pregnancy and the decrease in fibers during ripening.

was to establish a longitudinal distribution profile according to the weeks of gestation and postpartum. The cervical external os was gently wiped with rayon-tipped proctoscopic swabs before measurements were taken. The measuring site was selected at the 12 o'clock position. The R values that were calculated as the tissue collagen fluorescence counts at 390 nm divided by the counts at 340 nm (the reference peak for the excitation light) decreased progressively during the final 15 weeks of preg-

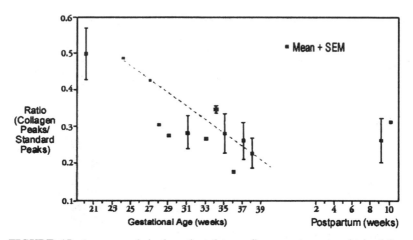

FIGURE 15. Average and single patient data on fluorescent spectra obtained from 40 nonpregnant and pregnant patients at various times of gestation and postpartum.

nancy (FIG. 15). So far, several hundred patients (including nonpregnant patients) have been recruited. Several of the subjects have been measured two or three times during their pregnancy and postpartum. The results show a gradual decrease of the fluorescence as pregnancy approaches term followed by a slow recovery during the postpartum period.[97]

We conclude that it is feasible to measure collagen fluorescence noninvasively from the surface of the external os of the rat and human cervix. The results of fluorescence measurements confirm our previous findings employing an invasive method to analyze cervical extensibility (FIG. 15) and other studies in the literature of cervical collagen content and cervical collagenase enzyme regulation. In view of the important role of collagen fibers and their turnover in the process of cervical function during pregnancy, the light-induced autofluorescence of cervical collagen could be a useful tool for evaluating cervical status and monitoring treatment strategies. The noninvasive measurements obtained with the collascope provide a good tool for the study of gestational changes in the human cervix. However, more human research is needed to reach a better understanding of how cervical collagen change progresses during human pregnancy and to investigate potential clinical applications of LIF.

POTENTIAL APPLICATIONS OF EMG AND LIF

Our preliminary data regarding abdominal recordings of uterine EMG activity and cervical LIF suggest that they could be extremely useful for a variety of obstetrical indications and problems (see TABLE 2). The potential benefits from the use of this method include the reduction in preterm delivery rate and improved perinatal outcome, the identification of treatment regimens, and a decrease in cesarean section rate. In addition, these methods can be used in research to define mechanisms that

TABLE 2. Uses and potential benefits of diagnostic devices

Clinical condition	EMG	LIF	Clinical use	Potential benefits	Percent use
Antepartum	+	+	Predict preterm delivery	Prevent preterm delivery and improve perinatal outcome	100
Early labor	+	+	Differentiate between false and true labor	Prevent unnecessary admissions	30
Preterm contractions	+	+	Determine need for tocolysis.	Prevent unnecessary use of tocolytics and decrease cost.	10
Cervical incompetence	+	+	Rule out the presence of subclinical uterine electrical activity. Detect abnormalities in cervical collagen content. Post-cerclage monitoring.	Better define candidates for cerclage. Better understanding of etiologies. More objective measure of cervical change.	1–3
Induction of labor	+	+	Predict success of induction.	Prevent unnecessary prolonged inductions.	20
Induction of labor	–	+	Predict need for cervical ripening. Determine whether more ripening is needed.	Prevent starting inductions when the cervix is not ready.	
Induction of labor	+	–	More objective and accurate analysis of uterine activity. Improved method to monitor and adjust oxytocin infusion.	Decrease numbers of cesarean sections due to inappropriate use of oxytocin.	
Augmentation of labor	+	–	More objective and accurate analysis of uterine activity. Better way to monitor and adjust oxytocin infusion.	Decrease numbers of cesarean sections due to inappropriate use of oxytocin.	50
Failure to progress	+	–	More objective and accurate analysis of uterine activity. Determine whether abnormal uterine activity is the cause.	Decrease numbers of cesarean sections due to inappropriate use of oxytocin.	15
Tocolysis	+	+	Predict success of tocolysis. More objective and accurate analysis of uterine activity. Improved method to monitor and adjust tocolytic therapy.	Prevent complications from tocolytics. Decrease time on tocolytics.	10
Noninvasive, *in vivo* measurements	+	+	No interference from surgical procedures or implantable devices. Continuous measurements over time in the same animal.	Define the mechanisms that regulate uterine and cervical function in term and preterm labor.	–
				Study different treatments to induce, augment, or inhibit these mechanisms	–

regulate normal and abnormal function of the uterus and cervix and ways to control them pharmacologically. Of the many potential applications for EMG and LIF outlined in TABLE 2, prediction of labor or when patients will enter the conditioning phase of parturition promises to yield the greatest results.

FUTURE STUDIES

Future studies with both transabdominal EMG measurements and LIF will focus on the ability to predict when labor (term or preterm) will occur following the measurements. Because EMG power density spectral analysis and LIF measurements differ between those in labor and those not in labor, it seems that detection of a transition period and prediction of when labor will occur is possible. At present we know from experience with induction of labor with antiprogestins that labor begins from 12 to 24 hours after treatment. Therefore we can assume that when we begin to see changes in EMG patterns and LIF that about the same amount of time is required. On the other hand, if signals are low, perhaps more than 24 hours will be needed; and conversely, if signals are high, labor should be expected in less than 24 hours.

ACKNOWLEDGMENT

This work was supported by National Institutes of Health Grant #HD37480.

REFERENCES

1. US PREVENTIVE SERVICES TASK FORCE. 1989. Guide to Clinical Preventive Services: An Assessment of the Effectiveness of 169 Interventions. Williams & Wilkins. Baltimore, MD.
2. VENTURA, S.J., J.A. MARTIN, S.C. CURTIN & T.H. MATTHEWS. 1997. Report of final natality statistics. Mon. Vital Stat. Rep. 45: 12.
3. BROWN, E.R. & M. EPSTEIN. 1984. Immediate consequences of preterm birth. In Preterm Birth: Causes, Prevention, and Management. F. Fuchs & P.G. Stubblefield, Eds.: 323. Macmillan Publishing. New York.
4. GOLDENBERG, R.L., S.P. CLIVER, J. BRONSTEIN, et al. 1994. Bed rest in pregnancy. Obstet. Gynecol. 84: 131–136.
5. MOU, S.M., S.G. SUNDERJI, S. GALL, H. HOW, et al. 1991. Multicenter randomized clinical trial of home uterine activity monitoring for detection of preterm labor. Am. J. Obstet. Gynecol. 165: 858–866.
6. WAPNER, R.J., D.B. COTTON, R. ARTAL, et al. 1995. A randomized multicenter trial assessing a home uterine activity monitoring device used in the absence of daily nursing contact. Am. J. Obstet. Gynecol. 172(3): 1026–1034.
7. DYSON, D.C., K.H. DANGE, J.A. BAMBER, et al. 1998. Monitoring women at risk for preterm labor. N. Engl. J. Med. 338: 15–19.
8. ANDERSEN, H.F., C.E. NUGENT, S.D. WANTY & R.H. HAYASHI. 1990. Prediction of risk for preterm delivery by ultrasonographic measurement of cervical length. Am. J. Obstet. Gynecol. 163(3): 859–867.
9. GUZMAN, E.R., C. HOULIHAN & A. VINTZILEOS. 1995. Sonography and transfundal pressure in the evaluation of the cervix during pregnancy. Obstet. Gynecol. Surv. 50(5): 395–403.
10. CHUNG, T.K.H., C.J. HAINES, D. KONG, et al. 1993. Transvaginal sonography in the diagnosis and management of cervical incompetence. Gynecol. Obstet. Invest. 36: 59–61.

11. IAMS, J.D., R.L. GOLDENBERG, P.J. MEIS, *et al.* 1996. The length of the cervix and the risk of spontaneous premature delivery. N. Engl. J. Med. **334:** 567–572.
12. COOK, C.M. & D.A. ELLWOOD. 1996. A longitudinal study of the cervix in pregnancy using transvaginal ultrasound. Br. J. Obstet. Gynecol. **103:** 16–18.
13. IAMS, J.D., J. PARASKOS, M.B. LANDON, *et al.* 1994. Cervical sonography in preterm labor. Obstet. Gyencol. **84:** 40–46.
14. LOCKWOOD, C.J., R. WEIN, R. LAPINKSI, *et al.* 1993. The presence of cervical and vaginal fetal fibronectin predicts preterm delivery in an inner-city obstetric population. Am. J. Obstet. Gynecol. **169(4):** 798–804.
15. NAGEOTTE, M.P., D. CASAL & A.E. SENYEI. 1994. Fetal fibronectic in patients at increased risk for premature birth. Am. J. Obstet. Gynecol. **170:** 20–25.
16. LOCKWOOD, C.J., R.D. MOSCARELLI, R. WEIN, *et al.* 1994. Low concentrations of vaginal fetal fibronectin as a predictor of deliveries occurring after 41 weeks. Am. J. Obstet. Gynecol. **171:** 1–4.
17. HELLEMANS, P., J. GERRIS & P. VERDONK. 1995. Fetal fibronectin detection for prediction of preterm birth in low risk women (see comments). Br. J. Obstet. Gynecol. **102:** 207–212.
18. IAMS, J.D., D. CASAL, J.A. MCGREGOR, *et al.* 1995. Fetal fibronectin improves the accurace of diagnosis of preterm labor (see comments). Am. J. Obstet. Gynecol. **173:** 141–145.
19. MCGREGOR, J.A., G.M. JACKSON, G.C. LACHELIN, *et al.* 1995. Salivary estriol as risk assessment for preterm labor: a prospective trial. Am. J. Obstet. Gynecol. **173:** 1337–1342.
20. COPPER, R.L., R.L. GODENBERG, M.B. DUBARD, *et al.* 1995. Cervical examination and tocodynamometry at 28 weeks' gestation: prediction of spontaneous preterm birth. Am. J. Obstet. Gynecol. **172:** 666–671.
21. KURIYAMA, H. 1961. Recent studies of the electrophysiology of the uterus. *In* Progesterone and the Defence Mechanism of Pregnancy. Ciba Foundation Study Group, Vol. **9:** 51–70. Little Brown. Boston.
22. CSAPO, A.I. 1962. Smooth muscle as a contractile unit. Physiol. Rev. **42:** 7–33.
23. MARSHALL, J.M. 1962. Regulation of activity in uterine smooth muscle. Physiol. Rev. **42:** 213–227.
24. OHKAWA, H. 1975. Electrical and mechanical interaction between the muscle layers of rat uterus and different sensitivities to oxytocin. Bull. Yamaguchi Med. Sch. **22:** 197–210.
25. KURIYAMA, H. & H. SUZUKI. 1976. Changes in electrical properties of rat myometrium during gestation and following hormonal treatments. J. Physiol. London **260:** 315–333.
26. KANDA, S. & H. KURIYAMA. 1980. Specific features of smooth muscle cells recorded from the placental region of the myometrium of pregnant rats. J. Physiol. London **299:** 127–144.
27. OSA, T. & T. FUJINO. 1978. Electrophysiological comparison between the longitudinal and circular muscles of the rat uterus during the estrous cycle and pregnancy. Jpn. J. Physiol. **23:** 197–209.
28. OSA, T., T. OGASAWARA & S. KATO. 1983. Effects of magnesium, oxytocin and prostaglandin F2 on the generation and propagation of excitation in the longitudinal muscle of rat myometrium during late pregnancy. Jpn. J. Physiol. **33:** 51–67.
29. BENGTSSON, B., E.M.H. CHOW & J.M. MARSHALL. 1984. Activity of circular muscle of rat uterus at different times in pregnancy. Am. J. Physiol. **246:** C216–C223.
30. KAWARABAYASHI, T. & J.M. MARSHALL. 1981. Factors influencing circular muscle activity in the pregnant rat uterus. Biol. Reprod. **24:** 373–379.
31. ANDERSON, G.F., T. KAWARABAYASHI & J.M. MARSHALL. 1981. Effect of indomethacin and aspirin on uterine activity in pregnant rats: comparison of circular and longitudinal muscle. Biol. Reprod. **24:** 359–372.
32. MARSHALL, J.M. 1959. Effects of estrogen and progesterone on single uterine muscle fibers in the rat. Am. J. Physiol. **197:** 935–942.
33. HONNEBIER, M.B., R.A. WENTWORTH, J.P. FIGUEROA & P.W. NATHANIEL. 1991. Temporal structuring of delivery in the absence of a photoperiod: preparturient myome-

trial activity of the rhesus monkey is related to maternal body temperature and depends on the maternal circadian system. Biol. Reprod. **45:** 617–625.

34. TAVERNE, M.A.M. & J. SCHEERBOOM. 1985. Myometrial electrical activity during pregnancy and parturition in the pigmy goat. Res. Vet. Sci. **38:** 120–123.
35. DUCSAY, C.A. & C.M. MCNUTT. 1989. Circadian uterine activity in the pregnant rhesus macaque: do prostaglandins play a role? Biol. Reprod. **40:** 988–993.
36. NATHANIELSZ, P.W., A. BAYLEY, E.R. POORE, *et al.* 1980. The relationship between myometrial activity and sleep state and breathing in fetal sheep throughout the last third of gestation. Am. J. Obstet. Gynecol. **138:** 653–659.
37. SUREAU, C., J. CHAVINIE & M. CANNON. 1965. L'electrophysiologie uterine. Bull. Fed. Soc. Gynecol. Obstet. **17:** 79–140.
38. DEMIANCZUK, N., M.E. TOWELL & R.E. GARFIELD. 1984. Myometrial electrophysiologic activity and gap junctions in the pregnant rabbit. Am. J. Obstet. Gynecol. **149:** 485–491.
39. VERHOEFF, A., R.E. GARFIELD, J. RAMONDT & H.C. WALLENBURG. 1986. Myometrial activity related to gap junction area in periparturient and in ovariectomized estrogen treated sheep. Acta. Physiol. Hung. **67:** 117–129.
40. FIGUEROA, J.P., S. MAHAN, E.R. POORE & P.W. NATHANIELSZ. 1985. Characteristics and analysis of uterine electromyographic activity in the pregnant sheep. Am. J. Obstet. Gynecol. **151:** 524–531.
41. SUREAU, C. 1956. Etude de l'activité électrique de l'utérus au cours du travail. Gynecol. Obstet. **555:** 153–175.
42. WOLFS, G.M.J.A. & M. VAN LEEUWEN. 1979. Electromyographic observations on the human uterus during labor. Acta. Obstet. Gynecol. Scand. Suppl. **90:** 1–62.
43. WOLFS, G.M.J.A. & H. ROTTINGHUIS. 1970. Electrical and mechanical activity of the human uterus during labour. Arch. Gynakol. **208:** 373–385.
44. LOPES, P., G. GERMAIN, G. BREART, *et al.* 1984. Electromyographical study of uterine activity in the human during labor induced by prostaglandin. Gynecol. Obstet. Invest. **17(2):** 96–105.
45. CSAPO, A. & H. TAKEDA. 1963. Electrical activity of the parturient human uterus. Nature **200:** 68.
46. CSAPO, A.I. 1981. Force of labour. *In* Principles and Practice of Obstetrics and Perinatology. L. Iffy & H.A. Kamientzky, Eds.: 761–799. John Wiley and Sons. New York.
47. CSAPO, A. & J. SAUVAGE. 1968. The evolution of uterine activity during human pregnancy. Acta. Obstet. Gynecol. Scand. **47:** 181.
48. BUHIMSCHI, C. & R.E. GARFIELD. 1996. Uterine contractility as assessed by abdominal surface recording of EMG activity in rats during pregnancy. Am. J. Obstet. Gynecol. **174:** 744–753.
49. BUHIMSCHI, C., M.B. BOYLE & R.E. GARFIELD. 1997. Electrical activity of the human uterus during pregnancy as recorded from the abdominal surface. Obstet. Gynecol. **90:** 102–111.
50. BUHIMSCHI, C., M.B. BOYLE, G.R. SAADE & R.E. GARFIELD. 1998. Uterine activity during pregnancy and labor assessed by simultaneous recordings from the myometrium and abdominal surface in the rat. Am. J. Obstet. Gynecol. **178:** 811–822.
51. DUCHÊNE, J., D. DEVEDEUX, S. MANSOUR & C. MARQUE. 1995. Analyzing uterine EMG: tracking instantaneous burst frequency. IEEE Eng. Med. Biol. **March/April:** 125–132.
52. MARQUE, C., J. DUCHÊNE, S. LECTERCQ, *et al.* 1986. Uterine EMG processing for obstetrical monitoring. IEEEE Trans. Biomed. Eng. **33:** 1182–1187.
53. GARFIELD, R.E. & C. YALLAMPALLI. 1994. Structure and function of uterine muscle. *In* The Uterus. T. Chard & J.G. Grudzinskas, Eds.: 54–93. Cambridge Reviews in Human Reproduction. Cambridge.
54. GARFIELD, R.E. 1994. Role of cell-to-cell coupling in control of myometrial contractility and labor. *In* Control of Uterine Contractility. R.E. Garfield & T.N. Tabb, Eds.: 40–81. CRC Press. Boca Raton, FL.
55. TEZUKA, N., M. ALI, K. CHWALISZ & R.E. GARFIELD. 1995. Changes in transcripts encoding calcium channel subunits of rat myometrium during pregnancy. Am. J. Physiol. **269**(Cell. Physiol. 38): C1008–C1017.

56. GARFIELD, R.E. & C. YALLAMPALLI. 1993. Control of myometrial contractility and labor. *In* Basic Mechanisms Controlling Term and Preterm Birth. K. Chwalisz & R.E. Garfield, Eds.: 1–28. Springer-Verlag. New York.

57. CHWALISZ, K. & R.E. GARFIELD. 1997. Regulation of the uterus and cervix during pregnancy and labor: role of progesterone and nitric oxide. Ann. N.Y. Acad. Sci. **828:** 238–253.

58. CHWALISZ, K. & R.E. GARFIELD. 1998. New molecular challenges in the induction of cervical ripening: nitric oxide as the final metabolic mediator of cervical ripening. Hum. Reprod. **13:** 101–104.

59. GARFIELD, R.E., G. SAADE, C. BUHIMSCHI, *et al.* 1998. Control and assessment of the uterus and cervix during pregnancy and labor. Hum. Reprod. In press.

60. CHWALISZ, K. & R.E. GARFIELD. 1994. Antiprogestins in the induction of labor. Ann. N.Y. Acad. Sci. **734:** 387–413.

61. CHALLIS, J.R., S.J. LYE & W. GIBB. 1997. Prostaglandins and parturition. Ann. N.Y. Acad. Sci. **828:** 254–267.

62. CASEY, M.L. & P.C. MACDONALD. 1997. The endocrinology of pregnancy. Ann. N.Y. Acad. Sci. **828:** 273–284.

63. DANFORTH, D.N. 1983. The morphology of the human cervix. Clin. Obstet. Gynecol. **26:** 7–13.

64. WOESSNER, J.F. & T.H. BREWER. 1963. Formation and breakdown of collagen and elastin in the human uterus during pregnancy and postpartum involution. Biochem. J. **89:** 75–82.

65. LEPPERT, P.C., S. KELLER, J. CERRETA & I. MANDL. 1982. Conclusive evidence of elastin in the uterine cervix. Am. J. Obstet. Gynecol. **142:** 179–182.

66. DANFORTH, D.N., A. VIES, M. BREEN, *et al.* 1986. The effect of pregnancy and labor on the human cervix: changes in collagen, glycoprotein and glycosaminoglycans. Am. J. Obstet. Gynecol. **120:** 641–651.

67. LIGGINS, G.C. 1981. Cervical ripening as an inflammatory reaction. *In* Cervix in Pregnancy and Labour: Clinical and Biochemical Investigation. D.A. Ellwood & A.B.M. Anderson, Eds.: 1–9. Churchill Livingstone. New York.

68. BRYANT, W.M., J.E. GREENWELL & P.M. WEEKS. 1968. Alterations in collagen organization during dilatation of the cervix uteri. Surg. Gynecol. Obstet. **126:** 27–39.

69. HARKNESS, M.L.R. & R.D. HARKNESS. 1959. Changes in the physical properties of the uterine cervix of the rat during pregnancy. J. Physiol. London **148:** 524–547.

70. KOKENYESI, R. & J.F. WOESSNER, JR. 1990. Relationship between dilatation of the rat uterine cervix and a small dermatan sulfate proteoglycan. Biol. Reprod. **42:** 87–97.

71. RAJABI, M.R., D.D. DEAN, S.N. BEYDOUN & J.F. WOESSNER, JR. 1988. Elevated tissue levels of collagenase during dilation of uterine cervix in human parturition. Am. J. Obstet. Gynecol. **139:** 971–976.

72. CHWALISZ, K., S.S. QING, G. NEEF & W. ELGER. 1987. The effect of the antigestagen ZK98.299 on the uterine cervix. Acta. Endocrinol. (Suppl.) **114:** 113–114.

73. CHWALISZ, K., S.S. QING, A. ESCH & W. ELGER. 1988. Cervical softening in nonpregnant guinea pigs. Acta. Endocrinol. (Suppl.) **25:** 1315.

74. CALDER, A.A., M.P. EMBREY & T. TAIT. 1977. Ripening of the cervix with extra-amniotic prostaglandin E_2 in viscous gel before induction of labour. Br. J. Obstet. Gynaecol. **84:** 264–268.

75. RATH, W., R. OSMERS, B.C. ADELMANN-GRILL, *et al.* 1993. Biochemical changes in the human cervical connective tissue after intracervical application of prostaglandin E_2. Prostaglandins **45:** 375–384.

76. LEPPERT, P.C. 1995. Anatomy and physiology of cervical ripening. Clin. Obstet. Gynecol. **38:** 267–279.

77. LEPPERT, P.C. 1998. The biochemistry and physiology of the uterine cervix during gestation and parturition. Prenat. Neonat. Med. **3:** 103–105.

78. ROBINSON, G., G.M. FILSHIE & M. CUST. 1991. Medical dilatation of the human cervix. *In* The Extracellular Matrix of the Uterus, Cervix and Fetal Membranes: Synthesis Degradation, and Hormonal Regulation. P.C. Leppert & J.F. Woessner, Eds.: 159–181. Perinatology Press. New York.

79. EKMAN, G., H. ALMSTRÖM, L. GRANSTRÖM, *et al.* 1991. Connective tissue in human cervical ripening. *In* The Extracellular Matrix of the Uterus, Cervix and Fetal Membranes: Synthesis Degradation and Hormonal Regulation. P.C. Leppert & J.F. Woessner, Eds.: 87–96. Perinatology Press. New York.

80. MORI, Y. & A. ITO. 1991. Cervical ripening: biochemical regulation. *In* The Extracellular Matrix of the Uterus, Cervix and Fetal Membranes: Synthesis, Degradation and Hormonal Regulation. P.C. Leppert & J.F. Woessner, Eds.: 77–86. Perinatology Press. New York.

81. LEPPERT, P.C. & S. YEH YU. 1991. Elastin and collagen in the human uterus and cervix: biochemical and histological correlation. *In* The Extracellular Matrix of the Uterus, Cervix and Fetal Membranes: Synthesis Degradation and Hormonal Regulation. P.C. Leppert & J.F. Woessner, Eds.: 59–67. Perinatology Press. New York.

82. YEH YU, S. & P.C. LEPPERT. 1991. The collagenous tissues of the cervix during pregnancy and delivery. *In* The Extracellular Matrix of the Uterus, Cervix and Fetal Membranes: Synthesis Degradation and Hormonal Regulation. P.C. Leppert & J.F. Woessner, Eds.: 68–76. Perinatology Press. New York.

83. KLINE, S.B., H. MENG & R.A. MUNSICK. 1995. Cervical dilation from laminaria tents and synthetic osmotic dilators used for 6 hours before abortion. Obstet. Gynecol. **86:** 931–935.

84. BOKSTRÖM, H. & N. WIQVIST. 1995. Prostaglandin release from human cervical tissue in the first trimester of pregnancy after preoperative dilatation with hygroscopic tents. Prostaglandins **50:** 179–188.

85. ROUBEN, D. & F. ARIAS. 1993. A randomized trial of extra-amniotic saline infusion plus intracervical foley catheter balloon versus prostaglandin E_2 vaginal gel for ripening the cervix and inducing labor in patients with unfavorable cervices. Obstet. Gynecol. **82:** 290–294.

86. PORRECO, R.P. & J.A. THORP. 1996. The cesarean birth epidemic: trends, causes, and solutions. Am. J. Obstet. Gynecol. **175:** 369–374.

87. UNDENFRIEND, S. 1962. Fluorescence Assay in Biology and Medicine, Vol. I. Academic Press. New York.

88. CANTOR, C.R. & P.R. SCHIMMEL. 1980. Biophysical Chemistry. W.H. Freeman. New York.

89. LAKOWICZ, J.R. 1986. Principles of Fluorescence Spectroscopy, 3rd print. Plenum Press. New York.

90. RAMANUJAM, N., M.F. MITCHELL, A. MAHADEVAN, *et al.* 1994. Fluorescence spectroscopy: a diagnostic tool for cervical intrepithelial neoplasia (CIN). Gynecol. Oncol. **52:** 31–38.

91. LAM, S., J.Y.C. HUNG, S.M. KENNEDY, *et al.* 1992. Detection of dysplasia and carcinoma in situ by ratio fluorometry. Am. Rev. Respir. Dis. **146:** 1458–1461.

92. COTHREN, R.M., R.R. RICHARDS-KORTUM, M.V. SIVAK, *et al.* 1990. Gastrointestinal tissue diagnosis by laser induced fluorescence spectroscopy at endoscopy. Gastrointest. Endosc. **36:** 105–111.

93. SCHOMAKER, K.T., J.K. FRISOLI, C.C. COMPTON, *et al.* 1992. Ultraviolet laser-induced fluorescence of colonic tissue: basic biology and diagnostic potential. Lasers Surg. Med. **12:** 63–78.

94. GLASSMAN, W., M. BYAM-SMITH & R.E. GARFIELD. 1995. Changes in rat cervical collagen during gestation and following antiprogesterone treatment as measured in vivo with light induced autofluorescence. Am. J. Obstet. Gynecol. **173:** 1550–1556.

95. FUJIMOTO, D. 1977. Isolation and characterization of a fluorescent material in bovine achilles tendon collagen. Biochem. Biophysics. Res. Commun. **76(4):** 1124–1129.

96. GLASSMAN, W.S., Q-P. LIAO, S-Q. SHI, *et al.* 1997. Fluorescence probe for cervical examination during various reproductive states. Proceedings of SPIE—Advances in Fluorescence Sensing Technology III. **2980:** 286–292.

97. OLSON, G., L. GOODRUM, E. MARTIN, *et al.* 1998. Noninvasive measurement of cervical collagen content in women approaching delivery. Am. J. Obstet. Gynecol. **178:** S91.

98. GARFIELD, R., W. MANER, E. MARTIN & G. SAADE. 2000. Prediction of parturition in humans using transabdominal uterine electromyographic activity recording. Am. J. Obstet. Gynecol. **182:** 536 (Abstr. 53).

Understanding Preterm Labor

JOHN R. G. CHALLIS,[a] STEPHEN J. LYE,[a] WILLIAM GIBB,[b] WENDY WHITTLE,[a] FALGUNI PATEL,[a] AND NADIA ALFAIDY[a]

[a]Departments of Physiology and Obstetrics & Gynaecology, University of Toronto, CIHR Group in Fetal and Neonatal Health and Development, CIHR Institute of Human Development, Child and Youth Health, Toronto, Canada

[b]Department of Obstetrics and Gynaecology, University of Ottawa, Ottawa, Canada

ABSTRACT: Increased uterine contractility at term and preterm results from activation and then stimulation of the myometrium. Activation can be provoked by mechanical stretch of the uterus and by an endocrine pathway resulting from increased activity of the fetal hypothalamic–pituitary–adrenal (HPA) axis. In fetal sheep, increased cortisol output during pregnancy regulates prostaglandin H synthase type 2 (PGHS2) expression in the placenta in an estrogen-independent manner, resulting in increased levels of PGE_2 in the fetal circulation. Later increases in maternal uterine expresssion of PGHS2 require elevations of estrogen and lead to increased concentrations of $PGF_2\alpha$ in the maternal circulation. Thus, regulation of PGHS2 at term is differentially controlled in fetal (trophoblast) and maternal (uterine epithelium) tissue. This difference may reflect expression of the glucocorticoid receptor (GR), but not estrogen receptor (ER), in placental trophoblast cells. In women, cortisol also contributes to increased PG production in fetal tissues through upregulation of PGHS2 (amnion and chorion) and downregulation of 15-OH PG dehydrogenase (chorion trophoblasts). The effect of cortisol on chorion expression of PGDH reverses a tonic stimulatory effect of progesterone, potentially through a paracrine or autocrine action. We have interpreted this interaction as a reflection of "progesterone withdrawal" in the primate, in relation to birth. Other agents, such as proinflammatory cytokines, similarly upregulate PGHS2 and decrease expression of PGDH, indicating the presence of several mechanisms by which labor at term or preterm may be initiated. These different mechanisms need to be considered in the development of strategies for the detection and management of the patient in preterm labor.

KEYWORDS: preterm labor; fetal hypothalamic–pituitary–adrenal axis; cortisol; progesterone withdrawal

INTRODUCTION

Preterm birth occurs in approximately 5 to 10% of all pregnancies. This figure may be higher in certain population groups and has not decreased over the past 20–30 years. Although some preterm births may be elective, approximately 30% occur in association with an underlying infectious process and about 50% are idiopathic

Address for correspondence: John R. G. Challis, University of Cambridge, Department of Obstetrics & Gynaecology, The Rosie Hospital, Robinson Way, Cambridge, England CB2 2SW. Voice: 416-978-2674; fax: 416-978-4940.

j.challis@utoronto.ca

preterm births of unknown cause. Preterm birth is associated with 70% of neonatal deaths and up to 75% of neonatal morbidity. Infants born preterm have an increased incidence of cerebral palsy, neurological handicap, and pulmonary disorders. The costs of caring for preterm babies in the United States has been estimated at around $8 billion annually. At present, there are no effective diagnostic indicators of preterm birth, and there are no effective treatments for this condition. Thus, the current direction of research remains to understand the underlying biochemistry of the birth process and to use that information to develop better diagnostic indicators and improve methods of therapeutic management.

PHASES OF PARTURITION

Uterine contractility during pregnancy and parturition can be divided into different phases.[1,2] Phase 0 of parturition corresponds to pregnancy, a time of relative uterine quiescence. Phase 1 of parturition is associated with *activation* of uterine function, wherein mechanical stretch or uterotrophic priming leads to upregulation of a cassette of genes required for contractions. These contraction-associated protein (CAP) genes includes connexin–43 (Cx43), the major protein of GAP junctions; agonist receptors; and proteins encoding ion channels. In phase 2 of parturition, the uterus can then be *stimulated* by uterotonins including prostaglandins, oxytocin, and corticotropin-releasing hormone (CRH). Phase 3 of parturition includes expulsion of the placenta and the involution process and has been attributed primarily to the effects of oxytocin.

Regulation of uterine quiescence during pregnancy (phase 0) has been discussed in several recent reviews.[1–4] Major effectors of myometrial relaxation, acting in a paracrine or endocrine fashion, include progesterone, relaxin, prostacyclin (PGI_2), parathyroid hormone–related peptide (PTH-rP), nitric oxide, and CRH, which may both inhibit and stimulate uterine contractility. These agents act in different ways, but in general result in increased intracellular levels of cyclic adenosine monophosphate (cAMP) or cyclic guanosine monophosphate (cGMP). These nucleotides inhibit intracellular calcium release and reduce the activity of the enzyme myosin light chain kinase (MLCK) that is required for shortening of the myofilaments. Several current strategies for managing preterm labor are directed at increasing intracellular cAMP and/or reducing the availability of calcium.

It is clear now that *activation* of myometrial function (phase 1) is driven through the fetal genotype and effected through two separate but interdependent pathways.[2] One involves activation of the fetal hypothalamic–pituitary–adrenal (HPA) axis. The second involves mechanical distension of the uterus, leading to stretch-related upregulation of CAP gene expression.

Maturation of fetal HPA function during late pregnancy is a consistent developmental change across species, including primates.[1–3] Extensive studies in fetal sheep have shown increased expression of CRH mRNA in parvocellular neurons of the paraventricular nucleus of the hypothalamus and of pro-opiomelanocortin (POMC) mRNA in the pars distalis of the fetal pituitary in late pregnancy. These changes correlate with increased concentrations of $ACTH_{1-39}$ in the fetal circulation. ACTH acts on the fetal adrenal to increase expression of key enzymes required for cortisol production (especially $P450_{C17}$) and to upregulate ACTH receptors in the fetal adrenal cortex. This allows enhanced binding and coupling to adenylate cyclase, resulting in increased sensitivity of the fetal adrenal gland to further stimulation by ACTH. Activation of the fetal HPA axis occurs in the presence of an adverse intrauterine enviroment, for example, with compromised uteroplacental blood flow and/or conditions of fetal hypoxemia. Fetal sheep made transiently hypoxemic had increased levels of hypothalamic CRH mRNA and pituitary POMC mRNA.[1] In late gestation, hypoxemia also led to increased levels of fetal adrenal ACTH receptor mRNA, consistent with increased overall responsiveness of the fetal HPA axis. When fetuses at two-thirds of term gestation were subjected to hypoxemia by repeated umbilical cord occlusion over several days, the adrenal cortisol response relative to the level of ACTH stimulation rose. Other experimental models of sustained, but episodic fetal hypoxemia produce similar fetal hormonal and cardiovascular responses and may result in shortened gestation length.

Increases in fetal HPA function in animal species such as sheep lead to changes in the placental output of progesterone before birth. During pregnancy, progesterone is required for uterine growth, but it simultaneously suppresses expression of CAP genes.[2] At term, in most animal species, the influence of progesterone on the myometrium declines, uterine stretch no longer stimulates uterine growth, and the increase in wall tension caused by continued fetal growth becomes translated into increased expression of CAP genes and myometrial activation. Mechanical stretch likely contributes to the greater incidence of preterm birth in pregnancies with multiple fetuses and may account for the higher incidence of preterm birth in pregnancies where the fetal size is large for gestational age. However, in women there does not appear to be a decline in circulating progesterone concentrations prepartum. We suggest below that this represents a mechanism to maintain relaxation of the lower uterine segment at the time of birth, while local antagonism of progesterone action in the fundal region of the uterus facilitates development of uterine contractions predominantly in that region.[1,2]

PROSTAGLANDINS AND PARTURITION

There is now compelling evidence that increased output of intrauterine prostaglandins (PGs) contributes to the drive toward myometrial contractility at term and preterm.[1,5] Studies in late pregnant sheep have helped clarify the endocrine pathways leading to altered PG output prepartum. In this species PGE_2 concentrations rise progressively in the fetal circulation over the last 15–20 days of gestation, corresponding temporally to the prepartum rise in fetal plasma cortisol and consistent with the suggestion of stimulatory effects of PGE_2 on the fetal HPA axis, as well as of cortisol on placental prostaglandin H synthase type 2 (PGHS2) gene expression.[1] $PGF_2\alpha$ rises in the maternal circulation, but only as a late event in pregnancy, coincident with the sharp prepartum rise in maternal free estradiol concentration. Thus, the possibility was raised that in late-gestation sheep, PGE_2 and $PGF_2\alpha$ were derived from different tissues within the pregnant uterus and their output was regulated by different control mechanisms.[6]

Previous studies had suggested that the prepartum rise of cortisol increased placental P450C17 expression, which allowed increased placental estrogen synthesis from C21 steroids. In turn, estrogen provoked increases in PG output. (See Challis *et al.*[1]) However, we found that placental PGHS2 mRNA and protein were detectable and increased before changes in placental P450C17 and that intra-fetal estradiol infusion had no stimulatory effect on placental PGHS2. Conversely, intra-fetal cortisol infusion for about 80 hours resulted in increased placental PGHS2 and fetal plasma PGE$_2$ concentrations even in the presence of an aromatase inhibitor. Therefore, this effect did not depend on the prepartum rise in placental estrogen output.[7] On the other hand, maternal uterine PGHS2 expression and PGF$_2\alpha$ output was attenuated by concurrent aromatase inhibition during cortisol infusion. These studies suggested that PGHS2 upregulation in placental trophoblasts could be stimulated directly by cortisol. We have now substantiated this conclusion using cultures of ovine placental trophoblasts treated with glucocorticoid *in vitro*. Regulation of PGHS2 in the maternal uterus required an increase in estrogen output, even during cortisol infusion. This finding is consistent with observations in nonpregnant sheep showing that estradiol treatment increases uterine PG output. In intact sheep at full term, the trophoblast cells express glucocorticoid receptor (GR) but not estrogen receptor (ER). Similarly, we found immunoreactive GR and GRα in the trophoblast cells, and the abundance of GRα protein was increased by cortisol infusion, in the presence or absence of aromatase inhibition (unpublished observations, W.L. Whittle). Therefore, it appears that the prepartum rise in fetal plasma cortisol increases GRα activity in the placenta and directly augments placental PG synthase. P450C17 protein levels were increased in animals treated with cortisol and with cortisol plus aromatase inhibition. Therefore P450C17 rises independently of the prepartum increase in estrogen. The results are consistent with the following sequence: cortisol upregulates placental PGHS$_2$ and the product PGE$_2$ stimulates placental P450C17, as suggested for other tissues including the adrenal gland. Definitive studies to prove this relationship of PGE$_2$ and P450C17 in the sheep placenta are still ongoing.

In women, prostaglandin production is discreetly compartmentalized within the tissues of the pregnant uterus.[1] PGE$_2$ is formed predominantly in amnion, and its output increases at the time of labor. Chorion and decidua also produce PGE$_2$. The presence in chorion of the enzyme 15-hydroxyprostaglandin dehydrogenase (PGDH) is presumed to cause metabolism of PGs generated in amnion and chorion, preventing their passage to the underlying tissues. Thus, in normal pregnancy those PGs that stimulate myometrial contractions are likely generated either within decidua or in the myometrium itself. In some cases of preterm birth, however, PGDH activity in chorion is diminished, the metabolic barrier reduced, and PGs generated within amnion or chorion could then provide the stimulus to myometrial contractions.[8] Studies on prostaglandin production from myometrium collected from women at the time of labor have led to divergent findings. Although some investigators have reported increased PG output, most reports have failed to demonstrate increased PG synthesis or PGHS activity in myometrium collected from women in labor at term or preterm.

Increased expression of PGHS2 occurs in response to a variety of growth factors including epidermal growth factor (EGF) and cytokines (interleukin-1, IL-1; tumor necrosis factor, TNF; and interleukin-6, IL-6).[5,9] The action of cytokines appears to be mediated through an NF-κB consensus sequence in the promoter region of PGHS2. This promoter also contains a cAMP response element and a glucocorticoid response element (GRE) at approximately 760 base pairs from the PGHS2 transcription start sign. Several years ago Gibb and colleagues[10,11] showed that human amnion cells maintained in monolayer tissue culture produced increased amounts of PGE_2 in a dose-dependent fashion in response to treatment with a synthetic glucocorticoid, dexamethasone. It remains unclear whether this action is on amniotic epithelium or fibroblast cells, since both contain glucocorticoid receptors (GR) and both have been reported to increase expression of PGHS2 upon glucocorticoid stimulation. However, in mixed cell cultures, the action of glucocorticoids is clearly dependent on interaction with GR and apparently requires activation of protein kinase C (PKC).

Proinflammatory cytokines also increase PGHS2 gene expression, mRNA, and protein levels and PG output by cultured amnion and chorion cells. Interestingly, antiinflammatory cytokines such as IL-10 attenuate the stimulatory effect of IL-1β on PGHS2 gene expression and activity.[12] Thus, *in vivo*, it is apparent that the relative amounts of eicosanoids and cytokines produced from an interactive cytokine–eicosanoid cascade will be critical in regulating the final response of the tissue and the level of prostaglandin produced.[9] These results also raise the interesting possibility that antiinflammatory cytokines might be used therapeutically to modulate the action of compounds such as IL-1.

PROSTAGLANDIN METABOLISM

Recently, it has become apparent that the biologically active levels of PG depend not only on rates of synthesis, but also on the rates of metabolism.[12] Normally, high levels of PGDH expressed in chorion trophoblasts would be expected to metabolize effectively PG generated within amnion or chorion. However, patients in preterm labor with an underlying infective process have markedly reduced numbers of trophoblasts in the chorion layer and dramatically reduced levels of PGDH activity.[8] In addition, approximately 15% of patients with idiopathic preterm labor had diminished expression of PGDH but normal presence of trophoblasts. PGDH activity is reduced modestly in chorion from patients at term, but is markedly diminished in myometrium and cervix of patients presenting in preterm labor. Thus, reduced prostaglandin metabolism appears to be an effective way of increasing prostaglandin levels that may then reach agonist PG receptors in a paracrine fashion. Furthermore, levels of matrix metalloproteinase (MMP)-9 in chorion are increased with preterm labor. Since this gelatinase enzyme contributes to the controlled degradation of collagen within the fetal membranes and MMP-9 activity is increased by PGE_2, this feed-forward cascade may also help explain the mechanism of preterm premature rupture of the membranes with MMP-9 as the predominant gelatinolytic activity.

Recent studies have been directed towards understanding the mechanism by which steroid hormones might regulate PGDH.[13] Surprisingly, these studies have also revealed a mechanism for local progesterone withdrawal within the human fetal membranes. Patel and colleagues[13] have shown that human chorionic PGDH gene expression and activity is inhibited by glucocorticoids (cortisol, betamethasone, and dexamethasone) and maintained in a tonic fashion by progesterone. Chorion trophoblasts express the enzyme 3β-hydroxysteroid dehydrogenase (3β-HSD) and have the capacity to produce their own progesterone from pregnenolone. Inhibition of

3β-HSD enzyme with the drug Trilostane inhibited progesterone output from chorion trophoblast cells and reduced PGDH mRNA levels. Replacement of progesterone or a synthetic progestagen restored PGDH activity. This effect could be blocked, in part, by a progesterone receptor antagonist. However, the action of progesterone to restore PGDH could also be blocked by a specific GR antagonist. This observation suggested that progesterone, produced locally within chorion, acts throughout pregnancy to maintain chorionic PGDH activity. It does so, however, through interacting with GR. At term, increased availability of endogenous cortisol would displace progesterone from GR, resulting in loss of the stimulation to PGDH and also a direct inhibitory effect on PGDH expression. This interaction, whereby the effects of progesterone are mediated through GR but can be opposed by increased output of glucocorticoid, may provide a mechanism for producing local progesterone withdrawal in the human uterus. It has been suggested elsewhere that this activity may be greater in the fundal area, thereby contributing to regionalized changes in uterine contractions.[1,14]

Surprisingly, we found that the biologically inactive corticosteroid, cortisone, was almost as effective as cortisol in inhibiting PGDH in chorion cells, but not in placental trophoblast cells.[12] In chorion, the action of cortisone could be blocked by a GR antagonist and was completely attenuated in the presence of the drug carbenexolone. This drug, an active ingredient of liquorice, inhibits the enzyme 11β-HSD-1. 11β-HSD-1 is abundantly expressed in chorion trophoblasts, and its predominant activity is to convert cortisone to cortisol. Thus, these cells have the potential to form cortisol locally from cortisone, in addition to forming progesterone locally from pregnenolone. Therapeutic regulation of PGDH, theoretically, could be accomplished by steroid hormones or by drugs that alter the levels of 11β-HSD-1.

CORTICOTROPIN-RELEASING HORMONE AND PRETERM LABOR

It is now well established that the concentrations of CRH in maternal blood rise progressively during human pregnancy.[15,16] This rise correlates with increased levels of CRH mRNA and CRH peptide in placental tissue.[17] In the circulation, CRH is largely associated with a high-affinity circulating CRH-binding protein (CRH-BP) produced in the liver, placenta, and also in other sites including the brain. CRH-BP effectively blocks the action of placental CRH on the maternal pituitary and on the myometrium. Near term, and in association with preterm labor, CRH-BP concentrations fall, coincident with the increase in circulating CRH.[16] Thus, it has been suggested that there is a substantial increase in free CRH concentrations in systemic plasma as a component of the trigger to the labor process.

Regulation of placental CRH output is multifactorial and has been reviewed extensively.[15] Briefly, CRH gene expression and CRH output by placental trophoblast cells is paradoxically increased by glucocorticoids. CRH output from placenta and fetal membranes also increases in response to prostaglandins, cytokines, and catecholamines and is decreased by nitric oxide and progesterone. Karalis and Majzoub[18] have suggested that the inhibitory effect of progesterone is exerted through binding to GR in trophoblast cells. At term, an increased level of cortisol is suggested to displace progesterone bound to GR, and this is reflected as an increase in CRH output. Thus the mechanism of interaction between progesterone and cortisol in the regulation of CRH is similar to that proposed for the regulation of PGDH.

The action of CRH on the intrauterine tissues and myometrium is effected through an extensive network of high-affinity CRH receptors with different specificities. There are two main classes of CRH receptor, CRH-R1 and CRH-R2. In myometrium, CRH acts by binding to CRH-R1, which is coupled to $G_{\alpha}s$, leading to stimulation of cAMP output. Thus the primary effect of CRH throughout pregnancy is likely to be one of uterine relaxation. The binding affinity of the CRH receptor in human myometrium increases during pregnancy, but then decreases before parturition. Studies by Grammatopoulos and Hillhouse[19,20] have suggested that oxytocin effects this change by upregulating a protein kinase C, which phosphorylates the CRH receptor protein, resulting in desensitization and loss of the inhibitory influence of CRH on myometrium. Therefore, the peptide CRH may act as an inhibitor or stimulant to the myometrium depending on the affinity and second messenger of the different receptor species.

The differential effects of CRH on the myometrium may also contribute to the regionalization of myometrial activity at term and in the preterm period. Stevens and colleagues[21] showed that the expression of CRH-R1 in myometrium collected from the lower uterine segment was higher in patients in labor compared to those not in labor. Furthermore, expression of CRH-R1 was substantially higher in the lower segment compared to fundal myometrium when paired samples of tissue from individual patients were examined. Thus at the time of labor, CRH may promote relaxation of the lower segment, but stimulate activity in the body of the uterus. This stimulatory action could be direct; it could also be indirect, since CRH stimulates output of prostaglandins by upregulating PGHS2 and downregulating PGDH in human fetal membranes.

There has been much interest recently in the possibility that elevations of maternal plasma CRH concentration may be used to predict which women are destined to enter preterm labor. McLean *et al.*[22] demonstrated elevated maternal plasma concentrations of CRH as early as 14–16 weeks of pregnancy in women who subsequently delivered preterm and lower concentrations of CRH in the plasma of women who delivered post-term. Korebrits *et al.*[23] found that maternal plasma CRH concentrations were elevated in patients at 28–32 weeks' gestation with an initial diagnosis of threatened preterm labor, who delivered within 48 hours. However, CRH concentrations were within the normal range in patients with the same initial diagnosis who proceeded to delivery at term. At the present time, it seems unlikely that a single measurement of maternal plasma CRH will provide an adequate means of predicting the patient who is at risk of preterm labor. However, we and others have suggested that a combination of biochemical tests including CRH and salivary estriol, combined with measurements of fibronectin, may be of sufficient sensitivity and specificity to be of clinical use.

BIRTH—AN INTEGRATED CASCADE?

From the preceding discussion, it should be apparent that birth, at term and preterm, results from processes leading to increased prostaglandin output. Glucocorticoids have a central role in those processes. Glucocorticoids also stimulate CRH

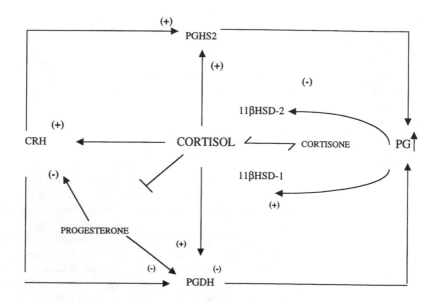

FIGURE 1. Cortisol (F) and prostaglandin (PG) interactions in the human fetal membranes. PGHS2, prostaglandin synthase type 2; PGDH, 15-hydroxyprostaglandin dehydrogenase; 11β-HSD-1, 11β-HSD-2, 11β-hydroxysteroid dehydrogenase Type 1, Type 2; CRH, corticotrophin-releasing hormone.

output within placenta and fetal membranes, and CRH similarly upregulates PGHS2 and downregulates PGDH. The effects of CRH may be modulated by the state of the CRH receptor. Oxytocin appears to play a key role in changing the affinity of CRH receptor interaction. Oxytocin could be derived from the systemic circulation, but also could be derived locally from chorion and/or decidua.

Increased levels of cortisol could be derived from the maternal circulation, for example in association with a maternal stress response or from the fetus following precocious activation of the fetal HPA axis. In addition, cortisol can be formed locally within chorion trophoblast cells from the inactive precursor cortisone. The expression of 11β-HSD-1 enzyme that effects this conversion increases in chorion trophoblasts progressively during human gestation. More recently, it has been shown (unpublished results, N. Alfaidy, J.R.G. Challis) that the activity of 11β-HSD-1 is increased significantly by prostaglandins through a mechanism that involves increased release of intracellular calcium and phosphorylation of the enzyme. In this way, increased production of prostaglandins (PGE_2, $PGF_2\alpha$) increased 11β-HSD-1 activity, leading to more cortisol formation from cortisone (FIG. 1). Cortisol, in turn, increases further PG production. It is evident that, with infection, other agents such as cytokines can intercede in this series of loops by stimulating PGHS2 and downregulating PGDH expression. It is also apparent that the mechanisms that predispose a woman to preterm labor almost certainly vary at different stages of gestation. The incidence of preterm birth in association with chorioamnionitis is higher earlier in pregnancy. Later in gestation, the fetal stress response may predominate. In this situation, fetal HPA activation increases fetal cortisol output, which in turn upregulates placental CRH expression. This is consistent with elevated concentrations of CRH in the umbilical cord plasma of fetuses with intrauterine growth restriction (IUGR). Recently, it has been shown that placental CRH also drives fetal adrenal steroidogenesis. This leads to increased production of DHEA from the fetal zone of the fetal adrenal gland. DHEA in turn is aromatized in the placenta to estrogen, thereby contributing to myometrial activation.

The ability to predict or diagnose the patient in preterm labor will be invaluable in selecting those women for whom prenatal corticosteroids should be administered to help promote fetal pulmonary maturity. There is increasing concern about the use of repeated corticosteroid administration at regular intervals to women who may not actually be at risk of preterm birth. Animal studies and human studies have now demonstrated detrimental effects of glucocorticoids on fetal growth, glucose homeostasis, cardiovascular function, and neural development. Clinically, the aim should be to restrict the use of corticosteroids and tocolytic treatment to those patients in whom preterm labor has been diagnosed. The purpose of continuing studies in this area will be to achieve those objectives.

ACKNOWLEDGMENTS

Work in the author's laboratory has been supported by the Canadian Institute of Health Research (CIHR) Group in Fetal and Neonatal Health and Development. We gratefully acknowledge support from the Parke-Davies Fellowship Trust of the University of Cambridge.

REFERENCES

1. CHALLIS, J.R.G., S.G. MATTHEWS, W. GIBB & S.J. LYE. 2000. Endocrine and paracrine regulation of birth at term and preterm. Endocr. Rev. **21:** 514–550.
2. LYE, S.K., C-W. OU, T.G. TEOH, *et al.* 1998. The molecular basis of labour and tocolysis. Fetal Matern. Med. Rev. **10:** 121–136.
3. LIGGINS, G.C. & G.D. THORBURN. 1994. Initiation of parturition. *In* Marshall's Physiology of Reproduction. G.E. Lamming, Ed.: 863–1002. Chapman and Hall. London, UK.
4. NORWITZ, E.R., J.N. ROBINSON & J.R.G. CHALLIS. 1999. The control of labor. N. Engl. J. Med. **341:** 660–666.
5. KNISS, D.A. 1999. Cyclooxygenases in reproductive medicine and biology. J. Soc. Gynecol. Invest. **6:** 285–292.
6. GYOMEREY, S., S.J. LYE, W. GIBB & J.R.G. CHALLIS. 2000. Fetal to maternal progression of prostaglandin H_2 synthase-2 expression in ovine intrauterine tissues during the course of labor. Biol. Reprod. **62:** 797–805.
7. WHITTLE, W.L., A.C. HOLLOWAY, S.J. LYE, *et al.* 2000. Prostaglandin production at the onset of ovine parturition is regulated by both estrogen-independent and estrogen-dependent pathways. Endocrinology **141:** 3783–3790.
8. SANGA, R.K., J.C. WALTON, C.M. ENSOR, *et al.* 1994. Immunohistochemical localization, mRNA abundance and activity of 15-hydroxprostaglandin dehydrogenase in placenta and fetal membranes during term and preterm labor. J. Clin. Endocrinol. Metab. **78:** 982–989.
9. KEELAN, J.A., T. SATO & M.D. MITCHELL. 1997. Interleukin (IL)-6 and IL-8 production by human amnion: regulation cytokines, growth factors, glucocorticoids, phorbol esters, and bacterial lipopolysacharide. Biol. Reprod. **57:** 1438–1444.

10. GIBB, W. & J.C. LAVOIE. 1990. Effects of glucocorticoids on prostaglandin formation by human amnion. Can. J. Physiol. Pharmacol. **68:** 671–676.
11. ECONOMOPOULOS, P., M. SUN, B. PURGINA & W. GIBB. 1996. Glucocorticoids stimulate prostaglandin H synthase type-2 (PGHS-2) in the fibroblast cells in human amnion cultures. Mol. Cell. Endocrinol. **117:** 141–147.
12. CHALLIS, J.R.G., F.A. PATEL & F. POMINI. 1999. Prostaglandin dehydrogenase and the initiation of labor. J. Perinat. Med. **27:** 26–34.
13. PATEL, F.A., V.L. CLIFTON, K. CHWALISZ & J.R.G. CHALLIS. 1999. Steroid regulation of prostaglandin dehydrogenase activity and expression in human term placenta and chorio-decidua in relation to labor. J. Clin. Endocrinol. Metab. **84:** 291–299.
14. SPAREY, C., S. ROBSON, J. BAILEY, et al. 1999. The differential expression of myometrial connexin-43, cyclooygenase-1 and –2 and $G_s\alpha$ proteins in the upper and lower segments of the human uterus during pregnancy and labor. J. Clin. Endocrinol. Metab. **84:** 1705–1710.
15. PETRAGLIA, F., P. FLORIO, C. NAPPI, & A.R. GENAZZANI. 1996. Peptide signaling in human placenta and membranes: autocrine, paracrine and endocrine mechanisms. Endocr. Rev. **17:** 156–186.
16. LINTON, E.A., A.V. PERKINS, R.J. WOODS, et al. 1993. Corticotropin releasing hormone-binding protein (CRH-BP); plasma levels decrease during the third trimester of normal human pregnancy. J. Clin. Endocrinol. Metab. **76:** 260–262.
17. FRIM, D.M., R.L. EMMANUEL, B.G. ROBINSON, et al. 1988. Characterization and gestational regulation of corticotropin-releasing hormone messenger RNA in human placenta. J. Clin. Invest. **82:** 287–292.
18. KARALIS, K. & J.A. MAJZOUB. 1995. Regulation of placental corticotrophin-releasing hormone by steroids—possible implication in labor initiation. Ann. N.Y. Acad. Sci. **771:** 551–555.
19. GRAMMATOPOULOS, D. & E.W. HILLHOUSE. 1999. Activation of protein kinase C by oxytocin inhibits the biological activity of the human myometrial corticiotropin-releasing hormone receptor at term. Endocrinology **140:** 585–594.
20. GRAMMATOPOULOS, D. & E.W. HILLHOUSE. 1999. Role of corticotrophin-releasing hormone in onset of labour. Lancet **354:** 1546–1549.
21. STEVENS, Y., J.R.G. CHALLIS & S.J. LYE. 1998. Corticotropin-releasing hormone receptor subtype 1 (CRH-R1) is significantly upregulated at the time of labor in the human myometrium. J. Clin. Endocrinol. Metab. **83:** 4107–4115.
22. MCLEAN, M., A. BISITS, J. DAVIES, et al. 1995. A placental clock controlling the length of human pregnancy. Nat. Med. **1:** 460–463.
23. KOREBRITS, C., M.M. RAMIREZ, L. WATSON, et al. 1998. Maternal corticotropin-releasing hormone is increased with impending preterm birth. J. Clin. Endocrinol. Metab. **83:** 1585–1591.

Ectopic Pregnancy

From Surgical Emergency to Medical Management

ANTHONY A. LUCIANO,[a] GERARD ROY,[b] AND EUGENIO SOLIMA[c]

[a]*Department of Obstetrics and Gynecology, University of Connecticut Health Center, Center for Fertility and Reproductive Endocrinology, New Britain General Hospital, New Britain, Connecticut 06050, USA*

[b]*Department of Obstetrics and Gynecology, University of Connecticut Health Center, Farmington, Connecticut, USA*

[c]*Department of Obstetrics and Gynecology, Ospedale Degli Infermi, Biella, Italy*

ABSTRACT: During the past 25 years, the incidence of ectopic pregnancy has progressively increased while the morbidity and mortality have substantially decreased, and the treatment has progressed from salpingectomy by laparotomy to conservative surgery by laparoscopy and more recently to medical therapy. This therapeutic transition from surgical emergency to medical management has been attributed to early diagnosis through the use of sensitive assays for hCG and the high definition of vaginal ultrasound. By using these sensitive diagnostic tools, we are now able to select those patients who are most likely to respond to medical management versus those who are at high risk of rupture and require surgery. Besides being less invasive and associated with significantly lower risks, medical therapy with methotrexate results in significant cost savings, which have been calculated to be approximately $3,000 per treated patient. Our goal is to identify those patients with ectopic pregnancy who are most likely to respond to methotrexate therapy and least likely to develop significant side effects. Recent studies have helped us define the predictors of success with methotrexate treatment in women with ectopic pregnancy. The reported success rates of treating ectopic pregnancy with methotrexate vary from 71% to 100%. The highest success rates have been reported from institutions that have detailed diagnostic and therapeutic protocols, readily available assays for serum hCG levels, high-resolution vaginal probe ultrasound, and support staff that can closely monitor clinical response. The importance of developing specific protocols to create a clinical environment that supports the effective use of medical therapy for ectopic pregnancy is confirmed by the associated cost savings, decreased morbidity, and patient preference. Modern diagnostic advances and minimally invasive treatments coupled with improved success rates for assisted reproductive technologies should reduce the morbidity and mortality associated with ectopic pregnancy and offer the affected couple a much more optimistic outlook for subsequent reproductive potential.

KEYWORDS: ectopic pregnancy; methotrexate; vaginal probe ultrasound; operative laparoscopy; laparotomy; salpingostomy; salpingectomy

Address for correspondence: Anthony A. Luciano, M.D., Professor of Obstetrics and Gynecology, University of Connecticut Health Center, Director of Center for Fertility and Women's Health, New Britain General Hospital, New Britain, CT 06050. Voice: 860-224-5469; fax: 860-224-5764.

aluciano@nbgh.org

INTRODUCTION

Ectopic pregnancy is a disaster in human reproduction. It is the result of a flaw in primate reproductive physiology that allows the conceptus to implant and develop outside the endometrial cavity, and it inevitably ends in the demise of the fetus. If not diagnosed and treated expeditiously, it may also take the life of the mother or, at the very least, compromise her future ability to reproduce. Although it has been recognized for over 400 years, ectopic pregnancy continues to be an ever-increasing affliction, affecting approximately 2% of all pregnancies.[1] The rising incidence of ectopic pregnancy in the past 25 years has been attributed to a number of factors including a greater prevalence of sexually transmitted disease, tubal sterilization and reversal, delayed childbearing, assisted reproductive technologies, and more successful clinical detection. There have been significant improvements, however, in the past decade in the ability to diagnose and treat this disease, thereby limiting its impact on the health of women.

Robert Lawson Tait, a British surgeon, is credited for performing the first successful laparotomy for ruptured tubal pregnancy in 1883.[2] At a time when ectopic pregnancy was associated with a >60% mortality rate, Tait lost only two patients of the first 42 that he operated on. By the 1920s immediate laparotomy and ligation of the bleeding vessels with removal of the affected tube had become the rule rather than the exception. This approach remained the standard of care until the late 1970s, when operative laparoscopy replaced lapartomy and salpingostomy replaced salpingectomy. During the past decade, the medical management of ectopic pregnancy has been successfully implemented, and in the future it may supplant the surgical treatment in the majority of cases.

EPIDEMIOLOGY

Until 1970, more than 80% of ectopic pregnancies were diagnosed after rupture, resulting in significant morbidity and mortality. With the excellent resolution obtained from pelvic ultrasound, the high sensitivity of radioimmunoassay for human chorionic gonadotropin (hCG), and the increased vigilance of the clinician, more than 80% of ectopic pregnancies can now be diagnosed before rupture. This has resulted in a tremendous decline in the mortality from ectopic pregnancy in the past two decades. As FIGURE 1 illustrates, in 1970 the case fatality rate was 35.5 per 10,000 ectopic pregnancies, which declined to 2.6 by 1992.[4] This >90% reduction in mortality occurred at a time when the overall incidence increased more than five-fold from 17,800 to 108,800.[1,5] Mortality from ectopic pregnancy, however, continues to be the number one cause of pregnancy-related death in the first trimester and accounts for approximately 9% of pregnancy-related deaths overall.[5] The risk for developing ectopic pregnancy is higher in black and other minority races (relative risk 1.6) and a disproportionate number of minority women, especially teenagers, die of the disease. Age, too, is an important risk factor, with increases of three- to fourfold noted in women 35–44 years of age compared to 15–24-year-old women.[5]

Theoretically, anything that impedes migration of the conceptus to the uterine cavity may predispose a woman to develop an ectopic gestation. These may be intrinsic anatomic defects in the tubal epithelium, hormonal factors that interfere with

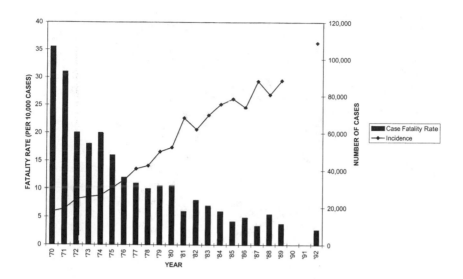

FIGURE 1. Case fatality rate and incidence of ectopic pregnancy (1970–1992). CDC data.

normal transport of the conceptus, or pathologic conditions that affect normal tube functioning. These risk factors are summarized in TABLE 1. Although factors such as progestin-containing IUD use at the time of conception and ovulation induction with clomiphene citrate may confer a higher relative risk, the most important explanation for the rising incidence of ectopic pregnancy is probably pelvic infection. High-risk behavior among teenagers and the decreasing age of coitarche have exposed more women to genital tract pathogens for a greater length of their reproductive years. The most common of these is now *Chlamydia trachomatis*, an organism that causes a range of clinical illness from asymptomatic cervicitis to salpingitis and frank pelvic inflammatory disease. Approximately 5–20% of cultures taken from women in the U.S. register positive for chlamydia, and numerous studies have shown the association between seropositivity for this organism and pelvic adhesive disease, salpingitis, tubal occlusion, and ectopic pregnancy.[6–8] Other organisms, such as *Neisseria gonorrhea,* are also frequently identified in cultures from patients with pelvic inflammatory disease, and with each episode the risk of tubal disease and ectopic pregnancy rises dramatically.[9,10] Effective vaccination against *Chlamydia trachomatis* is currently being explored. When it becomes clinically available, it will have a significant impact, not only on the incidence of ectopic pregnancy but also on the function and health of the reproductive system of women in the next generation.

SYMPTOMS

Besides the symptoms commonly associated with early pregnancy, women with ectopic pregnancy frequently experience pelvic pain and vaginal bleeding. (See TABLE 2.) The bleeding may range from light spotting to a heavy flow and may be

TABLE 1. Major contributing factors and associated relative risk for ectopic pregnancy

Risk factors	Relative risk
Current use of intrauterine devices	11.9
Use of clomiphene citrate	10.0
Prior tubal surgery	5.6
Pelvic inflammatory disease	4.0
Infertility	2.9
Induced abortion	2.5
Adhesions	2.4
Abdominal surgery	2.3
T-shaped uterus	2.0
Myomata	1.7
Progestin-only oral contraceptives	1.6

NOTE: Adapted from Marchbanks et al.[5]

the only sign of a pregnancy complication. First-trimester bleeding in itself is rather nonspecific, and up to 20% of women who subsequently have normal pregnancies may have this experience. Typically, women present to the emergency room with a complaint of pelvic pain as well, which may be sharp or cramping in nature. Unilateral rather than midline or diffuse pelvic discomfort should always increase the index of suspicion for tubal pregnancy. Shoulder pain is even more disconcerting, as it suggests phrenic nerve irritation from intraperitoneal blood beneath the diaphragm secondary to ruptured ectopic pregnancy. About one-third of patients with ectopic pregnancies experience syncope, which may be the result of a vaso-vagal response to visceral irritation and pain, or hypotension due to hypovolemia.[11] Oftentimes the symptoms of ectopic pregnancy may be difficult to distinguish from other complications of first-trimester pregnancy including spontaneous abortion, ruptured or bleeding corpus luteum cyst, and adnexal torsion. Nongynecological conditions such as urinary tract infection or calculi, diverticulitis, appendicitis, or other pathologic conditions of the bowel may also mimic the symptoms of ectopic pregnancy, further clouding the diagnosis and necessitating additional clinical evaluation. (See TABLE 3.)

PHYSICAL FINDINGS

The signs of ectopic pregnancy include lower abdominal tenderness with or without rebound and pelvic tenderness, usually much worse on the affected side. Abdominal rigidity, involuntary guarding, and severe tenderness as well as evidence of hypovolemic shock such as orthostatic blood pressure changes and tachycardia should alert the clinician to a surgical emergency that may occur in up to 20% of cases. On pelvic exam, the uterus may be slightly enlarged and soft, and there may be

TABLE 2. Signs and symptoms suggestive of ectopic pregnancy

Nausea, breast fullness, fatigue, interruption of menses

Lower abdominal pain, heavy cramping, shoulder pain

Uterine bleeding, spotting

Pelvic tenderness, enlarged, soft uterus

Adnexal mass, tenderness

Positive pregnancy test

Serum levels of hCG of <6000 mIU/ml at 6 weeks

Less than 66% increase in hCG titers in 48 hours

Serum progesterone <25 ng/ml

Aspiration of nonclotting blood on culdocentesis

Absence of gestational sac in the uterus by U/S when β-hCG titer exceeds discriminatory threshold

Gestational sac outside the uterus by U/S

TABLE 3. Differential diagnosis in cases of suspected ectopic pregnancy

Spontaneous abortion

Ruptured ovarian cyst

Corpus luteum hemorrhagicum

Adnexal torsion

Pelvic inflammatory disease

Endometriosis

Urolithiasis

Urinary tract infection

Appendicitis

Other lower gastrointestinal tract diseases

uterine or cervical motion tenderness suggesting peritoneal inflammation. An adnexal mass may be palpated, but it is usually difficult to differentiate from the ipsilateral ovary and is felt on the side opposite the ectopic pregnancy in 20% of cases.[11] Culdocentesis with the aspiration of nonclotting blood may also assist in making the diagnosis of ectopic pregnancy. A recent study found culdocentesis to be positive in 83% of ectopic cases. Nevertheless, its predictive values for ruptured versus nonruptured ectopic pregnancies were only 50% and 58%, respectively.[12] Although relatively easy to perform, culdocentesis may be quite painful and cannot exclude other sources of intraperitoneal bleeding such as corpus luteum hemorrhagicum. Its use has largely been supplanted by vaginal probe ultrasound, which can easily reveal free fluid in the abdomen and identify blood by its echogenic appearance.[13] In most cases where a surgical emergency is not apparent or when the patient is relatively asymptomatic but at high risk for ectopic pregnancy, further diagnostic tests may be necessary to confirm or exclude the diagnosis.

DIAGNOSIS

Serum Screens—Human Chorionic Gonadotropin

Awareness of the possibility of an ectopic pregnancy is the most important factor in its early detection. Therefore, the first step is to establish the diagnosis of pregnancy, which can now be done as early as 10 days after ovulation using the newer and more sensitive serum assays for the beta subunit of human chorionic gonadotropin (hCG). Urine test kits have also become sensitive and reliable enough to detect pregnancy before the first missed menses, but blood tests remain the gold standard and offer the convenience of being able to quantitate the hCG level from the same specimen. Once pregnancy has been confirmed, the serum hCG titer and the change in titers over subsequent days become important in managing the patient at risk.

In 1981 Kadar et al. discovered that in early normal gestations hCG levels double every 1.98 days.[14] Subsequent investigators have reported the doubling time to be dependent on gestational age, with 1.5 days for gestations less than 5 weeks and every 3.5 days at 7 or more weeks of gestation, or when levels exceed 10,000 mIU/ml.[15] In ectopic pregnancy, only one-third of patients show a normal serum hCG rise. In two-thirds of patients with ectopic gestations, hCG levels fail to double every two to three days, plateau, or decline over time. However, the finding of an abnormal hCG pattern allows only for the distinction from normal pregnancy. In fact, abnormal hCG pattern is consistent not only with ectopic gestation but also with intrauterine pregnancies that will ultimately end in abortion. Less than 25% of ectopic pregnancies have hCG concentrations of 6000 mIU/ml or greater at the initial evaluation, and pregnancies that demonstrate less than a 66% increase in hCG levels during a 48-hour period are either ectopic or aborting pregnancies. In very early pregnancy, 64% of women with ectopic pregnancy may initially have a normal doubling of serum hCG levels.[16] Thus, a normal rise in hCG levels does not reliably differentiate an ectopic from an intrauterine pregnancy. Using Kadar's criterion alone, 15% of normal uterine pregnancies would fall in the ectopic category, and 13% of the ectopic pregnancies would be missed. Besides being associated with lower titers and slower increases in the serum concentration of hCG than normal pregnancies, ectopics, after treatment, are also associated with significantly slower declines in serum hCG titers than spontaneous abortions and may take up to four weeks to return to zero.[17]

In summary, serum hCG levels are useful in (1) diagnosing pregnancy when positive, (2) identifying abnormal pregnancy (aborting or ectopic) when levels do not rise appropriately, and (3) monitoring the resolution of the ectopic gestation once therapy has been initiated. The major disadvantage in relying on following hCG titers to distinguish between normal and abnormal first-trimester pregnancies is the potential delay in diagnosis of ectopic pregnancy and its attendant morbidity. Hence the need for additional diagnostic tests, including serum progesterone levels and ultrasonographic studies.

Progesterone

There is little doubt that a single serum progesterone level can help differentiate ectopic from normal intrauterine gestation.[18,19] As yet, however, there is no consensus on one value that can be used to reliably differentiate normal from abnormal because of considerable overlap in progesterone levels between these two groups. A single serum progesterone value of 17.5 ng/ml is considered by McCord *et al.* to be the cut-off value between high-risk and normal pregnancy.[20] In their study, however, 8.3% of ectopic pregnancies were associated with a serum progesterone above the cut-off value. Using a progesterone value >25 ng/ml excluded ectopic pregnancy with 97.4% certainty in a large study by Stovall *et al.* Progesterone levels of 5 ng/ml or less indicate a nonviable pregnancy, ectopic or intrauterine, and exclude normal pregnancy with 100% sensitivity.[21] Although inexpensive, the usefulness of serum progesterone assays is limited because a significant number of women tested will fall in the indeterminate range between 5 and 25 ng/ml. Progesterone assays are also unreliable in differentiating viable from nonviable pregnancies in women who have conceived following ovulation induction or *in vitro* fertilization because of excessive progesterone production by multiple corpora lutea.

Numerous other serum and urine assays are currently being explored to distinguish normal from abnormal pregnancy. These include assays for pregnanediol glucoronide,[22,23] placental proteins,[24] creatinine kinase,[25] β-hCG core fragment,[26] and a quadruple serum screen including progesterone, estriol, hCG, and alpha feto-protein.[27] All of these assays are helpful in distinguishing ectopic from normal gestations, but it remains to be seen how reliably they will differentiate ectopic from abnormal intrauterine gestations. Of the tests mentioned above, only progesterone has had much clinical usefulness thus far. A recent study by Predanic found that elevated serum levels of Ca-125 greater than 112 IU/ml were useful in differentiating tubal abortion from viable ectopic pregnancy, but they are not helpful in its diagnosis.[28]

Ultrasound

Transabdominal

Currently, ectopic pregnancy can be detected earlier and more precisely with a combination of pelvic sonograms and measurements of serum hCG levels. Kadar *et al.* introduced two concepts to aid in the diagnosis of ectopic pregnancy: (1) The appearance of an intrauterine gestational sac by abdominal ultrasound correlates with a serum hCG level of 6,000–6,500 mIU/ml[28]; and (2) the doubling of hCG levels every 48 hours indicates a normal pregnancy. When the serum hCG level is above 6500 mIU/ml, the absence of an intrauterine sac strongly suggests an ectopic pregnancy. The absence of an apparent intrauterine sac with hCG levels below 6000 mIU/ml suggests an abnormal pregnancy—ectopic or spontaneous abortion.[29]

Transvaginal

Better and more accurate diagnostic results may now be obtained with high-frequency endovaginal transducers, which are capable of reliably visualizing a normal gestational sac in 98% of cases after the fifth week of pregnancy, when hCG levels are greater than 1000 mIU/ml (First International Reference Preparation).[30] The absence of an intrauterine gestational sac above this level should indicate an ec-

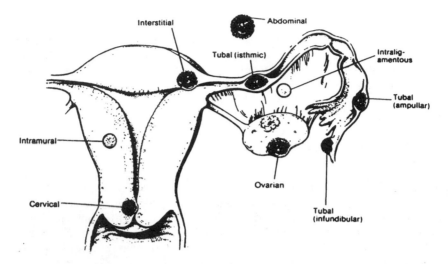

FIGURE 2. Sites of ectopic pregnancies (ampullary 92%, isthmic 4%, interstitial 2.5%, ovarian 0.4%, cervical 0.1%, others 1%).

topic pregnancy until proven otherwise. Vaginal probe U/S may reveal the presence of echogenic fluid, which is highly suggestive of ruptured ectopic pregnancy, and the presence of a decidual cyst (cast) indicates ectopic pregnancy in 80% of cases.[31] The experienced sonographer can usually differentiate this "single-ring" finding from an early intrauterine gestational sac, which has a characteristic "double-ring" sign of decidua around a chorionic sac.[32,33] The presence of a yolk sac inside a larger ring adds confidence to the diagnosis of intrauterine pregnancy, even if an embryo cannot be visualized.[34] Additionally, Yeh has described other signs of very early intrauterine gestation, even before an intrauterine sac is apparent, including an "intradecidual sign," which is an echogenic area within the thickened decidua seen as early as 25 days after the last menstrual period, and a "double-bleb sign" seen approximately two weeks later. This "double-bleb sign" is the first evidence of a developing embryo and is caused by an embryonic disc located between the amniotic and yolk sacs.[35] Endometrial stripe thickness has also been evaluated and in 97% of cases is suggestive of abnormal pregnancy, mostly ectopic, when less than 8 mm.[36]

The vast majority of ectopic pregnancies, about 95%, occur in the ampulla where fertilization takes place. However, they may occur anywhere along the tube, from fimbria to cornu, as well as extratubal sites such as the cervix, ovary, and abdominal cavity (FIG. 2); therefore, all of these areas must be screened.

In summary, the diagnosis of ectopic pregnancy can usually be established by the combination of serum hCG and progesterone levels and vaginal ultrasound evaluation. Abnormally rising serum hCG levels indicate an abnormal pregnancy, which may be either in the uterus or ectopic. Serum progesterone levels greater than 25 ng/ml indicate a normal pregnancy, unless conceived with assisted reproductive technologies. Serum progesterone levels between 5 and 25 ng/ml should heighten suspicion for an abnormal pregnancy either inside the uterus or ectopic. Serum progesterone levels below 5 ng/ml indicate a nonviable pregnancy, either intra- or extrauterine, which will most likely abort spontaneously. For pregnancies with serum hCG levels ≥1000 mIU/ml, the vaginal probe ultrasound will establish either the presence of an intrauterine pregnancy or not. If not in the uterus, the pregnancy is surely ectopic, whether or not it is visualized in an extrauterine site. Clinical correlation of these findings with respect to menstrual dating and ovulation pattern is especially helpful in achieving the correct diagnosis.

There may be situations, however, in which the hCG level is below the discriminatory threshold for vaginal ultrasound, there are no evident adnexal masses, and the patient is hemodynamically stable and without significant pain. In these cases, watchful waiting and assessment of hCG rise on an outpatient basis may be necessary. The patient should be asked to remain close to home and immediately report any worsening pelvic or shoulder pain, lightheadedness, tachycardia, or severe fatigue. Patients who are not compliant or have no one else at home who can assist them should be admitted until the diagnosis becomes clear. If the pregnancy is deemed nonviable by evidence of falling hCG levels or progesterone <5 ng/ml, or is otherwise unwanted, dilatation and curettage (D&C) with frozen section evaluation of uterine curettings may be useful.[37] If villi are present, the diagnosis of ectopic pregnancy may be ruled out. The only exceptions to this rule are cases of heterotopic pregnancies, which are becoming progressively more common with the expanding role of assisted reproductive technologies. If the D&C proves inconclusive, a diagnostic laparoscopy should be performed. The laparoscopy serves not only to make a definitive diagnosis but also to treat the ectopic pregnancy and associated intraperitoneal pathology if present.[38,39]

TREATMENT

Surgical Options

Salpingotomy versus Salpingectomy

The treatment options for ectopic pregnancies have broadened considerably in the past 10 years. Before this, laparatomy with salpingectomy was the standard practice. During the past 10 years, a more conservative surgical approach to unruptured ectopic pregnancy has been advocated to preserve tubal function. Several procedures have been successfully carried out, including linear salpingotomy, "milking" the pregnancy out of the distal ampulla, and removal of that segment of the fallopian tube which contains the ectopic gestation followed by reanastomosis. Recent reports from the literature indicate that the outcome in terms of either viable birth or repeat ectopic pregnancy are similar between the more aggressive surgical approach of salpingectomy, with or without oophorectomy, and the more conservative approach of salpingotomy.[40] Yet following an ectopic pregnancy, some patients have normal reproductive function, whereas others never achieve a successful pregnancy. It would be helpful to be able to recognize these different groups and implement the more conservative approach for the former and the more radical treatment for the latter, whose only viable option may be in assisted reproductive technologies.

In a retrospective study using multivariable analyses on a large number of patients, Pouly *et al.*[41] showed that the characteristics of the ectopic pregnancy, such as the size of hematosalpinx, the volume of hemoperitoneum, or tubal rupture, had no influence on the subsequent fertility potential. However, a positive history of salpingitis, previous ectopic pregnancy, previous tubal surgery, or the presence of adhesions on the contralateral tube significantly worsened the prognosis for subsequent successful pregnancy. Indeed, if two or more of these prognostic factors were present, the chances of a subsequent ectopic exceeded the chances of a successful pregnancy, which led the authors to suggest that such patients should be aggressively treated with bilateral salpingectomy and subsequent referral to IVF.

The status of the contralateral tube appears to be an important determinant of subsequent fertility potential.[40–43] When the contralateral tube and ovary were normal, Tumivaara and Kauppila reported a subsequent intrauterine pregnancy rate of 85% and only a 9% incidence of ectopic pregnancy, whether the surgery involved salpingectomy or salpingotomy. When the opposite tube was impaired, however, the subsequent intrauterine pregnancy rate was significantly lower, and the ectopic pregnancy rate was much higher, 46% and 52%, respectively.[40] Similar findings were obtained by Langer et al.,[42] who reported much lower subsequent intrauterine pregnancy rates when the opposite tube was involved with significant adhesions. In a different study, Marana et al. evaluated the contralateral tube by laparoscopy and salpingoscopy in patients with previous ectopic pregnancy. They did not find the presence of peritubal adhesions to be of prognostic value, but the status of the tubal mucosa evaluated by salpingoscopy was directly related to subsequent fertility. Indeed, 60% of patients with intra-ampullary adhesions but none of the patients with normal tubal mucosa subsequently experienced repeated ectopic pregnancy.[43]

It is clear from these studies that after an ectopic pregnancy, the subsequent prognosis varies significantly according to the patient's past medical history and the status of the contralateral tube. Therefore, at the time of laparoscopy, the patient's reproductive desires and past medical history should be known, and the pelvis should be thoroughly explored, with close examination of the contralateral tube, preferably by salpingoscopy. If the contralateral tube is abnormal and/or the medical history is positive for previous ectopic or tubal disease, she may best be served by salpingectomy (bilaterally) and referral to IVF. Trying to preserve severely compromised tubes does not increase the patient's chances of successful pregnancy; it only increases her subsequent chances of repeated ectopic pregnancy.

Laparoscopy

The contemporary surgical approach to the treatment of ectopic pregnancy is operative laparoscopy, which yields pregnancy rates comparable to those reported following laparotomy.[44–49] (See TABLE 4.) Reporting on their experience with the laparoscopic treatment of ectopic pregnancy, Bruhat et al. suggested in 1980 that the laparoscopic approach resulted in improved fertility rates because of reduced adhesion formation due to less peritoneal damage with laparoscopic surgery. Subsequent controlled animal studies[50] and clinical studies[51,52] confirmed the early impressions that laparoscopic surgery is associated with significant reductions in the extent of both *de novo* adhesion formation and re-formation. In a uniquely controlled and prospectively randomized study, Lundorff et al.[48] conducted a comparative analysis of adhesion formation following laparoscopic surgery versus laparotomy for the treatment of ectopic pregnancy. Tubal integrity and the extent of pelvic adhesions were assessed at second-look laparoscopy within 15 weeks of the initial surgical interven-

TABLE 4. Comparative results of conservative surgery for ectopic pregnancy by laparotomy versus laparoscopy

Authors	No. of Cases	% Intrauterine Pregnancy	% Ectopic Pregnancy
Laparotomy			
DeCherney and Kase[38]	49	40	12
Stromme[46]	45	71	15
Timonen *et al.*[47]	240	38	16
Vermesh *et al.*[45,a]	30	42	16
Lundorff *et al.*[48,a]	45	44	11
Total	**409**	**43**	**15**
Laparoscopy			
Pouly *et al.*[41]	118	64	22
DeCherney and Diamond[39]	79	62	16
Vermesh *et al.*[45,a]	30	50	6
Lundorff *et al.*[48,a]	42	52	7
Total	**267**	**60**	**16**

[a]Controlled and prospectively randomized to laparotomy versus laparoscopy.

tion. Although tubal patency did not differ between the two groups, patients who had been treated by laparotomy developed significantly more adhesions than those patients treated by laparoscopy. The authors concluded that the laparoscopic treatment of ectopic pregnancy results in less impairment of the pelvic status.

A similar study was published by Vermesh *et al.*,[45] who prospectively randomized patients with unruptured ectopic pregnancies to either laparoscopy or laparotomy and subsequently analyzed pregnancy rates, tubal patency by hysterosalpingogram, postoperative morbidity, length of hospital stay, duration of convalescence, and hospital cost. The authors found that, although the two surgical procedures were similarly safe and effective, the laparoscopic approach was more economical and required a shorter recovery period. Similarly, Brumsted *et al.*,[53] comparing the treatment of ectopic pregnancy by laparoscopy versus laparotomy, reported significantly shorter periods of convalescence (8.7 ± 7.8 days versus 25.7 ± 16.2 days, $p < 0.01$) and reduced postoperative analgesia requirements (0.84 ± 2.3 versus 4.64 ± 2.9 doses; $p < 0.01$) in the laparoscopy group compared to the laparotomy group.[40]

These data justify the following conclusions: (1) Laparoscopic treatment of ectopic pregnancy results in less postoperative adhesion formation and impairment of the pelvic status than occurs following laparotomy; (2) the laparoscopic approach is associated with significantly less blood loss and reduced analgesia requirements; and (3) reduced costs, hospitalization, and convalescence period are associated with laparoscopic surgery. Consequently, endoscopic surgery should be the preferred option in the surgical management of ectopic pregnancies. With adequate practice and surgical experience in operative laparoscopy and with the availability of proper instrumentation, most cases of ectopic pregnancy may be successfully treated by laparoscopy, regardless of size and location,[54] number of gestations,[55] and the presence or absence of tubal rupture.[56] However, in the critically ill patient, laparotomy may continue to have a role because of the swiftness with which it can allow access to the abdomen and subsequent control of hemorrhage.

In the surgical management of ectopic pregnancy, one must consider the patient's desire for further childbearing, which may determine whether or not valiant attempts to conserve tubal integrity and function should be made. In all instances, the couple should be fully informed of the possibility of laparotomy with salpingectomy or more extirpative surgery because of uncontrollable bleeding or other unexpected surgical findings. Even if neither tube can be saved, every effort should be made to preserve the uterus and at least one ovary to keep alive the hope for future pregnancy with the use of the now-successful technology of *in vitro* fertilization.[57]

Nonsurgical Treatment of Ectopic Pregnancy

Expectant Management

Recently, attention has been directed to the nonsurgical treatments of ectopic pregnancies, which include expectant management or the use of methotrexate. In view of the natural tendency of some ectopic pregnancies to terminate in tubal abortions or complete reabsorption, some investigators have questioned the necessity of surgery in very early cases. Instead, they suggest that some patients may be monitored by means of rising or falling serum levels of hCG until tubal abortion or reabsorption occurs.[58] Ylostalo *et al.* described a series of 83 patients managed expectantly in which 69% had spontaneous resolution of their ectopic pregnancies. To enter this study, patients had to have no evidence of rupture on vaginal ultrasound, decreasing hCG titers, and ectopic masses of less than 4 cm. These criteria were met by 26% of all ectopics managed during a two-year period, suggesting that for 18% of ectopics (69% of 26%), expectant management may be a viable option.[59] It has been suggested that expectant management may be the best way to preserve tubal function and fertility; however, following expectant management or salpingostomy, tubal patency rates have been reported to be the same.[60,61] In a prospective study of 30 patients whose ectopic pregnancy was treated expectantly, tubal patency of the affected tube was confirmed by hysterosalpingography in 93%, 825 subsequently conceived, and the rate of repeat ectopic pregnancy was 4.2%.[62] Investigators agree that lower initial hCG levels correlate strongly with successful spontaneous resolution. Trio *et al.* found that an initial hCG titer <1000 mIU/ml predicted successful outcomes for 88% of cases managed expectantly,[63] but no cut-off value has been found below which expectant management is uniformly safe. The real possibility of rupture despite low and declining serum levels of hCG[64] raise serious concerns regarding this management option, which may be appropriate only occasionally with very compliant patients. The adage that the sun must never set on a suspected ectopic may be old but not outdated.

Methotrexate

Methotrexate has been used extensively to treat hydatidiform mole; therefore, its activity against trophoblasts is well known. Since the late 1980s, systemic methotrexate has been employed to treat ectopic pregnancy with excellent results. The initial studies were done using methotrexate and leucovorin for the treatment of unruptured ectopic pregnancies in selected, stable patients. Subjects were treated with methotrexate 1 mg/kg intramuscularly, alternating with leucovorin 0.1 mg/kg intramuscularly every other day, for up to four doses of methotrexate. Patients were admitted to the hospital and closely monitored during therapy with complete blood and platelet counts, liver and renal function tests, and β-hCG levels.[65]

More recently, stable patients with ectopic masses less than 4 cm and no evidence of rupture have been treated with a single i.m. injection of methotrexate (50 mg/m^2) without leucovorin rescue.[66] This simplified regimen has been found to be safe and effective with rare adverse side effects. In a review of 17 studies involving 400 patients, single-dose methotrexate was found to be effective in approximately 92% of cases.[67] Some of these patients were administered additional doses of methotrexate when their serial quantitative β-hCG titers plateaued or kept rising. Three to seven days after receiving methotrexate, some patients may also experience pelvic pain, which may be caused by tubal abortion and can be confused with tubal rupture. In the presence of stable vital signs and serial normal hematocrits, these episodes are generally self-limited and do not warrant surgical intervention. The first quantitative β-hCG after giving methotrexate should not be obtained sooner than 4 days post treatment, as an initial increase in the hCG level is frequently noted, presumably due to trophoblast lysis.

Women most likely to respond to methotrexate therapy are thought to be those with small gestational sacs, lower serum concentrations of human chorionic gonadotropin and progesterone, and the absence of blood in the peritoneal cavity and fetal heart activity. However, a retrospective review of 360 consecutive cases of ectopic pregnancies treated with methotrexate revealed that neither the size of the gestation nor the presence of hemoperitoneum had any effect on the success rate. But high serum levels of serum chorionic gonadotropin (>10,000 IU/l) or progesterone (≥10 ng/ml) and the presence of fetal cardiac activity were associated with higher rates of failure of methotrexate therapy. The single most important factor associated with failure of treatment with a single-dose methotrexate protocol was high serum concentration of human chorionic gonadotropin.[68] Besides being less invasive and associated with significant lower risk, the treatment cost of ectopic pregnancy is significantly reduced by methotrexate therapy. In a retrospective study of 60 ectopic cases treated either surgically (laparotomy or laparoscopy) or with methotrexate, Stovall *et al.* reported the mean total charges for methotrexate to be $1,563 versus $6,626 and $8,001 for the laparoscopy- and laparotomy-treated patients, respectively.[69] In a more comprehensive study that accounted for the varying rates of resolution, complication, and side effects among women treated either with methotrexate or laparoscopic surgery, Morlock *et al.* found that the administration of methotrexate therapy for early unruptured ectopic pregnancy results in cost savings of approximately $3000 per treated patient.[70]

Although several studies have compared the relative therapeutic efficacy of systemic methotrexate versus surgery, only one study evaluated the relative impact on patients' health-related quality of life and patients' preference between these two therapeutic approaches. In a multicenter, randomized clinical trial conducted in the Netherlands, Nieuwkerk *et al.* found that patients treated with systemic methotrexate had more limitations in physical functioning, role functioning, and social functioning. They also had worse health perceptions, less energy, more pain, more physical symptoms, and a worse overall quality of life; furthermore, they were more depressed than surgically treated patients. This persistently more negative impact on patients' health-related quality of life may be explained by both the long-term persistence of the ectopic pregnancy and the prolonged treatment associated with the medical therapy.[71]

Oral methotrexate appears to be effective as well and, as more experience is gained, may become the preferred route of administration.[72] Other antineoplastic agents that are active against trophoblasts, such as dactinomycin,[73] may also be effective but have not been tried in any large studies and have no clear advantage over methotrexate.

The use of methotrexate to treat ectopic pregnancy is particularly attractive in patients who may be high surgical risks, such as cases of cornual pregnancy, incomplete resolution of surgically treated ectopic gestation, patients with gonadotropin-induced ovarian hyperstimulation syndrome, or patients suspected of having extensive intraperitoneal abdominal adhesions.[74]

Indeed, the first case of the successful use of methotrexate in ectopic pregnancy was reported by Tanaka et al. in a patient with a large cornual pregnancy diagnosed by laparoscopy, but because of the high risk of hemorrhage was treated medically.[75] Since his initial report in 1982, many investigators have described the successful use of methotrexate in unruptured interstitial pregnancy. This conservative, noninvasive management offers an attractive treatment alternative to cornual resection and avoids surgical trauma to the uterus. This could be of benefit in patients who desire to preserve fertility potential. Nevertheless, the risk of treatment failure, that is, uterine rupture, remains a dangerous possibility during systemic methotrexate treatment, especially in cases where regression of hCG levels is slow and the size of the gestational sac continues to increase during therapy. A recent review of the literature of the systemic methotrexate treatment for unruptured interstitial pregnancy, using single or multiple injection regimens, found that of 25 total reported cases, 20 were successful and 5 required surgical intervention. Of the five failures, two ruptured and required emergency surgery and three underwent scheduled operations for failure to respond, determined by inadequate hCG decline or persistent fetal cardiac activity.[71] Although different systemic regimens appear to be equally effective, for high-risk patients with cornual pregnancy, the multiple-dose regimen seems preferable under careful surveillance.

Systemic methotrexate therapy is contraindicated in patients who are hemodynamically unstable or have signs of bone marrow depression or liver or renal dysfunction, as evidenced by leukopenia and/or thrombocytopenia, elevated liver enzymes, or elevated serum creatinine, respectively.

COMBINED MEDICAL–SURGICAL THERAPY

Another treatment option for unruptured ectopic pregnancy is the local injection of methotrexate into the ectopic mass, either under the direction of ultrasound or at the time of diagnosis at laparoscopy. In a recent study by Kooi and Kock,[76] the authors were successful in 17 of 24 patients with a single injection. Seven patients required additional systemic injections, and one patient experienced tubal rupture 3 days after the initial injection. The local injection consisted of 10–20 ml of adrenaline at 1:80,000 dilution injected into the mesosalpinx with a 22-gauge needle, followed by 100 mg methotrexate injected into the tubal swelling. Leucovorin (15 mg) was given orally 30 hours after the administration of methotrexate. Subsequent systemic methotrexate injections were given intramuscularly at a dose of 50 mg every 2–4 days according to the patterns of serum hCG levels.

In a prospectively randomized study, Fernandez *et al.* compared the relative efficacy of methotrexate versus prostaglandin sulprostone (Nalador; Schering Laboratory, Lys-Lez- Lannoy, France), administered directly into the gestational sac or systemically by serial intramuscular injections on days 3, 5, and 7 after the day of diagnosis and local treatment, in 21 patients with an unruptured tubal pregnancy. Both therapies were equally effective. However, 34% of patients required laparoscopy for abdominal pain and hemorrhage (14%) or because of persistent rise in the serum levels of hCG (20%).[77]

More recently, Zilber *et al.* reported their experience in 48 patients with unruptured tubal pregnancy who were prospectively randomized to either laparoscopic salpingotomy or laparoscopic local methotrexate injection.[78] The authors found both methods equally effective and with balanced advantages/disadvantages for each treatment. The local methotrexate injection was associated with a shorter operation time and less need for surgical expertise, whereas the salpingotomy approach resulted in a shorter hospitalization and a reduced risk of persistent trophoblastic activity.

In a letter to the editor of *Fertility and Sterility*, Fernandez and Benifla describe their successful experience with treating 15 cases of cornual pregnancy with local injection of either methotrexate (1 mg/kg) or KCl. KCl was used when the cornual pregnancy was associated with a second intrauterine gestation (heterotopic). The injections were performed either by laparoscopy ($n = 6$) or under ultrasound guidance ($n = 9$) with complete resolution in 13 cases (86.6 %).[79]

Prophylactic methotrexate has been successfully used by Graczykowski and Mishell[80] to reduce the risk of persistent ectopic pregnancy. Following the resection of the ectopic pregnancy by salpingostomy, patients were randomly assigned either to methotrexate 1 mg/kg i.m. or control. The rate of persistent ectopic pregnancy was reduced from 14.5% in the control group to 1.9% in the study group.[80]

CONCLUSION

Ectopic pregnancy remains an ever-increasing health problem. Its incidence continues to rise, paralleling the progressive increase in the incidence of its etiologic factors, especially sexually transmitted diseases. Because of this, clinicians must be alert to the possibility of ectopic pregnancy in all women of reproductive age. Early confirmation of intrauterine pregnancy by measurement of serial hCG and transvaginal ultrasound when hCG levels reach 1000 mIU/ml in women with risk factors is essential. Use of serum progesterone in the symptomatic patient may also clarify the diagnosis, allowing prompt curettage and frozen section analysis for villi when the level is below 5 ng/ml and heightened suspicion when between 5 to 25 ng/ml.

Although the standard of care for ectopic pregnancy is currently surgical, medical therapy with methotrexate is becoming progressively more common and more desirable. Besides being less invasive and associated with significantly lower risks, the administration of methotrexate therapy for ectopic pregnancy results in significant cost savings, which Morlock et al.[70] have calculated to be approximately $3000 per treated patient. However, most studies have not considered the cost incurred to treat the side effects nor the complications and failure of the medical management, nor the quality of life and patients' preference. When successful, methotrexate treatment for ectopic pregnancy is very desirable from the economic, social, and patient perspective. However when medical therapy fails, the consequences may be quite catastrophic. Our goal is to identify those patients with ectopic pregnancy that are most likely to respond to methotrexate therapy and least likely to develop significant side effects. The elegant study by Lipscomb et al.[68] has clearly defined for us the predictors of success of methotrexate treatment in women with tubal ectopic pregnancy. When our patients with ectopic pregnancy present with low serum levels of hCG (<5000 IU/l) and progesterone (<10 ng/ml) and an absence of fetal cardiac activity, we can expect a success rate with single-dose methotrexate to exceed 90%. All other patients may best be served with surgical treatment.

It was pointed out by Creinin et al.[81] that institutions with the highest success rates with methotrexate therapy have in place a detailed diagnostic and therapeutic protocol, readily available assays for serum hCG levels, high-resolution vaginal probe ultrasound, and support staff that can closely monitor clinical response. The importance of developing specific protocols and creating a clinical environment that supports the effective use of medical therapy for ectopic pregnancy is confirmed by the associated cost savings, decreased morbidity, and patient preference.[71] It is indeed a small price to pay for the therapeutic transition "from surgical emergency to medical management" for the treatment of ectopic pregnancy. Modern diagnostic advances and minimally invasive treatments coupled with the improved success rates of assisted reproductive technologies should reduce the morbidity and the mortality associated with ectopic pregnancy and offer the affected couple a much more optimistic outlook for subsequent reproductive potential.

REFERENCES

1. Ectopic Pregnancy—United States, 1990–1992. Morbid. Mortal. Wkly. Rep. 1995. (Jan. 27) **44(3):** 46–48.
2. TAIT, R.L. 1884. Five cases of extra-uterine pregnancy operated upon at the time of rupture. Br. Med. J. **1:** 1250.
3. GOLDNER, T.E., H.W. LAWSON, Z. XIA & H.K. ATRASH. 1993. Surveillance for ectopic pregnancy—United States, 1970–1989. Morbid. Mortal. Wkly. Rep. CDC Surveillance Summaries **42(SS-6):** 73–85.
4. NCHS. 1994. Advanced report of final mortality statistics, 1992. US Department of Health and Human Services, Public Health Service, CDC (Monthly vital statistics report; Vol. 43, no. 6, Suppl.).
5. MARCHBANKS, P.A., J.F. ANEGER, C.B. COULMAN, et al. 1988. Risk factors for ectopic pregnancy: a population based study. JAMA **259:** 1823–1827.
6. SHEFFIELD, P.A., D.E. MOORE, L.F. VOIGT, et al. 1993. The association between Chlamydia trachomatis serology and pelvic damage in women with tubal ectopic gestations. Fertil. Steril. **60(6):** 970–975.
7. CHOW, J.M., M.L. YONEKURA, G.A. RICHWALD, et al. 1990. The association between Chlamydia trachomatis and ectopic pregnancy. JAMA **263(23):** 3164–3167.
8. MOORE, D.E., L.R. SPADONI, H.M. FOY, et al. 1982. Increased frequency of serum antibodies to Chlamydia trachomatis in infertility due to distal tubal disease. Lancet **2(8298):** 574–577.

9. WESTROM. L., L.P. BENGTSSON & P.A. MARDH. 1981. Incidence, trends, and risks of ectopic pregnancy in a population of women. Br. Med. J. (Clin. Res. Educ.) **282(6257):** 15–18.

10. JOESOEF, M.R., L. WESTROM, G. REYNOLDS, *et al.* 1991. Recurrence of ectopic pregnancy: the role of salpingitis. Am. J. Obstet. Gynecol. **165(1):** 46–50.

11. WECKSTEIN, L.N. 1985. Current perspective on ectopic pregnancy. Obstet. Gynecol. Surv. **40(5):** 259–272.

12. VERMESH, M., J.W. GRACZYKOWSKI & M.V. SAUER. 1990. Reevaluation of the role of culdocentesis in the management of ectopic pregnancy. Am. J. Obstet. Gynecol. **162:** 441–443.

13. NYBERG, D.A., M.P. HUGHES, L.A. MACK & K.Y. WANG. 1991. Extrauterine findings of ectopic pregnancy of transvaginal US: importance of echogenic fluid. Radiology **178(3):** 823–826.

14. KADAR, N., B.V. CALDWELL & R. ROMERO. 1981. A method of screening for ectopic pregnancy and its indications. Obstet. Gynecol. **58(2):** 162–166.

15. FRITZ, M.A. & S.M. GUO. 1987. Doubling time of hCG in early normal pregnancy: relationship to hCG concentration and gestational age. Fertil. Steril. **47(4):** 584–589.

16. SHEPHERD, R.W., P.E. PATTON, M.J. NOVY & K.A. BURRY. 1990. Serial data hCG measurements in the early detection of ectopic pregnancy. Obstet. Gynecol. **75:** 417–420.

17. KAMEAVA, M.M., M.L. TAYMOR, M.J. BERGER, *et al.* 1983. Disappearance of human chorionic gonadotropin following removal of ectopic pregnancy. Obstet. Gynecol. **62:** 486–488.

18. MATTHEWS, C.P., P.B. COULSON & R.A. WILD. 1986. Serum progesterone levels as an aid in the diagnosis of ectopic pregnancy. Obstet. Gynecol. **68(3):** 390–394.

19. GELDER, M.S., L.R. BOOTS & J.B. YOUNGER. 1991. Use of a single random serum progesterone value as a diagnostic aid for ectopic pregnancy. Fertil. Steril. **55(3):** 497–500.

20. MCCORD, M.L., D. MURAM, J.E. BUSTER, *et al.* 1996. Single serum progesterone as a screen for ectopic pregnancy exchanging specificity and sensitivity to obtain optimal test performance Fertil. Steril. **66:** 513–516.

21. STOVALL, T.G., F.W. LING, S.A. CARSON & J.E. BUSTER. 1992. Serum progesterone and uterine curettage in differential diagnosis of ectopic pregnancy. Fertil. Steril. **57(2):** 456–457.

22. LONG, C.A., N.S. WHITWORTH, H.M. MURTHY, *et al.* 1994. First-trimester rapid semiquantitative assay for urine pregnanediol glucuronide predicts gestational outcome with the same diagnostic accuracy as serial human chorionic gonadotropin measurements. Am. J. Obstet. Gynecol. **170(6):** 1822–1825.

23. SER, M.V., M VERMESH, R. ANDERSON, *et al.* 1988. Rapid measurement of urinary pregnanediol glucuronide to diagnose ectopic pregnancy. Am. J. Obstet. Gynecol. **159(6):** 1531–1535.

24. STABILE, I., F. OLAJIDE, T. CHARD & J.G. GRUDZINSKAS. 1994. Circulating levels of placental protein 14 in ectopic pregnancy. Br. J. Obstet. Gynaecol. **101(9):** 762–764.

25. DUNCAN, W.C., V.M. SWEETING, P. CAWOOD & P.J. ILLINGWORTH. 1995. Measurement of creatine kinase activity and diagnosis of ectopic pregnancy. Br. J. Obstet. Gynaecol. **102(3):** 233–237.

26. COLE, L.A., A. KARDANA, D.B. SEIFER & H.C. BOHLER, JR. 1994. Urine hCG β-subunit core fragment, a sensitive test for ectopic pregnancy. J. Clin. Endocrinol. Metab. **78(2):** 497–499.

27. GROSSKINSKY, C.M., M.L. HAGE, L. TYREY, *et al.* 1993. hCG, progesterone, alphafetoprotein, and estradiol in the identification of ectopic pregnancy. Obstet. Gynecol. **81**(5, Pt. 1): 705–709.

28. PREDANIC, M. 2000. Differentiating tubal abortion from viable ectopic pregnancy with serum Ca-125 and β-human chorionic gonadotropin determinations. Fertil. Steril. **73:** 5222–5225.

29. KADAR, N., G. DEVORE & R. ROMERO. 1981. Discriminatory hCG zone: its use in the sonographic evaluation for ectopic pregnancy. Obstet. Gynecol. **58(2):** 156–161.

30. CACCIATORE, B., U.L. STENMAN & P. YLOSTALO. 1990. Diagnosis of ectopic pregnancy by vaginal ultrasonography in combination with a discriminatory serum hCG level of 1000 IU/l (IRP). Br. J. Obstet. Gynaecol. 97(10): 904–908.
31. ACKERMAN, T.E., C.S. LEVI, E.A. LYONS, et al. 1993. Decidual cyst: endovaginal sonographic sign of ectopic pregnancy. Radiology 189(3): 727–731.
32. BRADLEY, W.G., C.E. FISKE & R.A. FILLY. 1982. The double sac sign of early intrauterine pregnancy: use in exclusion of ectopic pregnancy. Radiology 143(1): 223–226.
33. NYBERG, D.A., F.C. LAING, R.A. FILLY, et al. 1983. Ultrasonographic differentiation of the gestational sac of early intrauterine pregnancy from the pseudogestational sac of ectopic pregnancy. Radiology 146(3): 755–759.
34. NYBERG, D.A., L.A. MACK, D. HARVEY & K. WANG. 1988. Value of the yolk sac in evaluating early pregnancies. J. Ultrasound Med. 7(3): 129–135.
35. YEH, H.C. 1988. Sonographic signs of early pregnancy. Crit. Rev. Diagn, Imaging 28(3): 181–211.
36. SPANDORFER, S.D. & K.T. BARNHART. 1996. Endometrial stripe thickness as a predictor of ectopic pregnancy. Fertil. Steril. 66(3): 474–477.
37. SPANDORFER, S.D., A.W. MENZIN, K.T. BARNHART, et al. 1996. Efficacy of frozen section evaluation of uterine curettings in the diagnosis of ectopic pregnancy. Am. J. Obstet. Gynecol. 175: 603–605.
38. DeCHERNEY, A.H. & N. KASE. 1979. The conservative surgical management of unruptured ectopic pregnancy. Obstet. Gynecol. 54: 451–453.
39. DeCHERNEY, A.H. & M.P. DIAMOND. 1987. Laparoscopic salpingostomy for ectopic pregnancy. Obstet. Gynecol. 70: 948–950.
40. TUOMIVAARA, L. & A. KAPPILA. 1988. Radical or conservative surgery for ectopic pregnancy? A follow-up study of fertility of 323 patients. Fertil. Steril. 50: 580–583.
41. POULY, J.L., C. CHAPRON, H. MANHES, et al. 1991. Multifactorial analysis of fertility after conservative laparoscopic treatment of ectopic pregnancy in a series of 223 patients. Fertil. Steril. 56: 453.
42. LANGER, R., A. RATZIEL, R. RON-EL, et al. 1990. Reproductive outcome after conservative surgery for unruptured tubal pregnancy—a 15-year experience. Fertil. Steril. 53: 227–231.
43. MARANA, R., L. MUZII, M. RIZZI, et al. 1995. Prognostic role of laparoscopic salpingoscopy of the only remaining tube after contralateral ectopic pregnancy. Fertil. Steril. 63(2): 303–306.
44. POULY, J.L., H. MAHNES, G. MAGE, et al. 1986. Conservative laparoscopic treatment of 321 ectopic pregnancies. Fertil. Steril. 46: 1093–1097.
45. VERMISH, M., P.D. SILVA, G.F. ROSEN, et al. 1989. Management of unruptured ectopic gestation by linear salpingostomy: a prospective randomized clinical trial of laparoscopy versus laparotomy. Obstet. Gynecol. 73: 400–403.
46. STROMME, W.B. 1973. Conservative surgery for ectopic pregnancy. Obstet. Gynecol. 41: 251–254.
47. TIMONEN, S. & U. NIEMINEN. 1967. Tubal pregnancy choice of operative method of treatment. Acta Obstet. Gynecol. Scand. 46: 327–332.
48. LUNDORFF, P., J. THORBURN & B. LINDBLOM. 1992. Fertility outcome after conservative surgical treatment of ectopic pregnancy evaluated in a randomized trial. Fertil. Steril. 57: 998–1002.
49. BRUHAT, M.A., H. MAHNES, G. MAGE, et al. 1980. Treatment of ectopic pregnancy by means of laparoscopy. Fertil. Steril. 33: 411–414.
50. LUCIANO, A.A., D.B. MAIER, E.I. KOCH, et al. 1989. A comparative study of postoperative adhesions following laser surgery by laparoscopy versus laparotomy in the rabbit model. Obstet. Gynecol. 74: 220–224.
51. NEZHAT, C., M.D. METZER, F. NEZHAT & A.A. LUCIANO. 1990. Adhesion formation following reproductive surgery by videolaparoscopy. Fertil. Steril. 53: 1008–1011.
52. LUNDORFF, P., M. HAHLIN, B. KALLFELT, et al. 1991. Adhesion formation after laparoscopic surgery in tubal pregnancy: a randomized trial versus laparotomy. Fertil. Steril. 55: 911–915.

53. BRUMSTEAD, J., C. KESSLER, C. GIBSON, *et al.* 1988. A comparison of laparoscopy and laparotomy for the treatment of ectopic pregnancy. Obstet. Gynecol. **71:** 889–892.
54. NEZHAT, C. & F. NEZHAT. 1990. Conservative management of ectopic gestation— letter to the editor. Fertil. Steril. **53:** 382.
55. FRISHMAN, G.N., M.M. STEINHOFF & A.A. LUCIANO. 1990. Triplet tubal pregnancy treated by outpatient laparoscopic salpingostomy. Fertil. Steril. **54:** 934–935.
56. NEZHAT, F., W. WINER & C. NEZHAT. 1991. Salpingectomy via laparoscopy: a new surgical approach. J. Laparoendosc. Surg. **1:** 91–95.
57. LUCIANO, A.A. 1990. Ectopic pregnancy. *In* Current Therapy in Obstetrics and Gynecology. E.J. Quilling & F.P. Zuspan, Eds.: 226–229. Saunders. Philadelphia.
58. FERNANDEZ, H., J.D. RAINHORN & E. PAPIERNIK. 1988. Spontaneous resolution of ectopic pregnancy. Obstet. Gynecol. **71(2):** 171–173.
59. YLOSTALO, P., B. CACCIATORE, J. SJOBERG, *et al.* 1992. Expectant management of ectopic pregnancy. Obstet. Gynecol. **80(3, Pt. 1):** 345–348.
60. SHALEV, E., D. PELEG, A. TSABARI, *et al.* 1995. Spontaneous resolution of ectopic tubal pregnancy: natural history. Fertil. Steril. **63(1):** 15–19.
61. YLOSTALO, P., B. CACCIATORE, A. KOSKIMIES, *et al.* 1991. Conservative treatment of ectopic pregnancy. Ann. N.Y. Acad. Sci. **626:** 516–523.
62. RANTALA, M. & J. MAKINEN. 1997. Tubal patency and fertility outcome after expectant managemnt of ectopic pregnancy. Fertil. Steril. **68:** 1043–1046.
63. TRIO, D., N. STROBELT, C. PICCIOLO, *et al.* 1995. Prognostic factors for successful expectant management of ectopic pregnancy. Fertil. Steril. **63(3):** 469–472.
64. TULANDI, T., R. HEMMINGS & F. KHALIFA. 1991. Rupture of ectopic pregnancy in women with low and declining serum β-human chorionic gonadotropin concentrations. Fertil. Steril. **56:** 786–787.
65. STOVALL, T.G., F.W. LING & J.E. BUSTER.1989. Outpatient chemotherapy of unruptured ectopic pregnancy. Fertil. Steril. **51:** 435–438.
66. STOVALL, T.G., F.W. LING & L.A. GRAY. 1991. Single-dose methotrexate for treatment of ectopic pregnancy. Obstet. Gynecol. **77(5):** 754–757.
67. SLAUGHTER, J.L. & D.A. GRIMES. 1995. Methotrexate therapy. Nonsurgical management of ectopic pregnancy. West. J. Med. **162(3):** 225–228.
68. LIPSCOMB, G.H., M.L. McCORD, T.G. STOVALL, *et al.* 1999. Predictors of success of methotrexate treatment in women with tubal ectopic pregnancies. N. Engl. J. Med. **341:** 1974–1978.
69. STOVALL, T.G., D.D. BRADHAM, F.W. LING & M. NAUGHTON. 1994. Cost of treatment of ectopic pregnancy: single-dose methotrexate versus surgical treatment. J. Women's Health **3:** 445–450.
70. MORLOCK, R., J. LAFATA, E. LAFATA & D. EISENSTEIN. 2000. Cost-effectiveness of single-dose methotrexate compared with laparoscopic treatment of ectopic pregnancy. Obstet. Gynecol. **95:** 407–412.
71. NIEUWKERK, P.T., P.J. HAJENIUS, F. VAN DER VEEN, *et al.* 1998. Systemic methotrexate therapy versus laparoscopic salpingostomy in tubal pregnancy. Part II. Patient prefernces for systemic methotrexate. Fertil. Steril. **70:** 518–522.
72. HAJEENIUS, P.J., R.R. VOIGHT, S. ENGELSBEL, *et al.* 1996. Serum human chorionic gonadotropin clearance curves in patients with interstitial pregnancy treated with systemic methotrexate. Fertil. Steril. **66:** 723–728.
73. NEARY, B.A. & P.G. ROSE. 1995. Complete response of a persistent ectopic pregnancy to dactinomycin after methotrexate failure. A case report. J. Reprod. Med. **40(2):** 160–162.
74. KOOI, S. & H.C. KOCK. 1992. A review of the literature on the nonsurgical treatment of tubal pregnancies. Obstet. Gynecol. Surv. **47:** 739–749.
75. TANAKA, T., H. HAYASHI, T. KUTSUZAWA, *et al.* 1982. Treatment of interstitial ectopic pregnancy with methotrexate: report of a successful case. Fertil. Steril. **37:** 851–852.
76. KOOI, S. & H.C. KOCK. 1990. Treatment of tubal pregnancy by local injection of methotrexate after adrenaline injection into the mesosalpinx: a report of 25 patients. Fertil. Steril. **54:** 580–584.
77. FERNANDEZ, H., C. BATON, C. LELAIDER & R. FRYDMAN. 1991. Conservative management of ectopic pregnancy: prospective randomized clinical trial of methotrexate

versus prostaglandin sulprostone by combined transvaginal and systemic administration. Fertil. Steril. **55:** 746–750.
78. ZILBER, U., M. PANSKY, I. BUKOWSKY & A. GOLAN. 1996. Laparoscopic salpingostomy versus laparoscopic local methotrexate injection in the management of
unruptured ectopic gestation. Am. J. Obstet. Gynecol. **175:** 600–602.
79. FERNANDEZ, H. & J.L. BENIFLA. 1996. Medical treatment of cornual pregnancy. Fertil. Steril. **66:** 862.
80. GRACZYKOWSKI, J.W. & D.R. MISHELL. 1997. Methotrexate prophylaxis for persistent
ectopic pregnancy after conservative treatment by salpingostomy. Obstet. Gynecol.
89: 118–122.
81. CRENIN, M.D. & A.E. WASHINGTON. 1993. Cost of ectopic pregnancy management:
surgery versus methotrexate. Fertil. Steril. **60:** 963–969.

Laparoscopic Management of Adnexal Masses

The Opportunities and the Risks

TANJA PEJOVIC[a] AND FARR NEZHAT[b]

[a]Division of Gynecologic Oncology, Department of Obstetrics and Gynecology, Yale University School of Medicine, New Haven, Connecticut 06510, USA

[b]Division of Gynecologic Oncology, Mount Sinai School of Medicine, New York, New York 10029, USA

ABSTRACT: Suspected ovarian neoplasm is a common clinical problem affecting women of all ages. Although the majority of adnexal masses are benign, the primary goal of diagnostic evaluation is the exclusion of malignancy. It has been estimated that approximately 5–10% of women in the United States will undergo a surgical procedure for a suspected ovarian neoplasm during their lifetime. Despite the magnitude of the problem, there is still considerable disagreement regarding the optimal surgical management of these lesions. Traditional management has relied on laparotomy to avoid undertreatment of a potentially malignant process. Advances in detection, diagnosis, and minimally invasive surgical techniques make it necessary now to review this practice in an effort to avoid unnecessary morbidity among patients. Here, we review the literature on the laparosopic approach to the treatment of the adnexal mass without sacrificing the principles of oncologic surgery. We highlight potentials of minimally invasive surgery and address the risks associated with the laparoscopic approach.

KEYWORDS: adnexal masses; ovarian neoplasm; laparotomy

INTRODUCTION

Approximately 300,000 women are hospitalized annually in the United States because of adnexal masses.[1] For many years the traditional surgical treatment of the adnexal mass has been explorative laparotomy. Over the last decade, advances in laparoscopic techniques led to increased use of laparoscopy in gynecologic surgery. The main concern in the laparoscopic approach to adnexal mass management is the risk of undertreating ovarian cancer. With new diagnostic methods, such as CA-125, pelvic sonography including Doppler flow ultrasound, and intraoperative frozen section analysis, laparoscopic treatment of adnexal masses emerges as safe, offering a decreased risk in morbidity, mortality, and cost without compromising the care of the minority of the patients with adnexal malignancy.

Address for correspondence: Farr Nezhat, M.D., FACOG, Division of Gynecologic Oncology, Box 1173, Mount Sinai School of Medicine, 1 Gustav Levy Place, New York, New York 10029. Voice: 212-241-5994; fax: 212-987-6386.

farr.nezhat@mssm.edu

EVALUATION OF THE ADNEXAL MASS

Anatomically, the adnexa consist of the ovaries, fallopian tubes, broad ligament, and the structures within the broad ligament. The differential diagnosis of an adnexal mass is complex and includes lesions of infectious origin such as hydrosalpinx or tubo-ovarian abscess, functional cysts, endometriomas, and benign and malignant tumors of the ovary or tissues proximal to the adnexa.

The most important components in the evaluation of adnexal masses are the age of the patient, the history, the findings on physical examination, and the results of radiologic and laboratory studies. The patient's age is crucial in determining the probable etiology of an adnexal mass. In the newborn, small functional cysts, attributed to the presence of maternal hormones, are found occasionally, and these fully regress within the first months of life. In premenarchal and postmenopausal women, an adnexal mass is considered a highly abnormal finding, requiring immediate surgical exploration. The most frequent type of ovarian tumors in premenarchal girls and adolescents are germ cell tumors. Among these, benign cystic teratomas are most frequently found, but dysgerminomas and other germ cell tumors must be ruled out at surgical exploration.

In the reproductive-age period, the differential diagnosis is varied, and both benign and malignant tumors of multiple organs may occur. Benign masses include follicular cysts, corpus luteum cysts, endometriomas, polycystic ovary disease, and tubo-ovarian abscess. Ectopic pregnancy must always be ruled out in women of reproductive age. Leiomyomas, present in one-third of women, are an important part of differential diagnosis. Occasionally, extragenital lesions such as peritoneal or omental cysts, retroperitoneal lesions, or gastrointestinal disease are found, mimicking adnexal disease.

The overall risk of primary ovarian malignancy rises from 13% in premenopausal to 45% in postmenopausal women.[2] Many authors consider that any ovarian mass or any palpable ovary in postmenopausal woman requires surgical exploration.[3] Malignant ovarian tumors in this age group are usually epithelial in origin or metastatic from primary tumors of the breast, uterus, or gastrointestinal tract.

History

A complete history is essential for the diagnosis of an adnexal mass. The most common symptom is abdominal pain. The patient should be asked about onset of the pain, type, duration, localization, and relation to menstrual cycle. In premenopausal women, midcycle pain indicates ovulation. Pain following intercourse is suggestive of ruptured ovarian or corpus luteum cyst while pain during intercourse indicates endometriosis. Sudden onset of severe pain, sometimes associated with nausea and vomiting, is typical of torsion of adnexal mass. Any type of unilateral pain associated with positive urine β-hCG points toward diagnosis of ectopic pregnancy. Menstrual disturbances are an important part of the history. Dysmenorrhea or menorrhagia is suggestive of uterine leiomyomas. Bleeding in premenarchal girls with solid ovarian mass calls for ruling out a germ cell tumor. Epithelial ovarian tumors usually present with vague symptoms, frequently related to the gastrointestinal tract—dyspepsia, bloating, and constipation—whereas bleeding or sharp abdominal pain are rare.

Physical Examination

A complete physical examination with a focus on signs of neoplasm and infection is necessary to determine the cause of an adnexal mass. Pertinent findings include presence of enlarged peripheral lymph nodes and presence of pleural effusions and/ or ascites. The breast examination is particularly important in women with adnexal mass, as the ovary is a frequent location of metastasis for breast carcinoma.

Particular importance in detection and description of an adnexal mass is given to bimanual and rectovaginal examinations. Bimanual gynecologic examination is helpful in estimating the size, localization, mobility, and consistency of the mass. The rectovaginal examination allows for assessment of the cul-de-sac, rectum, posterior uterine surface, the uterosacral ligaments, and the parametria. Again, all elements of the history, including the patient's age, should be taken into account when interpreting findings at physical examination: in premenopausal patients a complex adnexal mass, cul-de-sac nodularity, and tender uterosacral ligaments suggest endometriosis, whereas similar findings in postmenopausal woman suggest ovarian malignancy.

Diagnostic Imaging Studies

Pelvic ultrasound is currently the most useful technique for diagnostic evaluation of the adnexal mass. Transvaginal ultrasound, developed in the late 1980s, allows use of increased frequencies and therefore provides better resolution than abdominal ultrasound.[4] Doppler flow imaging was the preferred technique of the early 1990s. The parameters of interest in ultrasound evaluation of adnexal mass are size, number of loculi, presence of papillary or solid excrescences within the mass, overall echo density, and pulsatility index (PI).

Findings that suggest malignancy include multiple loculations, gross septae, and papillary projections within the lumen of the cyst, wall nodules, or solid areas. However, no single gray-scale sonographic feature allows distinction between benign and malignant adnexal masses. Although initially Doppler flow ultrasonography seemed to hold promise in this regard, several studies assessing the value of this technique reported controversial results.[5]

A seminal work by Sassone et al.[6] evaluated an ultrasound scoring system to predict ovarian malignancy. Transvaginal sonographic pelvic images of 143 patients were correlated with surgico-pathologic findings. The variables included in the scoring system were the wall thickness of the adnexal cyst, the inner wall structure, presence and thickness of septa, and echogenicity. The scoring system was useful in distinguishing benign from malignant masses, with a sensitivity of 100%, a specificity of 83%, and positive and negative predictive values of 37 and 100%, respectively. A variety of other scoring systems have been proposed since with a sensitivity of 74–96% and a specificity of 23–80%. (For review see Grab et al.[7]) Most recently, Alcazar and Jurado developed a logistic model to predict malignancy based on menopausal status, ultrasound morphology, and color Doppler findings in 79 patients with adnexal masses.[8] The authors derived a mathematical formula to estimate preoperatively the risk of malignancy of a given adnexal mass in a simple and reproducible way. When this formula was applied prospectively, 56 of 58 (96.5%) adnexal masses were correctly classified.

The combination of sonomorphology and additional ovarian Doppler blood flow measurements has been suggested to improve specificity.[5] However, the comparisons of different studies have been complicated by the fact that no standard has been established for Doppler indices and cut-off values. While most authors prefer PI as a standard and consider PI < 1.0 to suggest malignancy, some authors use resistance index (RI) with varied cut-off values from 0.4 to 0.7 indicating malignancy.

In general, CT and MRI are not indicated routinely for evaluation of adnexal mass. CT is probably better suited for localization of metastasis because of its ability to evaluate the liver, omentum, mesentery and paraaortic region. The major limitation of CT in detecting early ovarian cancer is its inability to detect lesions less than 2 cm in diameter. MRI has not demonstrated any clear advantage over CT, but, because it does not use ionizing radiation, MR is useful in the evaluation of an adnexal mass in a pregnant patient. It may also be useful in further evaluation of adnexal masses detected by ultrasound but characterized as of "intermediate" nature. Grab et al. have investigated the accuracy of sonography versus MRI and positron emission tomography (PET) in 101 patient with asymptomatic adnexal mass who subsequently underwent laparoscopy.[7] Ultrasound evaluation established the correct diagnosis in 11 of 12 ovarian malignancies (sensitivity 92%) but with a specificity of only 60%. With MRI and PET, specificities improved to 84 and 89%, respectively, but sensitivities declined. When all modalities were combined, specificity was 85% and sensitivity 92% while accuracy was 86%. However, because negative PET or MR results do not rule out early-stage ovarian cancer or borderline malignancy, ultrasound remains the most important tool in detection of early ovarian neoplasms.

Tumor Markers

The most helpful laboratory studies in the evaluation of adnexal masses are the quantitative β-hCG, complete blood count (CBC) with differential, and, in selected cases, tumor markers. The quantitative β-hCG is essential in ruling out ectopic pregnancy. A CBC and differential are useful when an infectious cause for the adnexal mass is suspected. Tumor markers are indicated in some cases. In premenarchal girls or adolescents, when the possibility of a germ cell tumor is investigated, the tumor markers LDH, hCG, and α-fetoprotein are mandatory.

No single marker has been shown to be sufficiently sensitive or specific to contribute to the diagnosis of epithelial ovarian cancer. CA-125 is an exception that has been extensively studied. Still, CA-125 levels greater than 35 IU/ml have also been found in 1% of the normal population. Furthermore, serum CA-125 is an antigenic determinant found in both benign and malignant conditions. Benign conditions causing elevation of CA-125 include myoma, adenomyosis, benign ovarian tumors, liver disease, pelvic inflammatory disease, endometriosis, nonmalignant peritonitis, or pleural effusions. An elevated CA-125 is found in ovarian malignancies and in several other carcinomas, for example, cancer of the pancreas, colon, lung, and breast. Serum CA-125 is elevated in 80% of all patients with serous carcinoma of the ovary, but in only 50% of the patients with stage I disease.[9] As a diagnostic aid, CA-125 is most useful in postmenopausal women with an ultrasonographically suspicious pelvic mass. In that subgroup of patients, a level greater than 65 IU/ml has been shown to have a positive predictive value of 97%.[10] Changes in the level of CA-125 can be used as a reliable indication of response or progression according to various criteria, but it does not yet have a clear place in diagnosis or prognosis.[11]

Family History

The incidence of ovarian cancer in patients with no family history of the disease is 1 in 70 (1.4%). For the women with a single first-degree relative affected, the risk for ovarian cancer is increased three to four times over the risk in the general population. The 1994 NIH consensus conference on ovarian cancer did not recommend routine screening of these patients.[12] In families with multiple cases of ovarian cancer, the risk approaches the 50% probability observed in dominantly inherited syndromes. The women in the latter group have a 3–10% risk of having one of the three recognized forms of hereditary ovarian cancer syndrome: (i) the site-specific syndrome, (ii) the breast–ovarian cancer syndrome, and (iii) Lynch syndrome II. Women with site-specific syndrome tend to develop ovarian cancer at an age 10–20 years younger than those patients without a family history of ovarian cancer. Women with breast–ovarian cancer syndrome tend to have multiple relatives with breast and/or ovarian carcinoma. Those with Lynch syndrome II have a history of nonpolyposis colon cancer associated with history of breast, endometrial, or ovarian cancer. Germline mutations of *BRCA1* and *BRCA2* genes are implicated in the pathogenesis of hereditary ovarian cancer syndromes. Carriers of the *BRCA1* mutation have an 80% lifetime risk of developing breast cancer and a 45% risk of ovarian cancer. Germline *BRCA2* mutations predispose female carriers to an increased risk of ovarian cancer that is less pronounced than the risk associated with *BRCA1* mutations. It is recommended that those patients with hereditary ovarian cancer syndromes have annual rectovaginal examinations, CA-125 measurement, and transvaginal ultrasound until age 35 or the completition of childbearing. At that point, a prophylactic bilateral oophorectomy is recommended, but firm criteria for prophylactic oophorectomy have not been established.[13]

Screening

Because prognosis of ovarian cancer is strongly related to disease stage at the time of diagnosis, efforts are being made to improve early detection. Primary modalities include annual physical and gynecologic examination, pelvic ultrasound, tumor markers (CA-125), and genetic screening. Success has been reported with each modality, but inconsistencies between studies are common, and there is still no accepted screening standard.[14]

A large, randomized study to assess the feasibility of population screening using CA-125 values alone has been recently reported[15]: 21,935 postmenopausal women over the age of 45 were randomized into a control group or a three-year screening program consisting of CA-125 measurements which, if above 30 U/ml, were followed by pelvic ultrasound. If the volume of the ovary on ultrasound examination was larger than 8.8 ml, a gynecologic referral was made. Of 468 women with elevated CA-125 in the screening arm, 29 underwent surgery and 6 were diagnosed with ovarian cancer (0.055%). Three out of six were diagnosed with early-stage ovarian cancer. The positive predictive value (PPV) of the study was 21%, but it remained unclear whether there was any survival benefit. This study raises health economy and psychosocial issues and seems to confirm that screening of general population with CA-125 is not recommended.

Transvaginal ultrasound is another screening modality that is considered safe, time efficient, and well accepted by patients. Its greatest limitation is a low positive predictive value, as suggested by the inability of ultrasound to reliably distinguish between benign and malignant lesions. In a large and well-conducted study, Nagell *et al.* reported a PPV of 9.3%, indicating that 11 patients underwent surgery for benign adnexal mass for every ovarian malignancy detected.[16] Another major limitation of transvaginal screening is its failure to detect primary peritoneal carcinoma or ovarian malignancy in which ovarian size is normal.[16,17] On the other hand, Sato *et al.* reported the results of primary screening of 183,034 asymptomatic women and found 22 primary tumors and 2 metastatic tumors in 324 patients who underwent surgery, for a diagnostic rate of 0.047%.[18] Of the 22 primary tumors, 17 (77.3%) were stage I carcinomas. The percentage of the total number of carcinoma cases at stage I increased from 29.7% to 58.8% after the introduction of screening. It is unclear whether the encouraging results of this study may be related to different epidemiologic and biologic factors associated with ovarian cancer in Japan and the fact that the population examined already was undergoing screening for cervical carcinoma, or whether the suggested ultrasound algorithm may be reproducible in other studies.

TREATMENT

The Role of Laparoscopy

One of the major benefits of laparoscopic approach to all adnexal masses is avoiding overtreatment and unnecessary laparotomy. Most adnexal masses are benign, with malignancy found in only 7–13% of premenopausal and 8–45% postmenopausal patients.[19] The incidence of unsuspected ovarian cancer at laparoscopy has been shown to be only 0.04% in the 1990 survey of the American Association of Gynecologic Laparoscopists.[20] Further benefits of laparoscopic treatment of adnexal masses include shorter length of hospital stay,[21,22] decreased postoperative pain and recovery time,[23] less adhesion formation,[24] and lesser cost to the patient and the hospital.[25]

Accurate diagnosis at surgery is a key in management of adnexal masses. In the largest series of laparoscopically managed adnexal masses in women of reproductive age, Nezhat *et al.* reported that the most reliable indicators of malignancy were the combination of laparoscopic visualization of the whole peritoneal cavity and frozen section analysis.[26] Chapron *et al.* examined the accuracy of frozen section diagnosis in a series of 228 patients of whom 26 had suspicious adnexal masses at the time of laparoscopy. In all 26 patients frozen sections showed benign results, and in each case definitive histologic diagnosis confirmed the frozen section findings.[27] In a prospective study of 160 patients with adnexal masses treated at a gynecologic oncology service, Dottino *et al.* found a discrepancy between frozen section and final pathologic assessment in 3% of the cases.[28] It seems, therefore, that laparoscopy is a safe and reliable tool in the diagnosis and treatment of pelvic masses if performed cautiously and with the principles of cancer surgery kept in mind. Two important exceptions to the high accuracy of frozen section diagnosis are in very large tumors or tumors with borderline characteristics. In both cases accuracy depends on the relative risk of sampling bias. One solution to this problem is to remove entire adnexa and allow pathologic rather than surgical sampling.

Women of Reproductive Age

For the purpose of management, adnexal masses in this group of women can be divided into cystic and noncystic. Most of the simple cystic masses (50–90%) spontaneously resolve within two menstrual cycles. Medical management seems to offer no advantage over expectant management. Indications for surgery include size greater than 8–10 cm or growth on two subsequent scans, pain, worrisome personal or family history, failure to resolve within 2–6 months, and an incidentally found cyst while performing surgery for other indications. The principles of cancer surgery should apply to the treatment of benign-appearing cysts, because up to one-third of malignancies will retain a benign appearance.[29] Larger cysts, after excision from the ovary and placement in an endobag, may be ruptured to facilitate their removal without additional excisions or peritoneal contamination. Even larger cysts, which exceed the size of intracorporeal sacs, may be removed through minilaparotomy or colpotomy with excellent results.[30,31] Canis reported the results of a 12-year study of laparoscopically managed benign ovarian cysts that demonstrated a low complication rate of 1.5%, effectiveness of the procedure with a recurrence rate of 1.8%, and preservation of fertility after laparoscopic management.[32]

The role of laparoscopy in the management of noncystic masses has been a subject of controversy over the last decade.[33–36] According to the American Association of Gynecologic Laparoscopists, the majority of clinicians considers laparotomy to be the safest treatment of noncystic masses.[20] Maiman et al. reported that laparoscopic visualization might fail to identify cancer in one-third of the cases.[29] Wenzel et al. reported that 31 of 42 patients who underwent laparoscopic oophorectomy had a residual disease at subsequent staging laparotomy.[37] However, in both studies the use of frozen section analysis was minimal, and conversion to laparotomy was not performed in patients who were felt to have malignant or suspicious masses. On the other hand, in a French study conducted by Chapron et al., 11% of 228 masses evaluated preoperatively as "high risk" were found not to have features of malignancy during laparoscopy; all 26 were spared unnecessary surgery by obtaining frozen section diagnosis of excised adnexa.[27] Dottino et al. reported safe use of laparoscopy in 88% of 160 pre- and postmenopausal patients with suspicious adnexal masses.[28] All authors stress the importance of preoperative counseling, availability of immediate frozen section analysis, ability to convert to laparotomy immediately, and surgical expertise.[27,32]

Postmenopausal Women

The standard operative approach to adnexal masses in postmenopausal women has been explorative laparotomy to ensure adequate exposure for the treatment of ovarian cancer. Reports beginning in the late 1980s started to question this approach, observing that even in this group of patients there was a propensity for benign lesions,[38–40] and in some series up to 75% of tumors were histologically benign.[28,35,41] In the only prospective study, Dottino *et al.* reported that nearly 90% of cases were managed laparoscopically without appreciable increase in morbidity.[28] The same principles of careful visualization of the peritoneal cavity and obtaining the washings from the diaphragm, paracolic gutters, and pelvis before other surgical interventions were followed. Cystectomy in postmenopausal woman is not recommend; removal of the entire adnexa with frozen section diagnosis instead is warranted. Removal of a normal-appearing contalateral ovary should be performed according to preoperative consultation and past medical and family history when histology is benign.

Prior Nongynecologic Cancer

The primary question in patients with an adnexal mass and a history of previous non-gynecologic malignancy is whether the mass represents a new lesion, benign or malignant, or is a mark of metastatic disease. Although these patients seem to have *a priori* high risk of malignancy, Chi *et al.* found that even in this group 71% of the 34 patients had histologically benign masses.[33] Since one-third of the patients will be diagnosed with malignant disease, preoperative evaluation should include a CT scan, which allows comprehensive metastatic evaluation. Laparoscopy may be used in the diagnostic setting in certain cases, for example, if no tissue diagnosis can be obtained by fine needle aspiration. No prospective studies are available for this group; however, retrospective studies suggest that the initial laparoscopic approach decreases the number of laparotomies performed for benign disease.[33]

Ovarian Cancer

The most common indications for laparoscopy in patients with presumed or known ovarian malignancy include (i) laparoscopic staging of early-stage disease and (ii) second-look laparoscopy. Laparoscopy is a very attractive staging technique because of the magnification it provides and its ability to inspect the entire peritoneal cavity through a 10-mm incision. Preliminary data now suggest that in selected early ovarian cancers, an experienced laparoscopist can perform a complete staging procedure without compromising outcome.[28,35] Querleu described the first adequate laparoscopic surgical staging for ovarian carcinoma in 1993.[42] Subsequently, a few series have been reported on a small number of patients who underwent laparoscopic surgical staging for early-stage ovarian carcinoma. However, with only about 50 patients described in the English literature who have undergone surgical staging, and with no long-term follow-up, it remains unclear whether apparent early-stage ovarian cancer can be adequately staged laparoscopically. GOG is currently evaluating the role of laparoscopy in the staging of inadequately staged ovarian cancer, and this may help clarify the role of endoscopic staging of early-stage disease. Until more information is gained, laparoscopy should be reserved for well-designed clinical trials.

A second-look operation for ovarian carcinoma is the most accurate method of assessing the disease status in patients who have undergone staging and primary chemotherapy. Traditionally, operation is performed through a midline incision as a second-look laparotomy. The overall probability of finding persistent disease at the time of a second look is 50%. Although laparoscopy has certain advantages over laparotomy—primarily, better visualization of the diaphragm, superior view of the surface of the liver, and the ability to magnify even small lesions—controversial results were recently reported for laparoscopic second-look procedures. In a multi-center retrospective study of 192 patients with advanced ovarian cancer who underwent second-look surgery, Gaducci et al. reported a higher recurrence rate and shorter survival after negative laparoscopy compared with negative second-look laparotomy.[43] It is important to note there was no common therapy after negative second-look surgery in the group of 115 patients in the study, and the choices of treatment were based on personal preference. Clough et al. evaluated 20 patients who underwent laparoscopic second-look surgery followed by immmediate comparative laparotomy. The authors reported that the presence of postoperative adhesions and difficulties in visualization of mesentery and small bowel precluded safe and reliable laparoscopy.[44] (For a review, see also Canis et al.[45]) These data suggest that inadequate surgical procedures may be hazardous, but this may apply to laparotomy as well as laparoscopy. In contrast, when Abu-Rustum et al. compared the results of 31 second-look laparoscopies with those of 70 second-look laparotomies, they found similar rates of minimal residual disease for both laparotomy and laparoscopy.[46] Recurrence after a negative second-look operation was 14% with both laparoscopy and laparotomy, at a median follow-up time of 22 months.[46] Nezhat et al. reported a similar progression-free interval and survival in 25 patients undergoing second-look laparoscopy compared with 27 patients in the second-look laparotomy arm.[47] Overall, the postoperative morbidity after laparoscopic second-look surgery seems to be low, the hospital stay shorter, and intraoperative complications minimal if the surgery is performed by an experienced laparoscopist and if the requirements for safe conditions are satisfied.

Risks of Laparoscopy

The improvements in laparoscopic techniques raise the possibility of universal use of laparoscopy for initial diagnosis and treatment of almost all adnexal masses. However, this approach has been burdened by results of studies highlighting the risks of laparoscopy.[48,49] These risks include (i) failure to recognize ovarian malignancy or inability to directly proceed with laparotomy if cancer is diagnosed and subsequent delay in adequate treatment; (ii) cyst rupture and spillage; (iii) port site metastases, and (iv) intraperitoneal tumor dissemination.

The major concern raised in regard to minimal-access surgery is the risk of inappropriate management of ovarian cancer. Maiman et al. have shown that delays of four weeks from the initial diagnosis to the complete surgical staging of incidentally detected ovarian cancer have been shown to worsen outcome.[29] Alvarez et al. questioned whether there is a risk of disease progression if the treatment is delayed for even less than two weeks.[50] Kinderman et al. argued that even a delay of 8 days can allow tumor progression; however, in that study in 55% of the cases the tumor was ruptured or morcelated, possibly allowing for tumor progression.[51] A study by Kinderman indicates indirectly that inadequate surgical procedures may worsen diagnosis. This applies to both laparoscopy and laparotomy. In a study by Helawa et al., only 40% of the cancer cases were suspected at initial laparotomy.[52] Several other studies reported about 20% incidence in the upstaging of early ovarian cancer after inadequate initial laparotomy.[53]

Tumor spillage is a concern during both laparoscopic surgery and laparotomy. Spillage of tumor contents may be problematic in benign conditions such as pseudomyxoma peritonei or rupture of mature teratoma because of the consequent chemical peritonitis. Spillage of malignant cyst fluid is cause for upstaging in the FIGO system from Ia to Ic. Much of the support for this upstaging is based on retrospective, poorly controlled studies, using treatment options that are now considered suboptimal.[54,55] Dembo *et al.*, however, found that rates of relapse or prognosis were not influenced by intraoperative rupture of the tumor in properly staged patients.[56] These findings were confirmed by Sevelda *et al.* who found that 5-year survival, with or without intaroperative tumor rupture, was 76% for stage I disease.[57] An increasing amount of evidence indicates that intraoperative tumor spillage does not affect survival, whereas spontaneous preoperative tumor rupture has a negative influence on survival.[58] Still, in many cases upstaging is the decisive factor in determining the need for additional treatment, and therefore extreme caution should be taken to minimize the risk of spillage.

Abdominal wall metastases, also called port- or wound-site metastases, have been reported after both laparoscopy and laparotomy. The incidence of these complications has been 1% after laparotomy and mostly 1–2% after laparoscopy, with a single study reporting an incidence of 16%.[59,60] The most likely mechanism for port-site metastases seems to be direct contamination by the surgical procedure during tumor extraction or the postoperative withdrawal of contaminated ports and loss of abdominal insufflation, and these have been reported in colon and gallbladder surgery as well.[61] Chu *et al.* and Wang *et al.* described recurrence at port sites in a patient who underwent laparoscopic staging for cervical cancer.[62,63] Similar port-site recurrence was described after laparoscopic staging for endometrial cancer. Kadar reported his experience on 25 patients with gynecologic malignancy who underwent laparoscopic procedures. Port-site metastases were found in 4 of 25 patients.[64] All port-site metastases in this series were associated with advanced disease, and all were inoculated at the time of surgery and were not treated postoperatively. Although port/wound-site recurrences may be disfiguring and difficult to treat, there is no prospective evidence that port-site metastases worsen prognosis. In the only retrospective study addressing this issue, Kruitwagen *et al.* failed to find a significant survival difference between patients with and without abdominal wall metastasis after adjusting for age, stage, grade, and amount of residual disease after primary debulking.[60]

A number of animal studies suggest increased tumor dissemination after a CO_2 pneumoperitoneum.[48] Voltz *et al.* reported diffuse intraperitoneal tumor spread after laparoscopy in nude mice injected intraperitoneally with a human lung cancer cell line. The survival time was the shortest in the group of mice in which CO_2 was used, compared with heated CO_2 or helium.[65] Canis *et al.*[66] used immunocompetent rats injected intraperitoneally with rat ovarian carcinoma cells and divided them into four groups: one group served as a control, another underwent laparotomy, a third group had low-pressure pneumoperitoneum (4 mm Hg), and the fourth group was exposed to 10 mm Hg pneumoperitoneum. There was greater tumor growth after laparotomy than laparoscopy. In the high-pressure pneumoperitoneum group (10 mm Hg), tumors were disseminated more diffusely than in the low-pressure pneumoperitoneum (4 mm Hg) group. Wound metastases were larger and more frequent after laparotomy. As pointed out by Canis *et al.*,[48] one has to be cautious when interpreting results of animal studies. Important variables that must be taken into consideration before reaching conclusions include the animal model, choice of cell line for inoculation, postoperative immune situation, the pressure of pneumoperitoneum, and sample size (number of animals). Each detail of a model can influence the results, and very careful selection of all parameters needs to be performed in order to closely mimic the clinical situation.

However, a few reports also raised concerns regarding possible intraperitoneal tumor dissemination following laparoscopy in clinical situations. Canis *et al.* reported a case of pelvic dissemination found at a restaging procedure 3 weeks after initial adnexectomy for a well-differentiated serous adenocarcinoma of the ovary.[32] Two cases of peritoneal carcinomatosis were reported in patients with cervical carcinoma who underwent laparoscopic lumphadenectomy and had miscoscopically positive nodes.[63,67] Although one may argue that these findings are more indicative of tumor biology than a consequence of surgical approach, it would be prudent to introduce surgical measures to prevent tumor dissemination and port site contamination. Canis *et al.* propose careful selection of cases and minimal tumor manipulation to prevent intraperitoneal tumor spread as well as removal of all specimens using an endobag and removal of all ports while the abdomen is still insufflated, to prevent possible contamination of port sites as well as the immediate local treatment of the ports with a cytotoxic agent.[45]

CONCLUSION

With growing interest in operative laparoscopy in gynecology, the indications for its use are broadening. Once limited to a small number of premenopausal women with clinically clearly benign adnexal masses, an increasing trend toward a universal laparoscopic approach to all adnexal masses is evident. Indeed, laparoscopy is considered safe and effective in the initial surgical evaluation of adnexal masses when strict guidelines are used, frozen section analysis is available, and principles of cancer surgery respected. Inevitably, however, the increased use of minimal access surgery to evaluate and manage adnexal masses has raised concerns of potential risks for undertreating ovarian cancer. Results of experimental studies in this regard indicate both advantages and disadvantages for laparoscopic surgery in the setting of potentially malignant adnexal masses. The results of these studies should be taken into consideration, and surgical practices modified to prevent possible port-site recurrences or potential tumor dissemination. The improvements in laparoscopic techniques and video equipment offer the opportunity to use laparoscopy to perform ovarian cancer surgery, previously performed only by laparotomy. The indications for laparoscopy in this setting are mostly limited to staging of early or incompletely staged ovarian cancer and second-look surgery. We advocate the practice of reasonable laparoscopy, with all safety conditions fullfilled, preferably in well-designed prospective clinical trials to better define its role in the management of malignant adnexal masses.

REFERENCES

1. CURTIN, J.P. 1994. Management of the adnexal mass. Gynecol. Oncol. **55:** S42–46.
2. KOONINGS, P.P., K. CAMPBELL, D.R. MISHELL, JR. & D.A. GRIMES. 1989. Relative frequency of primary ovarian neoplasms: a 10-year review. Obstet. Gynecol. **74:** 921–926.

3. DiSAIA, P.J. & W.T. CREASMAN. 1997. Clinical Gynecologic Oncology. Mosby-Year Book Inc. St. Louis, MO.
4. KURJAK, A., M. PREDANIC, S. KUPESIC-UREK & S. JUKIC. 1993. Transvaginal color and pulsed Doppler assessment of adnexal tumor vascularity. Gynecol. Oncol. **50:** 3–8.
5. KURJAK, A., I. ZALUD & Z. AFIREVIC. 1991. Evaluation of adnexal masses with transvaginal color ultrasound. J. Ultrasound. Med. **10:** 295–297.
6. SASSONE, A., I. TIMOR-TRITCH, A. ARTNER, et al. 1991. Transvaginal sonographic characterization of ovarian disease: evaluation of a new scoring system to predict ovarian malignancy. Obstet. Gynecol. **78:** 7–11.
7. GRAB, D., F. FLOCK & I. STOHR. 2000. Classification of asymptomatic adnexal masses by ultrasound, magnetic resonance imaging, and positron emission tomography. Gynecol. Oncol. **77:** 454–459.
8. ALCAZAR, J.L. & M. JURADO. 1999. Prospective evaluation of a logistic model based on sonographic morphologic and color Doppler findings developed to predict adnexal malignancy. J. Ultrasound. Med. **18:** 837–842.
9. JACOBS, I., A.P. DAVIES, J. BRIDGES, et al. 1993. Prevalence screening for ovarian cancer in postmenopausal women by CA125 measurement and ultrasonography. Br. Med. J. **306:** 1030–1032.
10. BROOKS, S.E. 1994. Preoperative evaluation of patients with suspicious ovarian cancer. Gynecol. Oncol. **55:** 80–90.
11. MEYER, T. & G.S.J. RUSTIN. 2000. Role of tumor markers in monitoring epithelial ovarian cancer. Br. J. Cancer **82:** 1535–1538.
12. NATIONAL INSITUTES OF HEALTH. 1995. NIH Consensus Statement 1994. Ovarian cancer: screening, treatment, and follow-up. JAMA **273:** 491–497.
13. MORROW, C.P. & J.P. CURTIN. 1998. Etiology and detection of gynecologic cancer. In Synopsis of Gynecologic Oncology. C.P. Morrow & J.P. Curtin, Eds.: 1–16. Churchill Livingstone. Philadelphia.
14. BELL, R., M. PETTICREW & T. SHELDON. 1998. The performance of screening tests for ovarian cancer: results of a systematic review. Br. J. Obstet. Gynaecol. **105:** 1136–1147.
15. JACOBS, I.J., S.J. SKATES, N. MACDONALD, et al. 1999. Screening for ovarian cancer: a pilot randomized study. Lancet **353:** 1207–1210.
16. VAN NAGELL, J.R., P.D. DEPRIEST, M.B. REEDY, et al. 2000. The efficacy of transvaginal sonographic screening in asymptomatic women at risk for ovarian cancer. Gynecol. Oncol. **77:** 350–356.
17. LU, K.H., J.E. GARBER, D.W. CRAMER, et al. 2000. Occult ovarian tumors in women with *BRCA1* and *BRCA2* mutations undergoing oophorectomy. J. Clin. Oncol. **18:** 2728–2732.
18. SATO, S., Y. YOKOYAMA, T. SAKAMOTO, et al. 2000. Usefulness of mass screening for ovarian carcinoma using transvaginal ultrasonography. Cancer **89:** 582–588.
19. PARKER, W.H. & J.S. BEREK. 1994. Laparoscopic management of the adnexal mass. Obstet. Gynecol. Clin. N. Am. **21:** 79–92.
20. HULKA, J.T., W.H. PARKER, M.W. SURREY, et al. 1992. American Association of Gynecologists and Laparoscopists. Survey of management of ovarian masses in 1990. J. Reprod. Med. **37:** 599–602.
21. MAIS, V., S. AJOSSA, S. GUERRIERO, et al. 1996. Laparoscopic versus abdominal myomectomy: a prospective randomized trial to evaluate benefits in early outcome. Am. J. Obstet. Gynecol. **174:** 654–658.
22. MAIS, V., S. AJOSSA, B. PIRAS, et al. 1995. Treatment of nonendometriotic benign adnexal cyst. A randomized comparison of laparoscopy and laparotomy. Obstet. Gynecol. **86:** 770–774.
23. DAVISON, J., W. PARK & L. PENNEY. 1993. Comparative study of operative laparoscopy vs. laparotomy: analysis of the financial impact. Reprod. Med. **38:** 357–360.
24. LUNDORFF, P., J. THORBURN, M. HAHLIN, et al. 1991. Adhesion formation after laparoscopic surgery in tubal pregnancy: a randomized trial versus laparotomy. Fertil. Steril. **55:** 911–915.
25. MARUIRI, F. & A. AZZIZ. 1993. Laparoscopic surgery for ectopic pregnancies: technology assessment and public health implications. Technol. Steril. **59:** 487–498.

26. NEZHAT, F.R., C.H. NEZHAT, C.E. WELANDER & B. BENIGNO, B. 1992. Four ovarian cancers diagnosed during laparoscopic management of 1011 women with adnexal masses. Am. J. Obstet. Gynecol. **167:** 790–796.
27. CHAPRON, C., J.B. DUBUISSON, O. KADOCH, *et al.* 1998. Laparoscopic management of oraganic ovarian cysts: is there a place for frozen section in the diagnosis? Hum. Reprod. **13:** 324–329.
28. DOTTINO, P.R., D.A. LEVINE, D.L. RIPLEY & C.J. COHEN. 1999. Laparoscopic management of adnexal masses in premenopausal and postmenopausal women. Obstet. Gynecol. **93:** 223–228.
29. MAIMAN, M., V. SELTZER & J. BOYCE. 1991. Laparoscopic excision of ovarian neoplasms subsequently found to be malignant. Obstet. Gynecol. **77:** 563–765.
30. FLYN NILOFF, J.M. 1995. Minilaparotomy for the ambulatory management of ovarian cysts. Am. J. Obstet. Gynecol. **173:** 1727–1730.
31. TENG, F.Y., D. MUZSNAI & R. PEREZ. 1996. A comparative study of laparoscopy and colpotomy for the removal of ovarian dermoid cysts. Obstet. Gynecol. **87:** 1009–1013.
32. CANIS, M., J.L. POULY, A. WATTICZ, *et al.* 1997. Laparoscopic management of adnexal masses suspicious at ultrasound. Obstet. Gynecol. **89:** 679–683.
33. CHI, D.S., J.P. CURTIN & R.R. BARAKAT. 1995. Laparoscopic management of adnexal masses in women with a history of nongynecologic malignancy. Obstet. Gynecol. **86:** 964–968.
34. NEZHAT, C.T., S. KAYONCUS, C.H. NEZHAT, *et al.* 1999. Laparoscopic management of ovarian dermoid cysts: ten years' experience. J. Soc. Laparosc. Surg. **3:** 179–184.
35. CHILDERS, J.M., A. NASSERI & E.A. SURWIT. 1996. Laparoscopic management of suspicious adnexal masses. Am. J. Obstet. Gynecol. **175:** 1171–1179.
36. PARKER, W.H. 1995. The case for laparoscopic management of the adnexal mass. Clin. Obstet. Gynecol. **38:** 362–369.
37. WENZEL, R., R. LEHNER, P. HUSSLEIN & P. SEVELDA. 1996. Laparoscopic surgery in cases of ovarian malignancies: an Austrian-wide survey. Gynecol. Oncol. **63:** 57–61.
38. ANDOLF, E., C. JORGENSEN, E. SCALENIUS, *et al.* Ultrasound measurement of the ovarian volume. Acta Obstet. Gynecol. Scand. **66:** 387–392.
39. RULIN, M.C. & A.L. PRESTON. 1987. Adnexal mass in post menopausal women. Obstet. Gynecol. **70:** 578–581.
40. GRANBERG, S., M. WIKLAND & I. JANSSON, I. 1989. Microscopic characterization of ovarian tumors and the relation to the histologic diagnosis: criteria to be used for ultrasound evaluation. Gynecol. Oncol. **35:** 139–144.
41. SHALEV, E., S. ELIYAHU, D. PELEG & A. TSABARI. 1994. Laparoscopic management of adnexal cystic masses in postmenopausal women. Obstet. Gynecol. **83:** 594–596.
42. QUERLEU, D. 1993. Laparoscopic periaortic node sampling in gynecologic oncology: a preliminary experience. Gynecol. Oncol. **49:** 24–29.
43. GADDUCCI, A., E. SARTORI, T. MAGGINO, *et al.* 1998. Analysis of failures after negative second-look in patients with advanced ovarian cancer: an Italian multicenter study. Gynecol. Oncol. **68:** 150–155.
44. CLOUGH, K. B., J.M. LADONNE, C. NOS, *et al.* 1999. Second-look for ovarian cancer: laparoscopy or laparotomy. A prospective comparative study. Gynecol. Oncol. **72:** 411–417.
45. CANIS, M., R. BOTCHORISHVILLI, H. MANHES, *et al.* 2000. Management of adnexal masses: role and risks of laparoscopy. Semin. Surg. Oncol. **19:** 28–35.
46. ABU-RUSTUM, N.R., R.B. BARAKAT, P.L. SIEGEL, *et al.* 1996. Second-look operation for epithelial ovarian cancer: laparoscopy or laparotomy? Obstet. Gynecol. **88:** 549–553.
47. NEZHAT, F.R., J. RAHAMAN, P. DOTTINO, *et al.* 1999. Accuracy of second-look laparoscopy compared with second-look laparotomy in predicting recurrence and survival in advanced ovarian cancer. *In* Abstracts of the Global Congress of Gynecologic Endoscopy, 28th Annual Meeting of the American Association of Gynecologic Laparoscopists S146.
48. CANIS, M., R. BOTCHORISHVILLI, A. WATTIEZ, *et al.* 2000. Cancer and laparoscopy, experimental studies: a review. Eur. J. Obstet. Gynecol. Reprod. Biol. **91:** 1–9.

49. CHILDERS, J.M. 1999. The virtues and pitfalls of minimally invasive surgery for gynecologic cancer: an update. Curr. Opin. Obstet. Gynecol. **11:** 51–59.
50. ALVAREZ, R.D., L.C. KILGORE, E.E. PARTRIDGE, et al. 1993. Staging of ovarian cancer diagnosed during laparoscopy: accuracy rather than immediacy. South. Med. J. **86:** 1256–1258.
51. KINDERMAN, G., V. MAASSEN & W. KUHN. 1996. Laparoscopic management of ovarian tumors subsequently diagnosed as malignant: a survey form 127 German departments of obstetrics and gynecology. J. Pelvic Surg. **2:** 245–251.
52. HELAWA, M.E., G.V. KREPART & R. LOTOCKI. 1986. Staging laparotomy in early epithelial ovarian carcinoma. Am. J. Obstet. Gynecol. **154:** 282–286.
53. STIER, E.A., R.B. BARAKAT, J.P. CURTIN, et al. Laparotomy to complete staging of presumed early ovarian cancer. Obstet. Gynecol. **87:** 737–740.
54. SAINZ DE LA CUESTA, R., B.A. GOFF, A.F. FULLER, et al. 1994. Prognostic importance of intraoperative rupture of malignant ovarian epithelial neoplasms. Obstet. Gynecol. **84:** 1–7.
55. WEBB, M.J., D.G. DECKER, E. MUSSEY & T.J. WILLIAMS. 1973. Factors influencing survival in stage I ovarian cancer. Am. J. Obstet. Gynecol. **116:** 222–228.
56. DEMBO, A.J., M. DAVY, A.E. STENWIG, et al. 1990. Prognostic factors in patients with stage I epithelial ovarian cancer. Obstet. Gynecol. **75:** 263–272.
57. SEVELDA, P., C. DITTTRICH & H. SALZER. 1989. Prognostic value of the rupture of capsule in stage I epithelial ovarian carcinoma. Gynecol. Oncol. **35:** 321–322.
58. SJOVALL, K., B. NILSSON & N. EINHORN. 1994. Different types of rupture of the tumor capsule and the impact on survival in early ovarian carcinoma. Int. J. Gynecol. Cancer **4:** 333–336.
59. CHILDERS, J.M., K.A. AQUA, E.A. SURWIT, et al. 1994. Abdominal wall tumor implantation after laparoscopy for malignant conditions. Obstet. Gynecol. **84:** 765–769.
60. KRUITWAGEN, R.F.P.M., B.M. SWINKELS, K.G.G. KEYSER, et al. 1996. Incidence and effect on survival of abdominal wall metastases at trocar puncture sites following laparoscopy or paracentesis in women with ovarian cancer. Gynecol. Oncol. **60:** 233–237.
61. PAOLUCCI, V., B. SCHAELF, M. SCHNEIDER & C. GUTT. 1999. Tumor seeding following laparoscopy: international survey. World J. Surg. **23:** 989–997.
62. CHU, K., S. CHANG, F. CHEN, et al. 1997. Laparoscopic surgical staging in cervical cancer—preliminary experience among Chinese. Gynecol. Oncol. **64:** 49–53.
63. WANG, P.H., C.C. YUAN, K.C. CHAO, et al. 1997. Squamous cell carcinoma of the cervix after laparoscopic surgery: a case report. J. Reprod. Med. **42:** 801–804.
64. KADAR, N. 1997. Port-site recurrences following laparoscopic operations for gynecologic malignancies. Br. J. Obstet. Gynecol. **104:** 1308–1313.
65. VOLTZ, J., V. PAOLUCCI, B. SCHAEFF, et al. 1998. Laparoscopic surgery: the effects of insufflation gas on tumour-induced lethality in nude mice. Am. J. Obstet. Gynecol. **178:** 793–795.
66. CANIS, M., R. BOTCHORISHVILLI, A. WATTIEZ, et al. 1998. Tumor growth and dissemination after laparotomy and CO_2 pneumoperitoneum: a rat ovarian cancer model. Obstet. Gynecol. **92:** 104–108.
67. COHN, D.E., H.K. TAMIMI & B.A. GOFF. 1997. Intraperitoneal spread of cervical cancer after laparoscopic lymphadenectomy. Obstet. Gynecol. **89:** 864–865.

Laparoscopic Myomectomy

Fertility Results

JEAN-BERNARD DUBUISSON, CHARLES CHAPRON, ARNAUD FAUCONNIER, AND KATAYOUN BABAKI-FARD

Service de Chirurgie Gynécologique Clinique Universitaire Baudelocque, Hôpital Cochin, 123, Boulevard Port-Royal, 75014 Paris, France

ABSTRACT: The appearance of uterine myomas has been linked to infertility. It has been suggested that surgical management of myomas by laparoscopic myomectomy improves fertility rates in these group of patients. In this paper we initially describe specific aspects of the surgical technique of laparoscopic myomectomy including the set-up, precise technique for hysteroromy, enucleation of the myoma, suturing of the uterus, and extraction of the myoma. We detail recent findings that demonstrate improved fertility rates in women undergoing laparoscopic myomectomy. We recommend that, when criteria for selection of patients is strictly adhered to and patients present with no other associated infertility, laparoscopic myomectomy be used to increase the implantation rate.

KEYWORDS: laparoscopic myomectomy; uterine myoma; fertility; laparotomy

INTRODUCTION

The frequency at which myomas occur during the period when patients are sexually active is estimated at between 30 and 40%. Although it is difficult to state categorically that myomas are responsible for infertility, several elements indicate that they do bear some responsibility: the pregnancy rate is lower in patients with myomas,[1–3] and, in cases of medically assisted procreation (IVF), the implantation rate is lower in patients presenting interstitial myomas.[4–6]

Surgical management of myomas depends on their number and their location. Myomas with a mostly intracavity development should be dealt with by hysteroscopy, and these constitute a specific group that we will not discuss in this paper. Interstitial and subserous myomas can be operated either by laparotomy or by laparoscopy. Laparoscopic myomectomy is a technique that has been properly validated,[7,8] in that the indications have been established clearly: two or fewer in number, 8 cm or less in diameter. In this paper we will look at fertility after laparoscopic myomectomy. To begin with, we present the essential points concerning the laparoscopic surgical technique, after which we discuss the fertility results.

Address for correspondence: Prof. Jean-Bernard Dubuisson, Service de Chirurgie Gynécologique, Clinique Universitaire Baudelocque, C.H.U. Cochin, 123, Boulevard Port-Royal, 75014 Paris, France. Voice: 01-58-41-18-81; fax: 01-40-51-77-62.

jean-bernard.dubuisson@cch.ap-hop-paris.fr

OPERATING TECHNIQUES

The current technique for laparoscopic myomectomy is well established and will not be described.[7,8] Instead, we would like to clarify certain points that will make this technique easier, avoid complications, and avoid conversion to laparotomy.

The set-up is of prime importance. The first step is uterine cannulation with a blunt curet and two tenaculum forceps attached to each other such that the uterus can be manipulated to provide anteversion, retroversion, lateralization, and rotation. If the myoma is large, the laparoscope should be inserted several centimeters above the umbilicus in order to obtain a panoramic view of the pelvis. Similarly the accessory trocars should be inserted sufficiently high on the abdomen to provide an easy approach to the myomas for the laparoscopic instruments.

A precise technique should be used for the hysterotomy. It should be direct in order to keep dissection time and bleeding to a minimum. It should be vertical for posterior myomas in order to allow easier suturing by means of a curved needle fitted into a needle holder introduced via the midline trocar. The hysterotomy should be transverse or oblique for anterior myomas, for easier suturing using a curved needle in a needle holder introduced via one of the lateral trocars. The incision is made using a monopolar electrode (curved scissors, for example). We do not feel that the use of lasers is indicated in this situation. Hysterotomy is not the best indication for the harmonic scalpel because its coagulation or section effect is slow and it does not achieve perfect hemostasis of the big veins surrounding the myoma.

After the hysterotomy, the myoma is enucleated using the curved scissors along the cleavage plane of the pseudocapsule, with a minimum of coagulation. Unwarranted coagulation causes tissue necrosis, which can affect the quality of healing.[9] Hydrodissection is of no help for cleavage in this situation.

The uterine suture is made along one or two planes. It consists of bringing the entire thickness of the edges of the myomectomy site together to prevent the formation of hematomas. We use large, curved needles for this (30 or 40 mm) swaged to Vicryl (1, 0, 00) to make simple separate or U-shaped stitches. If additional seroserosa suturing is needed, we use finer suture material (Vicryl 00 or 000).

At this point, extraction takes place with electric morcellation. The 10/12-mm suprapubic accessory trocar allows the morcellator to be inserted. Electric morcellation avoids cutting the myoma with the cold knife via the abdominal wall and thus avoids enlarging one of the supra pubic incisions, which often gives displeasing cosmetic results. If no electric morcellator is available, or it proves inefficient because the myoma is too hard, extraction by posterior colpotomy is a solution that is both elegant and rapid.

FERTILITY RESULTS

We have already reported our fertility results after laparoscopic myomectomy for a series of 91 patients.[10] Detailed results are given in TABLE 1. The rate of patients achieving pregnancy is 53.1% (43 patients). These 43 patients obtained 51 pregnancies. The rate of ongoing intrauterine pregnancy is 80.4% (41 patients). The ectopic

TABLE 1. Descriptive analysis of reproductive outcome after laparoscopic myomectomy

	Without associated factors No. (%)	With associated factors No. (%)	Total population No. (%)
Patients operated	25	66	91
Patients assessed	24 (100.0)	57 (100.0)	81(100.0)
Women pregnant	17 (70.8)	26 (45.6)	43 (53.1)
Total pregnancies	20 (100.0)	31(100.0)	51(100.0)
Pregnancy outcome			
EP	0 (0.0)	1 (3.2)	1 (2.0)
Miscarriage	5 (25.0)	4 (12.9)	9 (17.6)
Delivery	13 (65.0)	24 (77.4)	37 (72.6)
Ongoing IUP	2 (10.0)	2 (6.5)	4 (7.8)
Mode of conception			
Spontaneous	17 (85.0)	14 (45.2)	31 (60.8)
Stimulation	3 (15.0)	5 (16.1)	8 (15.7)
Insemination	0 (0.0)	2 (6.4)	2 (3.9)
IVF	0 (0.0)	10 (32.3)	10 (19.6)

ABBREVIATIONS: EP, ectopic pregnancy; IUP, intrauterine pregnancy; IVF, *in vitro* fertilization.
SOURCE: From Dubuisson *et al.*[10] Used with permission.

pregnancy rate for this series is low (1 patient, 2%). The pregnancy rate obtained in this series of infertile patients using *in vitro* fertilization (IVF) techniques is 20% (10 cases). Detailed study of the results enables the two populations to be distinguished according to whether any other factors are associated with the myomas.

For patients with no associated infertility factor, that is, patients for whom the only reason found to explain the infertility was myoma, the results are very encouraging with a high percentage of patients achieving pregnancy at 70.8% (17 patients). Twenty pregnancies were achieved by these 17 patients. These results are significantly higher than those for patients presenting infertility factors associated with the myomas (45.6%: 26 patients; 31 pregnancies). Similarly, the way in which these pregnancies were achieved differed, depending on whether other associated infertility factors were involved. When there were no associated infertility factors, all the pregnancies were obtained spontaneously (17 cases, 85%) or with the help of stimulation (3 cases, 15%). No pregnancy in this group was obtained by assisted reproductive techniques (ART). It is quite a different matter for the group of patients with associated infertility factors. One-third of the pregnancies obtained (32.3%, 10 cases) used IVF. The rate of spontaneous pregnancies was only 45.2% (14 patients), and the rate of pregnancies after ovarian stimulation was 16.1% (5 patients)(TABLE 1).

DISCUSSION

Laparoscopic myomectomy, which has now been described by several authors,[11–13] is now a completely validated technique.[8] The indications have been established clearly,[8] and the risk of complications assessed.[7] The specific point that is the subject of much debate in the literature is the quality of the uterine scar after laparoscopic myomectomy. Several cases of uterine rupture have been reported.[14–16] For our part, on the basis of a series of over 100 births after laparoscopic myomectomy, the uterine rupture rate is 1%.[17] It is important to stress that, although there is indeed a risk, it is not at all specific to laparoscopic myomectomy. Cases of uterine rupture have been reported after hysteroscopic resection,[18] myolysis,[19] and even myomectomy by laparotomy.[20]

Concerning fertility, we feel the following points are essential:

- Although it is important to stress that the indications for laparotomy and for laparoscopic surgery for myomectomy are completely different, the fertility results observed after each of these techniques are comparable.[21,22] The results are reported in detail in TABLE 2. Given that the advantages of laparoscopic surgery compared with laparotomy are now fully accepted, myomectomy should be carried out by operative laparoscopy if the indications are acceptable. The advantages of operative laparoscopy have been confirmed by a randomized, prospective trial by Mais et al.[23]

- The most important outcome is the excellent pregnancy rates obtained for those infertile patients with no other associated factor to explain their infertility. This prompts us to propose myomectomy for these patients, including when the myoma is small. One of the reasons that we have decided to ablate these small myomas is that, during follow-up of these patients, we have observed an increase in volume detected by successive ultrasound scan.

- The results after myomectomy for infertile women with other associated infertility factors are far less favorable, both in our experience and as reported by others.[21] This does not imply that myomectomy should be avoided by these patients. Publications addressing the question of implantation after IVF in patients with or without interstitial myoma show that patients with no myoma have a very distinct advantage.[5] Consequently, the goal of the myomectomy will essentially be to optimize the results of ART, rather than to hope for a spontaneous pregnancy.

- One of the problems specific to myomectomy, regardless of the approach (laparotomy or laparoscopic surgery), is frequency of postoperative adhesions.[24] In our experience, after laparoscopic myomectomy the proportion of patients presenting adhesions is 36% (16 out of 45).[25] It must be borne in mind that, although the rate after laparoscopic myomectomy appears more favorable than that observed after myomectomy by laparotomy, the indications differ according to the operative technique. In our daily practice this considerable risk of postoperative adhesions means we offer, but do not impose, a second-look laparoscopy to patients who desire pregnancy. Any adhesions are corrected during this inspection. The second advantage of a sec-

TABLE 2. Main myomectomy series for infertility published since 1960

Author	Year	No. with infertility	No. without associated factor[a]	Percent of conception among infertile women	Percent of conception among women without associated factor
Laparoscopy					
Hasson *et al.*	1992	17		65	
Miller *et al.*	1996	40		75	
Daraï *et al.*	1997	44	29	39	48
Dubuisson *et al.*	1998	81	24	53	71
Total laparoscopy		**182**	**53**	**56**	**58**
Laparotomy					
Stevenson	1964	52		58	
Malone *et al.*	1968	75		49	
Loeffler *et al.*	1970	23		39	
Babaknia *et al.*	1978		67		51
Ranney *et al.*	1979	25	9		
Berkeley *et al.*	1983	25	6	36	16
Garcia *et al.*	1984	17	17	53	53
Rosenfeld	1986	23	23	65	65
Starks	1988	32		63	
Gatti *et al.*	1989	30	20	43	67
Gehlbach *et al.*	1993	37	9	51	
Tulandi *et al.*	1993	26	25	67[b]	
Acien *et al.*	1996	20	4	50	100
Total laparotomy		**359**	**155**	**53**	**57**

[a]Definition varies depending on the authors.
[b]Cumulative probability of conception at one year (number of pregnancies not communicated).
SOURCE: The authors are referenced in the article by J.B. Dubuisson *et al.*[10]

ond-look laparoscopy is the possibility of carrying out a methylene blue test to check tube permeability and, above all, the quality of the uterine scar. The existence of a uterine fistula or dehiscence of the myomectomy scar is an important risk factor for uterine rupture.[13,15]

CONCLUSION

Laparoscopic myomectomy is a validated and reproducible technique. The fertility results obtained in patients presenting no other associated infertility factor are very much in favor of surgery. If the criteria for selection are properly applied (number and size of the myomas), the operation should be carried out by laparoscopic surgery. The advantage is less clear for patients presenting associated factors for infertility. Before considering medically assisted procreation, we recommend laparoscopic myomectomy with the aim of increasing the implantation rate.

REFERENCES

1. ROSS, R.K., M.C. PIKE, M.P. VESSEY, et al. 1986. Risk factors for uterine fibroids: reduced risk associated with oral contraceptives. Br. Med. J. **293:** 359–362.
2. PARAZZINI, F., E. NEGRI, C. LA VECCHIA, et al. 1996. Reproductive risk factors and risk of uterine fibroids. Epidemiology **7:** 440–442.
3. CRAMER, D.W., A.M. WALKER & I. SCHIFF. 1979. Statistical methods in evaluating the outcome of infertility therapy. Fertil. Steril. **32:** 80–86.
4. FAHRI, J., J. ASHKENAZY, D. FELDBERG, et al. 1995. Effect of uterine leiomyomata on the results of in-vitro fertilization treatment. Hum. Reprod. **10:** 2576–2578.
5. STOVALL, D., S. PARRISH, B. VAN VOORHIS, et al. 1998. Uterine leiomyomata reduce the efficacy of assisted reproduction cycles: results of a matched follow-up study. Hum. Reprod. **13:** 192–197.
6. ELDAR-GEVA, T., S. MEAGHER, D.L. HEALY, et al. 1998. Effect of intramural, subserosal, and submucosal uterine fibroids on the outcome of assisted reproductive technology treatment. Fertil. Steril. **70:** 687–691.
7. DUBUISSON, J.B., C. CHAPRON & L. LEVY. 1996. Difficulties and complications of laparoscopic myomectomy. J. Gynecol. Surg. **12:** 159–165.
8. DUBUISSON, J.B., C. CHAPRON, A. FAUCONNIER, et al. 1997. Laparoscopic myomectomy and myolysis. Curr. Opin. Obstet. Gynecol. **9:** 233–238.
9. ELKINS, T.E., T.G. STOVALL, J. WARREN, et al. 1987. A histologic evaluation of peritoneal injury and repair. Obstet. Gynecol. **70:** 225–228.
10. DUBUISSON, J.B., A. FAUCONNIER, C. CHAPRON, et al. 2000. Reproductive outcome after laparoscopic myomectomy in infertile women. J. Reprod. Med. **45:** 23–30.
11. DUBUISSON, J.B., F. LECURU, H. FOULOT, et al. 1991. Myomectomy by laparoscopy: a preliminary report of 43 cases. Fertil. Steril. **56:** 827–830.
12. HASSON, J.M., C. ROTMAN, N. RANA, et al. 1992. Laparoscopic myomectomy. Obstet. Gynecol. **80:** 884–888.
13. NEZHAT, C., F. NEZHAT, S.L. SILFEN, et al. 1991. Laparoscopic myomectomy. Int. J. Fertil. **36:** 275–280.
14. HARRIS, W.J. 1992. Uterine dehiscence following laparoscopic myomectomy. Obstet. Gynecol. **80:** 545–546.
15. DUBUISSON, J.B., X. CHAVET, C. CHAPRON, et al. 1995. Uterine rupture during pregnancy after laparoscopic myomectomy. Hum. Reprod. **10:** 1475–1477.
16. FRIEDMANN, W., R.F. MAIER, A. LUTIKUS, et al. 1996. Uterine rupture after laparoscopic myomectomy. Acta Obstet. Gynecol. Scand. **75:** 683–684.
17. DUBUISSON, J.B., A. FAUCONNIER, J.V. DEFFARGES, et al. 2000. Pregnancy outcome and deliveries following laparoscopic myomectomy. Hum. Reprod. **15:** 869–873.
18. YARON, Y., M. SHENHAV, A.J. JAFFA, et al. 1994. Am. J. Obstet. Gynecol. **170:** 786–787.
19. ARCANGELI, S. & M.M. PASQUARETTE. 1997. Gravid uterine rupture after myolysis. Obstet. Gynecol. **89:** 857.
20. GOLAN, D., A. AHARONI, R. GONON, et al. 1990. Early spontaneous rupture of the post myomectomy gravid uterus. Int. J. Gynecol. Obstet. **31:** 167–170.
21. VERCELLINI, P., S. MADDALENA, O. DE GIORGI, et al. 1999. Determinants of reproductive outcome after abdominal myomectomy for infertility. Fertil. Steril. **72:** 109–114.
22. BULETTI, C., D. DE ZIEGLER, V. POLLI, et al. 1999. The role of leiomyomas in infertility. J. Am. Assoc. Gynecol. Laparosc. **6:** 441–445.

23. MAIS, V., S. AJOSSA, S. GUERRIERO, *et al.* 1996. Laparoscopic versus abdominal myomectomy: a prospective randomized trial to evaluate benefits in early outcome. Am. J. Obstet. Gynecol. **174:** 654–658.
24. TULANDI, T., C. MURRAY & M. GURALNICK. 1993. Adhesion formation and reproductive outcome after myomectomy and second-look laparoscopy. Obstet. Gynecol. **82:** 213–215.
25. DUBUISSON, J.B., A. FAUCONNIER, C. CHAPRON, *et al.* 1998. Second-look after laparoscopic myomectomy. Hum. Reprod. **13:** 2102–2106.

Management of Deep Endometriosis

CHARLES CHAPRON AND JEAN-BERNARD DUBUISSON

Assistance Publique – Hôpitaux de Paris (AP-HP), Service de Chirurgie Gynécologique, Clinique Universitaire Baudelocque, CHU Cochin Saint Vincent de Paul, 75014 Paris, France

ABSTRACT: Deep endometriosis is defined as an endometriotic lesion that penetrates the retroperitoneal space for a distance of ≥5 mm. Deep endometriosis is extremely active, occurs in phase with eutopic endometrium, evolves progressively with age, and is most often located in the pouch of Douglas, the rectovaginal septum, the uterosacral ligaments, and occasionally in the uterovesical fold. These lesions are associated with pelvic pain, the intensity of which is proportional to the depth of penetration. It is clear that choice of treatment depends on the location of the endometriotic lesion. In this paper we describe our methods for the initial diagnosis and subsequent treatment of deep endometriosis. These include consultation and clinical examination protocols, use of rectal endoscopic ultrasonography (EUS), magnetic resonance imaging (MRI), and transvaginal ultrasonography techniques in diagnosis and surgical treatment approaches.

KEYWORDS: deep endometriosis; eutopic endometrium; rectal endoscopic ultrasonography; magnetic resonance imaging; transvaginal ultrasonography

INTRODUCTION

The idea that endometriosis is capable of penetrating the retroperitoneal space is universally accepted.[1] Deep endometriosis is defined as an endometriotic lesion penetrating the retroperitoneal space to a depth of 5 mm or more.[2] These lesions are responsible for pain, the intensity of which is proportional to the depth to which the lesions penetrate.[2] The most frequent locations for deep endometriosis are the vesico-uterine pouch, the uterosacral ligaments, and the pouch of Douglas.[1] Retroperitoneal lesions may be located in the posterior pelvis, in which case deep endometriotic lesions are found involving the uterosacral ligaments or the rectovaginal septum or the rectum. In the anterior pelvis deep endometriotic lesions are present in the form of lesions to the bladder. The clinical findings, symptoms, and means of treatment vary according to the location of the lesions. In this study we present our approach for diagnosis and treatment of patients presenting with deep pelvic endometriosis.

Address for correspondence: Professeur Charles Chapron, Service de Chirurgie Gynécologique, Clinique Universitaire Baudelocque, CHU Cochin Saint Vincent de Paul, 123 Boulevard Port Royal, 75014 Paris, France. Voice: 01-58-41-19-14; fax: 01-58-41-18-70.
charles.chapron@cch.ap-hop-paris.fr

DEEP PELVIC ENDOMETRIOSIS: DIAGNOSTIC APPROACH

Clinical Examination

In these situations the most prominent symptom is pelvic pain. This can take several forms: dysmenorrhea, deep dyspareunia, or chronic pelvic pain. Associated with this "typical" pain, and depending on where the lesions are located, functional symptoms may be observed involving the urinary tract (dysuria, urinary infection, sometimes hematuria) or the bowel (rectal tenesmus and sometimes rectorrhagia). The essential characteristic of these "associated" types of pain is their monthly cyclic pattern.

During speculum examination, the presence of bluish lesions indicates a diagnosis of endometriosis. In our experience these bluish lesions are often absent, notably when the uterosacral ligaments are affected. In other words, when no lesions suggesting endometriosis are present at speculum examination, this can in no way be taken to mean that the diagnosis of deep pelvic endometriosis can be eliminated. In our experience, the presence of lesions visible at speculum examination is more frequent when the rectovaginal septum is involved than in cases of infiltration of the uterosacral ligaments.

The presence of a nodule must be sought during the vaginal examination. If possible, the examination should take place near the time of menstruation—ideally, during menstruation.[3] Although the most usual lesion observed is a nodule, this is not a hard and fast rule. In certain cases, less obvious signs need to be detected, such as a lateral deviation of the cervix[4] or asymmetric uterosacral ligaments appearing irregular, hardened, and taut.[5] The essential sign is that firm palpation of these lesions gives rise to pain identical to that of the deep dyspareunia that the patient describes.

Additional Investigations

The purpose is to establish a precise map of the deep pelvic endometriotic lesions. We consider this map indespensable for two reasons: (i) the conditions for the operative procedure are dictated by the site and extension of the lesions, and (ii) for the operation to be a success, the lesions must be radically excised. Performing pelvic ultrasound examination by the transvaginal route is excellent for a workup of the ovary and uterus but, in our experience, seems to be inferior for the diagnosis and workup of posterior pelvic lesions (uterosacral ligaments, recto-vaginal fascia).

When there is a suspicion of deep posterior pelvic endometriosis, we find two further means of investigation useful:

- *Rectal endoscopic ultrasonography* (EUS): Rectal EUS is reliable in the evaluation of rectovaginal endometriosis[6] and enables infiltration of the bowel wall to be diagnosed.[6,7] This information is essential, because it has a direct effect on the surgical technique to be used for exeresis.

- *Magnetic resonance imaging* (MRI): the great advantage of this means of investigation is that it offers the possibility of a complete workup of the pelvis in a single procedure. This is important in daily practice because lesions of the posterior compartment (uterosacral ligaments, rectovaginal septum, rectum) may be associated with anterior lesions (bladder).[8] Although MRI seems to be able to diagnose deep endometriosis of uterosacral ligaments (USL),[9] it lacks sensitivity in detecting rectal endometriosis without rectal distension.[9] Preliminary results show that MRI appears to be less reliable than rectal EUS when searching for the presence of bowel infiltration.[10,11] Further studies are needed nevertheless to clarify the indications for these two means of investigation in the workup for deep posterior pelvic endometriosis.

When deep endometriosis presents in an anterior location, in other words in cases of bladder endometriosis, we find three means of investigation helpful:

- *Cystoscopy*: Bear in mind that negative results do not preclude this diagnosis.[12,13] In addition to its advantages for diagnosis, cystoscopy makes it possible to check where the lesion is located relative to the ureteral meati. This factor must be taken into account when deciding on the operative technique.

- *Transvaginal ultrasonography*[14] and *MRI*[9]: As in the case of posterior lesions, the great advantage of MRI is that the whole pelvis can be explored. MRI is helpful for diagnosing small bladder lesions and assessing the depth to which these lesions penetrate into the bladder wall.[15] In this context, further studies are needed to specify the respective roles for these two means of investigation.

DEEP PELVIC ENDOMETRIOSIS: TREATMENT APPROACH

Surgical exeresis is the treatment of choice for deep pelvic endometriosis.[16,17] How the operation is approached depends on where the lesions are located. For bladder endometriosis, the treatment of reference is partial cystectomy. This can be achieved perfectly well in most cases by laparoscopic surgery.[8,18] Nevertheless, in certain situations the operation should take place via laparotomy. Two examples of such circumstances are (1) the need, due to the location of the lesions, to reimplant the ureters and carry out associated partial cystectomy and (2) the presence of bowel involvement associated with the bladder endometriosis lesions, justifying a specific surgical procedure during the same anesthesia.

In cases of deep posterior pelvic endometriosis, different techniques have been proposed.[19–24] For deep endometriosis infiltrating the uterosacral ligaments, exeresis can be treated by laparoscopic surgery.[5] Depending on how far the lesions extend, ureterolysis and dissection of the lateral rectal fossa may be needed. If the rectovaginal septum is involved, the surgical technique is different and uses both the laparoscopic and the vaginal approaches.[25] During the laparoscopic phase, the rectum is freed from the nodule after prior dissection of the lateral rectal fossae. The purpose of this dissection is to pass beneath the endometriotic nodule and to leave it attached to the posterior vaginal wall. This is then followed by laparoscopic colpotomy, after which exeresis of the lesion is completed by the vaginal route. In this case, unlike that of deep endometriosis infiltrating the uterosacral ligaments, ablation of the endometriotic nodule requires exeresis of part of the posterior vaginal wall. The vagina is then sutured via the vagina. The final phase of the operation consists of meticulous laparoscopic examination. When the bowel wall is infiltrated, although in certain carefully selected cases treatment can be carried out by laparoscopy,[26,27] the treatment of reference remains laparotomy. This is particularly true when resection and anastomosis are needed, because bowel lesions are multifocal in a considerable proportion of cases.[28]

Although in this context the treatment of first intention must be surgery, this does not mean to say that there is no place for medical treatment. The main indications, in our opinion, for medical treatment in cases of deep pelvic endometriosis are the following:

(1) *When there is doubt concerning the diagnosis.* If the painful functional symptoms disappear under medical treatment, this is highly suggestive of an endometriotic origin for the pain.[29] This test treatment enables potentially dangerous surgical procedures to be avoided in certain difficult diagnostic situations, where it is not clear that they would be beneficial. Recurrence of pain after surgical treatment correctly carried out is also a formal indication for medical prescription, rather than recommending repeated pelvic surgery.

(2) *When counterindications or important risk factors exist for difficult and dangerous surgical procedures.* In certain situations medical treatment can be useful in enabling surgical treatment to be deferred as required. Further studies are needed to establish whether there is an advantage to prescribing medical treatment before or after surgery, either to make the operation simpler or to help prevent the risk of recurrence.

CONCLUSION

Deep pelvic endometriosis gives rise to symptoms involving pain, dominated by deep dyspareunia and functional symptoms that follow a monthly menstrual cycle, the character of which is governed by the location of the lesions (bladder, rectum). It is essential to establish the extent of these lesions during the workup. The goal of this workup is to map out the deep endometriotic lesions exactly. The treatment of first intention remains surgery, because in most cases medical treatment will only be palliative. How successful the treatment is depends on how radical surgical exeresis can be. The details of the surgical procedure are dictated by the location and extension of the lesions. Further studies are needed to clarify the appropriateness and modalities of medical treatment for pre- and postoperative use.

REFERENCES

1. CORNILLIE, F.J., D. OOSTERLYNCK, J.M. LAUWEREYNS & P.R. KONINCKX. 1990. Deeply infiltrating endometriosis: histological and clinical significance. Fertil. Steril. **53:** 978–983.
2. KONINCKX, P.R., C. MEULEMAN, S. DEMEYERE, *et al.* 1991. Suggestive evidence that pelvic endometriosis is a progressive disease, whereas deeply infiltrating endometriosis is associated with pelvic pain. Fertil. Steril. **55:** 759–765.
3. KONINCKX, P.R., C. MEULEMAN, D. OOSTERLYNCK & F.J. CORNILLIE. 1996. Diagnosis of deep endometriosis by clinical examination during menstruation and plasma CA-125 concentration. Fertil. Steril. **65:** 280–287.
4. PROPST, A.M., K. STORTI & R.L. BARBIERI. 1998. Lateral cervical displacement is associated with endometriosis. Fertil. Steril. **70:** 568–570.
5. CHAPRON, C. & J.B. DUBUISSON. 1996. Laparoscopic treatment of deep endometriosis located on the uterosacral liagments. Hum. Reprod. **11:** 868–873.

6. FEDELE, L., S. BIANCHI, A. PORTUESE, *et al.* 1998. Transrectal ultrasonography in the assessment of rectovaginal endometriosis. Obstet. Gynecol. **91:** 444–448.
7. CHAPRON, C., I. DUMONTIER, B. DOUSSET, *et al.* 1998. Results and place of rectal endoscopic ultrasonography for patients with deep pelvic endometriosis. Hum. Reprod. **13:** 2266–2270.
8. CHAPRON, C. & J.B. DUBUISSON. 1999. Laparoscopic management of bladder endometriosis. Acta. Obstet. Gynecol. Scand. **78:** 887–890.
9. KINKEL, K., C. CHAPRON, C. BALLEYGUIER, *et al.* 1999. Magnetic resonnance imaging characteristics of deep endometriosis. Hum. Reprod. **14:** 1080–1086.
10. OHBA, T., H. MIZUTANI, T. MAEDA, *et al.* 1996. Evaluation of endometriosis in uterosacral ligaments by trans rectal ultrasonography. Hum. Reprod. **11:** 2014–2017.
11. SCHRÖDER, J., M. LÖHNERT, J.M. DONIEC & P. DOHRMANN. 1997. Endoluminal ultrasound diagnosis and operative management of rectal endometriosis. Dis. Colon Rectum **40:** 614–617.
12. VERCELLINI, P., M. MESCHIA, O. DE GORGI, *et al.* 1996. Bladder detrusor endometriosis: clinical and pathogenetic implication. J. Urol. **155:** 84–86.
13. SAVOCA, G., L. TROMBERTTA & S. TRIOANO. 1996. Echographic, MRI and CT features in cases of bladder endometriosis. Arch. Ital. Urol. Androl. **68:** 193–196.
14. FEDELE, L., E. PIAZZOLA, R. RAFFAELLI & A. PROTUESE. 1997. Preoperative assessment of bladder endometriosis. Hum. Reprod. **12:** 2519–2522,
15. BALLEYGUIER, C., C. CHAPRON, K. KINKEL, *et al.* 2001. Modalities and results of magnetic resonance imaging for patients with bladder endometriosis. In press.
16. KONINCKX, P.R. & D.C. MARTIN. 1995. Surgical treatment of deeply infiltrating endometriosis. *In* Endometriosis: Current Understanding and Management. R.W. Shaw, Ed.: 264–281. Blackwell Science Ltd. Oxford.
17. GARRY, R. 1997. Laparoscopic excision of endometriosis: the treatment of choice? Br. J. Obstet. Gynaecol. **104:** 513–515.
18. NEZHAT, C., F. NEZHAT, C.H. NEZHAT, *et al.* 1995. Urinary tract endometriosis treated by laproscopy. Fertil. Steril. **66:** 920–924.
19. WOOD, C., P. MAHER & D. HILL. 1993. Laparoscopic removal of endometriosis in the pouch of Douglas. Austr. N.Z.J. Obstet. Gynecol. **33:** 295–299.
20. DONNEZ, J., M. NISOLLE, F. CASANAS-ROUX, *et al.* 1995. Rectovaginal septum, endometyriosis or adenomyosis: laparoscopic management in a series of 221 patients. Hum. Reprod. **10:** 630–635.
21. REDWINE, D.B. 1991. Conservative laparoscopic excision of endometriosis by sharp dissection: life table analysis of reoperation and persistent or recurrent disease. Fertil. Steril. **56:** 628–634.
22. MARTIN, D.C. 1988. Laparoscopic and vaginal colpotomy for the excision of infiltrating cul de sac endometriosis. J. Reprod. Med. **33:** 806–808.
23. REICH, H., F. MCGLYNN & J. SALVAT. 1991. Laparoscopic treatment of cul-de-sac obliteration secondary to retrocervical deep fibrotic endometriosis. J. Reprod. Med. **36:** 516–522.
24. CHAPRON, C., J.B. DUBUISSON, X. FRITEL, *et al.* 1999. Operative management of deep endometriosis infiltrating the uterosacral ligaments. J. Am. Assoc. Gynecol. Laparosc. **6:** 31–37.
25. CHAPRON, C., S. JACOB, A. FAUCONNIER, *et al.* 2001. Laparoscopically assisted vaginal management of deep endometriosis infiltrating the rectovaginal septum. Acta Obstet Gynecol. Scand. **80:** 349–354.
26. NEZHAT, C., F. NEZHAT & E. PENNINGTON. 1992. Laparoscopic treatment of infiltrative rectosigmoid colon and rectovaginal septum endometriosis by the technique of videolaparoscopy and CO_2 laser. Br. J. Obstet. Gynaecol. **99:** 664–667.
27. REDWINE, D.B., M. KONING & D.R. SHARPE. 1996. Laparoscopically assisted transvaginal segmental resection of the rectosigmoid colon for endometriosis. Fertil. Steril. **65:** 193–197.
28. REDWINE, D.B. 1999. Ovarian endometriosis: a marker for more extensive pelvic and intestinal disease. Fertil. Steril. **72:** 310–315.
29. HURD, W.W. 1998. Criteria that indicate endometriosis is the cause of chronic pelvic pain. Obstet. Gynecol. **92:** 1029–1032.

Cancer and Pregnancy

WILLIAM T. CREASMAN

Department of Obstetrics and Gynecology, Medical University of South Carolina, Charleston, South Carolina 29425, USA

ABSTRACT: Carcinoma of the cervix is the most frequently diagnosed cancer in pregnancy. Still, it is an unusual situation. An abnormal Pap smear during pregnancy is a much more common occurrence and fortunately one that can be managed conservatively. Although definitive treatment for intraepithelial disease can be delayed until the postpartum period, diagnostic evaluation should be done when the abnormal Pap smear is present. Invasive cancer management is dependent on gestational age of the fetus. Pregnancy affords an excellent opportunity to screen for cervical neoplasia.

Keywords: cancer; cervical carcinoma; pregnancy

INTRODUCTION

Carcinoma of the cervix is the most frequently diagnosed cancer in pregnancy; still, it is an unusual situation. An abnormal Pap smear during pregnancy is a much more common occurrence and fortunately one that can be managed conservatively. Although definitive treatment for intraepithelial disease can be delayed until the postpartum period, diagnostic evaluation should be done when the abnormal Pap smear is present. Invasive cancer management depends on the gestational age of the fetus. Pregnancy affords an excellent opportunity to screen for cervical neoplasia.

CERVICAL CANCER

Pregnancy was once thought to have deleterious effects on the outcome and management of cervical cancer. Current opinion indicates that, in essence, they are coincidental findings.

Pregnancy may dictate the timing of therapy, but it has no effect on the prognosis or the fetus. Although carcinoma of the uterine cervix is the most frequently diagnosed cancer in pregnancy, it is still an unusual finding. The overall incidence ranges from 1 to 13 cases in 10,000 pregnancies; however, in large referral maternity hospitals, the incidence may be 1 per 1000–2500 deliveries. In large cancer referral centers, about 1% of women who have carcinoma of the cervix are pregnant at the time of diagnosis.

Address for correspondence: William T. Creasman, M.D., Department of Ob/Gyn, Medical University of South Carolina, 96 Jonathan Lucas Street, Suite 634, Charleston, SC 29425. Voice: 843-792-4509; fax: 843-792-0533.

Creasman@musc.edu

Carcinoma of the cervix, irrespective of whether or not the patient is pregnant, is highly curable if diagnosed in an early stage.[1] Pregnancy offers an added opportunity for cancer surveillance and screening. Although several decades ago an abnormal Pap smear in pregnancy was thought to be due to the pregnancy itself and not to a cervical abnormality, currently the reliability of cervical cytology is as valid in the pregnant patient as in the nonpregnant patient and should be evaluated accordingly.

Vaginal bleeding is the most common symptom in carcinoma of the cervix, whether or not the patient is pregnant. Unfortunately, this symptom often appears only with far-advanced disease. As much as 30% of reported patients had no symptoms when the diagnosis of cervical cancer was established.[2] When this does occur during pregnancy, investigation is imperative and the situation should not automatically be attributed to pregnancy. Examination during the first trimester will not lead to abortion or to premature labor in the third trimester. Added precautions may be necessary because of the pregnancy, but attention to them should not be postponed for fear of interfering with the pregnancy. An incomplete evaluation can lead to a dangerous delay in diagnosis.

In more than half the asymptomatic patients in one study,[2] the only abnormality was an abnormal Pap smear. Colposcopic examination, although usually more time consuming because of the larger area of the cervix, needs to be evaluated irrespective of the pregnancy. It is just as accurate in the pregnant as in the nonpregnant patient.

The age of patients with carcinoma of the cervix spans the reproductive years. Studies have indicated that an age range of 19–46 years with a mean of 33 years and the age at diagnosis had no influence on the prognosis of the patient within a given stage of cancer. Several reports have noted that survival of patients with carcinoma of the cervix associated with pregnancy was similar to that of nonpregnant patients with carcinoma of the cervix.[2,3]

In like manner, parity is not considered a prognostic factor in cervical cancer, but it has been implicated as a causative factor. Although early coital activity appears to be an important etiologic factor, early pregnancy and multiparity in many instances go hand in hand. The average parity for carcinoma of the cervix in the pregnant patient was 5.4. In a similar age group of patients who were not pregnant, the average parity was 3.5.[2] A more advanced lesion was not found with increasing parity and therefore did not influence prognosis.

Time of diagnosis in regard to gestational age may have a major impact on treatment options. It is therefore imperative to make a diagnosis as early as possible, with cervical cytology being a routine part of the initial work-up of a pregnant patient if she has not had one in the recent past. Although it is said that over 90% of adult women in the United States have been screened at least once, only about two-thirds of them have a Pap smear on a regular basis and that could be every 3 years or more. The guidelines, as noted by the American College of Obstetricians and Gynecologists, of yearly Pap smears should be followed for the pregnant patient as well.[4]

Intraepithelial Lesions

A patient with an abnormal Pap smear on prenatal evaluation should be evaluated as if she were not pregnant, with several exceptions. When cytologic study indicates some level of dysplasia, it is our opinion that these patients should undergo colposcopy. In some instances, this is technically easier to perform in the early part of the

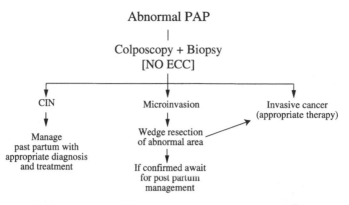

FIGURE 1. Management of abnormal PAP in pregnancy. From DiSaia and Creasman.[1] Used with permission.

second trimester than in the first trimester, as the pregnancy produces eversion of the cervix, making it easier to evaluate. The increased volume of the everted cervix with its multiple clefts makes the process more time consuming. Because of eversion, the entire transformation zone is usually apparent, and the chances of overlooking an endocervical lesion are minimal. If an abnormality on the cervix is identified colposcopically, we prefer to biopsy this area for documentation. If the physician who is involved in the pregnancy management of the patient and has expertise in colposcopy feels comfortable with his or her impression of the likely histology with colposcopy alone, it is acceptable not to perform a biopsy during pregnancy. In most cases a biopsy specimen should probably be taken. Certainly, the pregnant cervix is more apt to bleed than the nonpregnant cervix, but it can usually be controlled with Monsel's solution. Rarely is a suture required to stop the bleeding. Endocervical curettage is not performed. If only intraepithelial disease is noted on cytology, colposcopic evaluation, and biopsy, the patient can be followed throughout her pregnancy, be allowed to deliver vaginally, and be managed routinely postpartum (FIG. 1). We prefer to obtain one or two subsequent Pap smears during pregnancy, depending on when the initial evaluation is performed. It has not been our practice to repeat colposcopy. Postpartum, the cervix is reevaluated with cytology and colposcopy. In many instances, a lesion may not be found and the patient can be followed with cytology. Progression during pregnancy to invasive cancer has not been encountered. If, however, cytology, colposcopy, or biopsy suggests a microinvasive lesion, further evaluation is required. Some suggest that this is the only indication for conization in pregnancy (as in the nonpregnant patient). Classic conization in pregnancy can have disastrous effects with significant bleeding and even termination of pregnancy. We have found that a so-called "wedge" of the affected portion of the cervix gives the necessary information with much less chance of significant side effects. Injection of the lesion with a dilute solution of pitressin also helps with hemostasis. If <3 mm of invasion is present with clear surgical margins, the patient can be handled much as those with intraepithelial lesions. The patient can be followed expectantly throughout the pregnancy, and there is no contraindication to vaginal delivery. In many in-

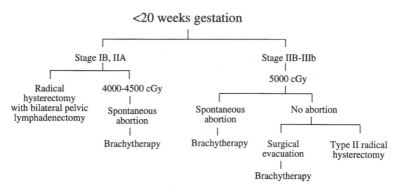

FIGURE 2. Therapy for cancer at <20 weeks' gestation. From DiSaia and Creasman.[1] Used with permission.

stances, this treatment may be adequate, particularly if the patient desires future fertility and if more definitive treatment postpartum is not indicated. One may want to do a classic conization postpartum before the final decision is made. Simple hysterectomy as definitive therapy is usually sufficient in these patients in whom subsequent fertility is not an issue. However, if greater depth of invasion is noted on the wedge or on conization, the patient may need more aggressive management. If conization is done during pregnancy, it should be "flat" instead of the classic cone.

Invasive Carcinoma

Although there are no hard and fast rules concerning length of gestation and treatment, it is accepted that if a patient is at <20 weeks of gestation, definitive therapy for cancer should be performed and the pregnancy ignored. The obvious exceptions depend on the patient's desires and the risk she is willing to take. In early stage disease (Stage IB–IIA), unless there are contraindications, radical hysterectomy and pelvic lymphadenectomy are the treatment advocated by many. The clinical decision of whether hysterotomy for technical reasons is necessary prior to definitive surgery is usually made intraoperatively. Radiation therapy, as in the nonpregnant patient, appears to be just as efficacious as radical surgery. External radiation can commence, and the pregnancy is usually aborted by 3,000-4,000 cGy. Brachytherapy can then be applied at the completion of external irradiation. In a small number of patients, abortion will not have occurred prior to completion of external radiation, and evacuation of the uterus will be required (Fig. 2). In late stage disease (Stage IIB or greater), radiation therapy should commence when the diagnosis is made.

After 20 weeks of gestation, allowing the patient to go to term before definitive therapy for the cervical cancer is an option, realizing that there may be a delay of as much as 3 months or longer before primary treatment of the cancer can be performed. Sood and Sorosky,[5] in a review of the literature, identified 63 patients with Stage IA-II disease who had a delay of up to 32 weeks before definitive therapy was performed. Only one patient with Stage IB2 adenocarcinoma of the cervix had a recurrence and died from disease; all the rest were without disease at the time of the

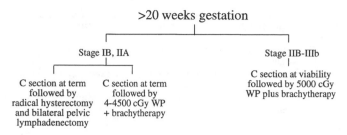

FIGURE 3. Therapy for cancer at >20 weeks' gestation. From DiSaia and Creasman.[1] Used with permission.

report.[5] Tewari and associates[6] reported on two patients with carcinoma of the cervix associated with pregnancy whose diagnosis was made early in the pregnancy. In both instances, suggested therapy would have interrupted the pregnancy. It was refused and neoadjuvant chemotherapy was given during the pregnancy, allowing the fetus to mature. Chemotherapy caused the clinical lesion to decrease in size, allowing the pregnancy to proceed. After delivery, definitive surgery was done. In the patient with a large Stage IIA cancer, recurrence and subsequent death resulted. The other patient with a Stage IB2 cancer is alive and well 2 years after surgery. Both infants are normal. Chemotherapy after the first trimester is well tolerated, exerts no detrimental effects on the fetus, and may be an option in selected cervical cancer patients who may be pregnant. A decision about optimal time of delivery must be made in concert with the maternal-fetal specialist. Although data suggest that the route of delivery, even in clinical cervical cancer, has no impact on either mother or fetus, most suggest cesarean section as the preferred mode of delivery. At least theoretically, there is less chance of bleeding from the trauma of the cervix dilating or even failing to dilate. In early stage disease, cesarean section followed by radical surgery can be performed in the same setting with no more morbidity than surgery in the nonpregnant patient. In advanced disease (Stage IIB or greater), standard radiation therapy is given. External therapy can commence immediately postpartum (FIG. 3). Episiotomy site recurrence of squamous cell carcinoma of the cervix after vaginal delivery has been reported. Although this is a rare site of recurrence, it has occurred even in early stage disease, and careful monitoring of the perineum in the immediate postoperative period is appropriate.

Even with a greater number of pregnant patients seeking care earlier in their gestation and with cancer surveillance being performed, many investigators note that a considerable number of patients will not have their cancer diagnosed until the third trimester or even postpartum. Surprisingly, patients with advanced lesions are being diagnosed 3–6 months postpartum after a normal vaginal delivery without intrapartum diagnosis and with no unusual intra- or postpartum complications.

REFERENCES

1. DISAIA, P.J. & W.T. CREASMAN. 1997. Clinical Gynecologic Oncology, 5th Ed. C.V. Mosby. St. Louis.
2. CREASMAN, W., F. RUTLEDGE & G. FLETCHER. 1970. Carcinoma of the cervix associated with pregnancy. Obstet. Gynecol. **36:** 495.

3. NISHER, J. & H. ALLEN. 1986. Carcinoma of the cervix in pregnancy. *In* Cancer in Pregnancy — Therapeutic Guidelines. H. Allen & J. Nisher, eds. Futura. Mount Kisco, NY.
4. AMERICAN COLLEGE OF OBSTETRICIANS AND GYNECOLOGISTS. Committee Opinion 152. March 1995. Washington, DC.
5. SOOD, A.K. & J.I. SOROSKY. 1998. Invasive cervical cancer complicating pregnancy. Obstet. Gynecol. Clin. N. Am. **25:** 343.
6. TEWARI, K., F. CAPPUCCINI, A. GAMBINO, *et al.* 1998. Neoadjuvant chemotherapy in the treatment of locally advanced cervical carcinoma in pregnancy. Cancer **82:** 1529.

Uterine Transplantation, Abdominal Trachelectomy, and Other Reproductive Options for Cancer Patients

GIUSEPPE DEL PRIORE,[a] J. RICHARD SMITH,[b] DEBORAH C.M. BOYLE,[c] DAVID J. CORLESS,[d] FARIS B.P. ZACHARIA,[e] DAVID A. NOAKES,[f] THOMAS DIFLO,[a] JAMES A. GRIFO,[a] AND JOHN J. ZHANG[a]

[a]NYU School of Medicine, New York, New York 10016, USA

[b]Chelsea and Westminster Hospital, London, UK

[c]Watford General Hospital, Watford, UK

[d]Leighton Hospital, Crewe, UK

[e]West Middlesex Hospital, London, UK

[f]Royal Veterinary College, Hatfield, UK

ABSTRACT: More and more women with cancer issues are now raising fertility concerns as survival improves and childbearing is delayed. Pregnancy is no longer contraindicated in cancer patients including breast and endometrial cancer survivors. In fact, survival in patients treated for breast cancer who subsequently become pregnant is actually higher than that in patients who do not become pregnant. "Therapeutic" abortions are no longer recommended. Assisted reproductive technology (ART) have been associated with ovarian neoplasms, but the association is probably not causal. Neither ART nor hormone replacement is contraindicated in cancer patients. Our institution is very supportive of patients and the difficult decisions cancer survivors face. Using a program of counseling and close collaboration between oncologists, perinatologists, and reproductive endocrinologists, informed patients are offered every possible option, including ART and uterine transplantation, to achieve their family planning objectives.

KEYWORDS: fertility; cancer; transplant

INTRODUCTION

A generation ago, women with gynecologic cancer had little to hope for and even less to look forward to. Survival was poor and expectations low. However, due to small but significant advances, such cancers are no longer a death sentence. Our greater treatment successes combined with the social phenomenon of later childbearing has presented us with an enviable problem. More and more women with cancer issues are now raising fertility concerns.

Address for correspondence: Dr. Giuseppe Del Priore, NYU School of Medicine, 550 First Avenue, Room NB 9E-2, New York, NY 10016. Voice: 212 263-2353; fax: 212-283-8251.
gd5@nyu.edu

GYNECOLOGIC CANCERS 2001: CURRENT STATUS

Breast Cancer

Breast cancer is still the leading cancer concern for women in the United States. Hopefully it may not remain so for long if recent trends continue. Breast cancer incidence and mortality have been declining in the United States since the late 1980s.[1,2] Some of this is due, at least in part, to better screening and earlier detection. Most cases of breast cancer in the United States are now detected by mammography.[3,4] Most of these cases are in the *in situ* stage with an impressive 97% survival and cure. In addition, although the peak age of breast cancer diagnosis is later in life, approximately 10–20% of breast cancer patients are of childbearing age. The end result is that 5–10% of breast cancer patients become pregnant each year.[5]

Pregnancy is no longer contraindicated in breast cancer patients. Survival in patients treated for breast cancer who subsequently become pregnant is actually higher than it is in patients who do not become pregnant.[6,7] Older studies were severely limited by not controlling for confounders and not recognizing the latency period between diagnosis and exposure to causative agents. For instance, they often failed to distinguish between cancers diagnosed during pregnancy and other pregnancy events. Cancers diagnosed during pregnancy are obviously unrelated to the pregnancy as a causative factor. "Therapeutic" abortions are no longer prescribed, because recent data indicate that they are not therapeutic and the recommendation has always appeared to patronize women and their ability to set their own priorities.[8] Optimal timing of conception after breast cancer treatment is uncertain. The current consensus is to wait between 6 and 24 months before attempting to conceive.[9] Timing of conception may appear even more difficult if assisted reproductive technology (ART) is contemplated.

ART has been associated with human neoplasms, although the association is probably not causal.[10,11] Nevertheless, patients and physicians continue to be nervous when employing ART in cancer patients. Our institution is very supportive of patients and the difficult decisions cancer survivors face. Using a formal program of counseling and close collaboration between oncologists, perinatologists, and reproductive endocrinologists, informed patients are offered every possible option to achieve their family planning objectives.

An illustrative, but by no means unique, case involved a woman with her attorney husband who had been treated unsuccessfully for 5 years before coming to NYU. Her father had died from breast cancer before the age of 50. She was diagnosed with stage IA, grade 1, ovarian cancer during her first laparoscopy at NYU and was treated with unilateral oophorectomy. Two years later, she successfully delivered twins and completed a hysterectomy and oophorectomy. She remains free of disease on estrogen replacement therapy (ERT) until this patient is ready to schedule the recommended bilateral mastectomy.

Neither ART nor ERT is contraindicated in this type of patient. Given the probable presence of an inherited mutation, her cancers were (i.e., ovarian) and are (i.e., breast) inevitable. ART allowed her to live her life as she decided. Certainly, in a patient with cancer (ovarian, in this case) quality of life is paramount. Achieving her family planning objectives immensely satisfied this patients quality of life issues with no definitive increase in cancer risk. In fact, successful ART is associated with a reduction in breast and ovarian cancer diagnosis.[12]

Although a selective estrogen receptor modulator may delay the diagnosis of her breast cancer, ERT is the only intervention of this type associated with a reduced risk of breast cancer death.[13–15] Consistent with the beneficial effects of estrogens, prolonged exposure to selective estrogen receptor modulators may actually worsen breast cancer survival.[16] Evidence of an estrogen benefit in breast cancer is increasing. Another multicentered national randomized clinical trial is currently underway using conjugated equine estrogen in breast cancer patients.[17–20] There are numerous other trials attempting to exploit the favorable prognosis of breast cancers associated with estrogen use.

Ovarian Cancer

Women with a family history of breast cancer are often at increased risk for ovarian cancer. Ovarian cancer has long been perceived as a silent killer; however, the current 5-year survival is double that of a generation ago.[21] The prognosis is very good for early stage disease with 90% of stage I cancer patients surviving 5 years or more. Patients with the best prognosis usually do not present with the typical signs of ovarian cancer to a gynecologic oncologist. Instead, a community gynecologist encounters them as an unexpected finding in a younger patient presenting with pain and an adnexal mass. Often in these situations fertility issues are unknown or undecided.

Treatment under these circumstances is best deferred until a definitive pathologic diagnosis can be made. Frozen section should not be used as an indication for castration of a young person except in the clearest situation of advanced epithelial ovarian cancer. Tertiary referral centers such as ours would even consider fertility preservation in relatively advanced ovarian cancer under the right circumstances. Although successful pregnancies have been reported after the diagnosis and treatment of advanced ovarian cancer, it should be considered carefully.[22] The worse potential surgical outcome in a younger patient with unclear fertility plans is to have a hysterectomy, bilateral oophorectomy, and omentectomy, but not thorough paraaortic lymph node dissection. Too often this staging procedure is omitted because of the unavailability of a trained gynecologic oncologist. This is the most important part of the surgical management of ovarian cancer, given that the high paraaortic nodes near the renal vessels are the most likely site of occult metastatic disease.[23,24] Therefore, if paraaortic nodes are not sampled, certainly then an apparently normal uterus and normal contralateral ovary should not be removed for the sake of "staging."

Once the diagnosis is confirmed by final pathologic review, a repeat operation may be necessary to determine the need for additional chemotherapy treatment. If the diagnosis is clear at the initial surgery and the patient desires future fertility, unilateral salpingoophorectomy and staging biopsies are acceptable. Cystectomies have sometimes been performed for a presumed benign cyst in an ovarian cancer patient when the diagnosis was not suspected. Although these patients have done well, the recurrence risk is higher than that of unilateral patients with salpingo-oophorectomy. However, long-term survival may not be any different.[25]

Spontaneous pregnancy is certainly not contraindicated after a diagnosis of ovarian cancer. ART, however, may be more difficult to consider because of its association with ovarian cancer.[11] This association is probably not causal.[10] In fact, successful treatment with ART is associated with reduced evidence of ovarian cancer. ART is perhaps most difficult to consider in infertility patients with a genetic predispostion for ovarian cancer. This issue has already been addressed herein.

ERT in menopausal patients with ovarian cancer should be encouraged for all the usual benefits. Quality of life considerations may be the most important indication. In patients with a potentially fatal cancer and a shortened life expectancy, short-term symptomatic relief is perhaps more important than long-term theoretical benefits or concerns. Fortunately, a randomized trial has proved that ERT patients with ovarian cancer have no negative impact on overall survival.[26]

Ovarian transplantation has been considered since at least the end of the nineteenth century. There are unconfirmed reports of success possibly based on chance alone. In one case, the surgeon reportedly removed both ovaries but not the right fallopian tube. He then transplanted "...a small piece of the patient's diseased ovary..." back into the retained tube. Menses and subsequent pregnancy resulted. Around the same time, further attempts to repeat the operation in other women all failed. Animal models, however, have succeeded in all aspects of ovarian transplantation. These include fresh and frozen transplants with successful folliculogenesis, resumption of normal endocrine function, normal conception, and normal birth.[27,28]

Our institution has an ongoing research protocol to achieve the same results in humans. We are investigating transplantation as well as *in vitro* replication of normal ovarian function. Potential advantages include a "natural" alternative for ERT and no need for embryo cryopreservation with resultant orphan embryos. Potential obstacles include the risk of reintroducing malignant cells (e.g., breast cancer patients harboring occult ovarian metastases) or potentially malignant cells (e.g., mutation carriers).

Endometrial Cancer

Endometrial cancer appears to immediately contraindicate future fertility. Fortunately, these patients can also exercise some reproductive options. Nearly 15% of endometrial cancer patients are of reproductive age. Our group always has a patient with endometrial cancer in some stage of conception. Many of these patients are diagnosed as part of their infertility evaluation and not because of symptoms; therefore, they are usually at an early stage with a good prognosis. After appropriate counseling, these patients are treated with prolonged high-dose progestins. However, we make it clear that our recommendation is always laparoscopic vaginal hysterectomy and staging throughout the alternative therapy with progestins.

Before prescribing progestins, we perform a tumor assessment, including an MRI of the pelvis. MRI is better than sonography, CT scan, and hysteroscopy for assessing endometrial disease status. MRI is the most accurate predictor of tumor size and depth of invasion.[29] If the tumor is small, well differentiated, and appears not to invade the uterus, we prescribe 12 weeks of high-dose megestrol. After the initial trial, a repeat office biopsy is performed.

We prefer to use any aspiration suction biopsy device along with an endometrial brush biopsy device (Tao Brush, Cook Ob-Gyn). In studies conducted at NYU, the positive and negative predictive value of the two tests combined and used simultaneously during a single office visit is 100%.[30,31] We may repeat a D&C once after the initial diagnosis of endometrial cancer; however, since the goal is fertility preservation, repeated D&Cs may reduce fertility secondary to endometrial scarring (i.e., Asherman's syndrome) and should be avoided.

We do not use hysteroscopy in the management of endometrial cancer. Hysteroscopy has been replaced by sonography, which is more accurate and less invasive, according to well-done randomized trials.[32,33] We also conducted a study on the role of hysteroscopy specifically in diagnosing endometrial cancer.[34] We found that hysteroscopy actually reduced the likelihood of correctly diagnosing endometrial cancer. The sensitivity was only 27% with a negative predictive value of 25%. An even greater concern is that of other investigators recently reporting that hysteroscopy may actually worsen the prognosis of patients with endometrial cancer.[35]

If this regimen of nonsurgical management is successful, we allow these patients to conceive usually with the help of ART. At delivery, the placenta is sent to pathology with the history of endometrial cancer noted. The endometrium is sampled intrapartum and again postpartum with the two office biopsy devices noted earlier. Once again we recommend hysterectomy and will consider cesarean hysterectomy or postpartum hysterectomy. Until the patient is ready for that decision, the two office biopsy techniques are performed at least every 6 months. Again, we try to avoid D&C with general anesthesia, as it may lead to impaired fertility and adds nothing to the combined sensitivity, specificity, and positive and negative predictive value of the noninvasive testing along with the two office biopsy techniques (i.e., aspiration and brush biopsy).

Cervical Cancer

For most of the world's women, cervical cancer is more important than any of the other gynecologic malignancies. Cervical cancer has, until now, always resulted in loss of fertility. Fortunately, there are more and more options for this large group of women.

Surgical conservation of the uterine fundus is now routinely performed either abdominally or vaginally.[36,37] This procedure has been reported for over 50 years, but has lately become very popular, because advances in laparoscopy have enabled surgeons to perform laparoscopic lymph node dissection. We prefer the vaginal route but have developed the abdominal route as an alternative if pelvic anatomy contraindicates the transvaginal approach. Both have reports indicating high survival and remarkable conception rates. A complete technical description of the procedures is available in most up-to-date surgical atlases.[38]

Radiation with chemotherapy is increasingly used for advanced cervical cancers. Although effective therapy, radiation causes ovarian failure quickly in most patients. Oophoropexy to reposition the ovaries out of the pelvis before radiation can reduce the incidence of ovarian failure but not eliminate it. Ovarian function is documented in as many as 75% of patients but in as few as 0% following ovarian transposition.[39] Fertility after pelvic radiation also depends on the type of cancer. In younger women classically affected with germ-cell tumors, 80% conception rates have been reported. These rates are probably overly optimistic for the cervical cancer patient. Because of the intense dose and location of the radiation treatment for cervical cancer, conceptions are exceedingly rare.[40] To preserve fertility, initial chemotherapy may be used to convert a nonsurgical case from radiation to radical trachelectomy.

As a last resort, uterine transplantation is fast becoming an option. This operation has already been successfully reported in an actual patient.[41] The first successful technique was reported in 1966 using dogs.[42] The vessels around the uterus and ovaries were isolated, divided, and then reanastomosed, with subsequent uterine function. Recently, a group from the University of California at San Diego has reported their techniques and successes performing orthotopic uteroovarian transplants in rats.[43] In brief, the uteroovarian block is dissected out with the entire pelvic circulation intact. The aorta and vena cava of the graft are used for the vascular supply. They are anastomosed to the infrarenal aorta and vena cava of the recipient. The success rate for this procedure was reasonable.

Our group is actively engaged in this line of rodent research. Our preliminary research in a porcine model has demonstrated that uterine arteries when transected and anastomosed, function normally at the suture line during pregnancy. A series of 12 radical abdominal trachelectomies undertaken in Hungary similarly demonstrated that the uterus supplied by only two of its original six arteries remained viable (L. Ungar, personal communication). Laboratory study of the vascular anatomy of the human pelvis in cadavers has identified suitable vessels for anastomosis during uterine transplantation.

CONCLUSION

Many of the aforementioned issues involve controversial or experimental interventions. Undoubtedly, with additional research some of the questions raised will become irrelevant, only to be replaced by equally controversial interventions. Throughout this evolution, it is helpful to remember how different individuals and cultures view the importance of fertility. At the start of the third millennium, childbirth worldwide continues to cause the death of approximately 493,000 women each year from such conditions as hemorrhage (123,000 deaths), sepsis (74,000 deaths), pregnancy-induced hypertension (62,000 deaths), obstructed labor (38,000 deaths), and others.[44] Instead of actual numbers of individuals affected, Western journals prefer to report "relative risks" and "odds ratios." Although they are reported by the media with great drama, relative risk can never fully communicate the risks and benefits of ART intervention. A relative risk of 2 or a doubling of the risk of cancer with ART may seem important to the lay public until they realize how rare the underlying outcome is.[45] Certainly, nothing discussed in this article comes anywhere near the risk of "natural" childbearing as experienced by the majority of the world's population.

There are, without question, risks in having a family under any circumstance. Patients with a history of cancer or with active disease add an extra measure of anxiety to the process for all concerned. However, the actual magnitude of the excess or attributable risk is probably small. Most women are willing to accept some risk to achieve their goal. In fact, there may be some advantages to conception for certain cancer patients (e.g., those with breast cancer). Throughout all these issues, physicians must focus on the patient's objectives. We have not even begun to grapple with the consequences of our actions on the subsequent generation. Do our responsibilities end with the patient or her offspring?

Cancer patients have options and time (although often limited). Physicians should urge family planning, not accidents, and discuss fertility issues with their cancer patients.

REFERENCES

1. GARFINKEL, L. & M. MUSHINSKI. 1999. U.S. cancer incidence, mortality and survival: 1973-1996. State Bull. Metrop. Insur. Co. **80:** 23–32.
2. WINGO, P.A., L.A. RIES, H.M. ROSENBERG, *et al.* 1998. Cancer incidence and mortality, 1973–1995: a report card for the U.S. Cancer **82:** 1197–1207.
3. EVANS, W.P., 3RD, A.L. STARR & E.S. BENNOS. 1997. Comparison of the relative incidence of impalpable invasive breast and ductal carcinoma in situ in cancers detected in patients older and younger than 50 years of age. Radiology **204:** 489–491.
4. WUN, L.M., E.J. FEUER & B.A. MILLER. 1995. Are increases in mammographic screening still a valid explanation for trends in breast cancer incidence in the United States? Causes Control **6:** 135–144.
5. BERNIK, S.F., T.R. BERNIK, B.P. WHOOLEY & M.K. WALLACK. 1998. Carcinoma of the breast during pregnancy: a review and update on treatment options. Surg. Oncol. **7:** 45–49.
6. KROMAN, N., M.B. JENSEN, M. MELBYE, *et al.* 1997. Should women be advised against pregnancy after breast-cancer treatment? Lancet **350:** 319–322.
7. VELENTGAS, P., J.R. DALING, K.E. MALONE, *et al.* 1999. Pregnancy after breast carcinoma: outcomes and influence on mortality. Cancer **85:** 2424–2432.
8. MICHELS, K.B. & W.C. WILLETT. 1996. Does induced or spontaneous abortion affect the risk of breast cancer? Epidemiology **7:** 521–528.
9. GEMIGNANI, M.L., J.A. PETREK & P.I. BORGEN. 1999. Breast cancer and pregnancy. Surg. Clin. N. Am. **79:** 1157–1169.
10. DEL PRIORE, G., K. ROBISCHON & W. PHIPPS. 1995. Risk of ovarian cancer after treatment for infertility. N. Engl. J. Med. **332:** 1300.
11. ROSSING, M.A., J.R. DALING, N.S. WEISS, *et al.* 1994. Ovarian tumors in a cohort of infertile women. N. Engl. J. Med. **331:** 771–776.
12. VENN, A., L. WATSON, F. BRUINSMA, *et al.* 1999. Risk of cancer after use of fertility drugs with in-vitro fertilization. Lancet **354:** 1586–1590.
13. COLLABORATIVE GROUP ON HORMONAL FACTORS IN BREAST CANCER. 1997. Breast cancer and hormone replacement therapy: collaborative reanalysis of data from 51 epidemiological studies of 52,705 women with breast cancer and 108,411 women without breast cancer. Lancet **350:** 1047–1059.
14. JERNSTROM, H., J. FRENANDER, M. FERNO & H. OLSSON. 1999. Hormone replacement therapy before breast cancer diagnosis significantly reduces the overall death rate compared with never-use among 984 breast cancer patients. Br. J. Cancer **80:** 1453–1458.
15. FOWBLE, B., A. HANLON, G. FREEDMAN, *et al.* 1999. Postmenopausal hormone replacement therapy: effect on diagnosis and outcome in early-stage invasive breast cancer treated with conservative surgery and radiation. J. Clin. Oncol. **17:** 1680–1688.
16. FISHER, B., J. DIGNAM, J. BRYANT, *et al.* 1996. Five versus more than five years of tamoxifen therapy for breast cancer patients with negative lymph nodes and estrogen receptor-positive tumors. J. Natl. Cancer Inst. **88:** 1529–1542.
17. LERNER-GEVA, L., A. TOREN, A. CHETRIT, *et al.* 2000. The risk for cancer among children of women who underwent *in vitro* fertilization. Cancer **88:** 2845–2847.
18. COBAU, C.D., K. DECLERCQ, D. NEUBERG, *et al.* 1996. A randomized trial of megestrol acetate with or without premarin in the treatment of potentially responsive metastatic breast cancer. A Study of the Eastern Cooperative Oncology Group (E2185). Cancer **77:** 483–489.
19. VASSILOPOULOU-SELLIN, R., L. ASMAR, G.N. HORTOBAGYI, *et al.* 1999. Estrogen replacement therapy after localized breast cancer: clinical outcome of 319 women followed prospectively. J. Clin. Oncol. **17:** 1482–1487.

20. VASSILOPOULOU-SELLIN, R. & R.L. THERIAULT. 1994. Randomized prospective trial of estrogen-replacement therapy in women with a history of breast cancer. J. Natl. Cancer Inst. Monogr. **16:** 153–159.
21. GURSKI, K.J. & G. DEL PRIORE. 1997. Gynecologic malignancies. *In* The Rochester Manual: Practical Patient Care. K. Illig & W. Cowles Husser, eds. Laennec Publishing. Cedar Grove, NJ.
22. MILLER, D.M., T.G. EHLEN & E.A. SALEH. 1997. Successful term pregnancy following conservative debulking surgery for a stage IIIA serous low-malignant-potential tumor of the ovary: a case report. Gynecol. Oncol. **66:** 535–538.
23. WALTER, A.J. & J.F. MAGRINA. 1999. Contralateral pelvic and aortic lymph node metastasis in clinical stage I epithelial ovarian cancer. Gynecol. Oncol. **74:** 128–129.
24. SAKAI, K., T. KAMURA, T. HIRAKAWA, *et al.* 1997. Relationship between pelvic lymph node involvement and other disease sites in patients with ovarian cancer. Gynecol. Oncol. **65:** 164–168.
25. MORRIS, R.T., D.M. GERSHENSON, E.G. SILVA, *et al.* 2000. Outcome and reproductive function after conservative surgery for borderline ovarian tumors. Obstet. Gynecol. **95:** 541–547.
26. GUIDOZZI, F. & A. DAPONTE. 1999. Estrogen replacement therapy for ovarian carcinoma survivors: a randomized controlled trial. Cancer **86:** 1013–1018.
27. MEIROW, D. 1999. Ovarian injury and modern options to preserve fertility in female cancer patients treated with high dose radio-chemotherapy for hemato-oncological neoplasias and other cancers. Leuk. Lymphoma **33:** 65–76.
28. SHAW, J.M., S.L. COX, A.O. TROUNSON & G. JENKIN. 2000. Evaluation of the long-term function of cryopreserved ovarian grafts in the mouse: implications for human applications. Mol. Cell Endocrinol. **161:** 103–110.
29. FREI, K.A., K. KINKEL, H.M. BONEL, *et al.* 2000. Prediction of deep myometrial invasion in patients with endometrial cancer: clinical utility of contrast-enhanced MR imaging: a meta-analysis and Bayesian analysis. Radiology **216:** 444–449.
30. YANG, G.C. & L.S. WAN. 2000. Endometrial biopsy using the Tao Brush method. A study of 50 women in a general gynecologic practice. J. Reprod. Med. **45:** 109–114.
31. DEL PRIORE, G., R. WILLIAMS, C.B. HARBATKIN, *et al.* 2001. Endometrial brush biopsy for the diagnosis of endometrial cancer. J. Reprod. Med. **46:** 439–443.
32. CICINELLI, E., F. ROMANO, P.S. ANASTASIO, *et al.* 1995. Transabdominal sonohysterography, transvaginal sonography, and hysteroscopy in the evaluation of submucous myomas. Obstet. Gynecol. **85:** 42–37.
33. KARLSSON, B., S. GRANBERG, P. HELLBERG & M. WIKLAND. 1994. Comparative study of transvaginal sonography and hysteroscopy for the detection of pathologic endometrial lesions in women with postmenopausal bleeding. J. Ultrasound Med. **13:** 757–762.
34. DEL PRIORE, G., S. FEINSTEIN, F.S. WILLIAMS & A. LIU. 2000. Accuracy of hysteroscopic visual impression for diagnosing endometrial complex atypical hyperplasia or cancer. Internat. J. Gynecol. Obstet. **70:** 57.
35. ZERBE, M.J., J. ZHANG, R.E. BRISTOW, *et al.* 2000. Retrograde seeding of malignant cells during hysteroscopy in presumed early endometrial cancer. Gynecol. Oncol. **79:** 55–58.
36. SMITH, J.R., D.C.M. BOYLE, D.J. CORLESS, *et al.* 1997. Abdominal trachelectomy. A new surgical technique for the conservative management of cervical carcinoma. Br. J. Gynaecol. Obstet. **104:** 1196–1200.
37. ROY, M. & M. PLANTE. 1998. Pregnancies after radical vaginal trachelectomy for early-stage cervical cancer. Am. J. Obstet. Gynecol. **179:** 1491–1496.
38. BOYLE, D.M., L. UNGARS, G. DEL PRIORE & J.R. SMITH. 2001. Radical abdominal trachelectomy. *In* Gynaecological Oncology: An Atlas of Investigation and Surgery. J.R. Smith, G. Del Priore, J.P. Curtin & J. Monaghan, Eds. Martin Dunitz, London, UK, and Mosby, St. Louis, MO.
39. CHAMBERS, S.K., J.T. CHAMBERS, R. KIER & R.E. PESCHEL. 1991. Sequelae of lateral ovarian transposition in irradiated cervical cancer patients. Int. J. Radiat. Oncol. Biol. Phys. **20:** 1305–1308.

40. MARTIN, X.J., F. GOLFIER, P. ROMESTAING & D. RAUDRANT. 1999. First case of pregnancy after radical trachelectomy and pelvic irradiation. Gynecol. Oncol. **74:** 286–287.
41. KANDELA, P. 2000. Letter to the editor. Lancet **356:** 838.
42. ERASLAN, S., R.J. HAMERNIK & J.D. HARDY. 1966. Replantation of uterus and ovaries in dogs, with successful pregnancy. Arch. Surg. **92:** 9–12.
43. LEE, S., L. MAO, Y. WANG, *et al.* 1995. Transplantation of reproductive organs. Microsurgery **16:** 191–198.
44. SCIARRA, J.J. 1993. Reproductive health: a global perspective. Am. J. Obstet. Gynecol. **168:** 1649–1654.
45. DEL PRIORE, G., P. ZANDIEH & M.J. LEE. 1997. Treatment of continuous data as categorical variables in obstetrics and gynecology. Obstet. Gynecol. **89:** 351–354.

Role of Exogenous and Endogenous Hormones in Endometrial Cancer

Review of the Evidence and Research Perspectives

ARSLAN AKHMEDKHANOV,[a,b] ANNE ZELENIUCH-JACQUOTTE,[b] AND PAOLO TONIOLO[a,b]

[a]Department of Obstetrics and Gynecology and [b]Department of Environmental Medicine, New York University School of Medicine, New York, New York 10016, USA

ABSTRACT: Endometrial carcinoma is the most common cancer of the female reproductive organs in the United States. International comparisons reveal that the incidence of endometrial cancer vary widely between different countries with the highest rates observed in North America and Northern Europe, intermediate rates in Eastern Europe and Latin America, and lowest rates in Asia and Africa. International variation in endometrial cancer rates may represent differences in the distribution of known risk factors, which include obesity, postmenopausal estrogen replacement, ovarian dysfunction, diabetes mellitus, infertility, nulliparity, and tamoxifen use. Most of the risk factors for endometrial cancer can be explained within the framework of the unopposed estrogen hypothesis, which proposes that exposure to estrogens unopposed by progesterone or synthetic progestins leads to increased mitotic activity of endometrial cells, increased number of DNA replication errors, and somatic mutations resulting in malignant phenotype. Although the impact of exogenous hormone replacement was intensively studied during the last two decades, less is known about the effects of endogenous hormones in endometrial cancer. A review of available experimental, clinical, and epidemiologic data suggests that in addition to estrogens, other endogenous hormones, including progesterone, androgens, gonadotropins, prolactin, insulin, and insulin-like growth factors, may play a role in the pathogenesis of different histopathologic types of endometrial cancer.

KEYWORDS: androgens; cancer; endogenous hormones; endometrial cancer; exogenous hormones; hormones; progesterone

INTRODUCTION

Adenocarcinoma of the endometrium is the most common carcinoma of the female reproductive organs and ranks fourth in total cancer incidence among women in the United States. In 2000, the American Cancer Society estimated that 36,100 new cases of endometrial cancer had been diagnosed in the United States and that about 6,500 women had died from the disease.[1] The majority (86%) of cases of

Address for correspondence: Dr. Arslan Akhmedkhanov, Department of Obstetrics and Gynecology, New York University School of Medicine, 550 First Avenue, NB 9E2, New York, NY 10016. Voice: 212-263-7763; fax: 212-263-8887.
akhmea01@med.nyu.edu

endometrial cancer arise after the age of 50, and the age-specific incidence peaks at 75–79 years (109.1 per 100,000), according to U.S. Surveillance, Epidemiology, and End Results (SEER) Program data.[2]

In the United States, the age-adjusted incidence in Caucasian women reached its highest point around 1975 (33.8 per 100,000), coinciding with a peak of estrogen sales for postmenopausal replacement use.[3] Since 1975, when the first reports on the association between exogenous estrogen use and increased risk of endometrial cancer appeared,[4,5] the incidence has declined substantially. By 1997, it was 23.1 per 100,000, or about 30% less than that in the mid-1970s. From 1973–1997, the age-adjusted mortality declined by 50% in U.S. White women under 50 years and by 26% in women 50 years and older.

During the same period, the age-adjusted incidence among U.S. Black women (15 per 100,000) was 70% lower than that in White women and has remained relatively constant. In contrast, the annual age-adjusted mortality from uterine cancer was almost twice as high in U.S. Blacks (6.2 per 100,000) as in U.S. whites (3.6 per 100,000). The excessive mortality experienced by U.S. Black women compared to Caucasian women may represent a different distribution of epidemiological risk factors correlated with socioeconomic, behavioral, and genetic susceptibility characteristics of African-American women.[6]

International comparisons show that incidence rates of endometrial cancer vary widely between countries.[7] Generally, the rates are highest in North America and Northern Europe, intermediate in Eastern Europe and Latin America, and lowest in Asia and Africa (FIG. 1). International differences in endometrial cancer incidence rates may be related to ample variations in body weight, the use of hormone replacement therapy, reproductive characteristics, such as age at menarche and parity, and endogenous estrogen levels.

Analyses of age-specific incidence curves reveal three distinctive patterns characterizing populations at high, intermediate, and low risk of endometrial cancer (FIG. 2). In populations with the highest rates (e.g., U.S. [Whites] and Switzerland), rates increase steadily from age 35 to age 60 with a slower increase thereafter until they peak at 75 years (between 100 and 120 per 100,000) and subsequently decline. In populations with intermediate rates (e.g., U.S. [Blacks] and the Netherlands), rates increase steeply until age 55–60 (between 60 and 80 per 100,000) and then tend to flatten out and decline after 70 years. In populations with the lowest rates (e.g., China and Japan), incidence rates peak earlier, at the age of 55 years (20 per 100,000), and subsequently decline (FIG. 2).

RISK AND PROTECTIVE FACTORS

Epidemiological research has identified several risk factors for endometrial adenocarcinoma. These include age,[8,9] obesity,[10–12] estrogen therapy in ovarian dysgenesis,[13,14] postmenopausal estrogen replacement,[4,5,15] diabetes mellitus,[16–18] ovarian dysfunction,[19,20] early menarche,[21,22] late menopause,[23,24] infertility,[25,26] nulliparity,[27,28] and, more recently, tamoxifen use.[29,30]

The use of estrogen-progestin combination type of oral contraceptives is reported to decrease a woman's risk of endometrial cancer[23,27,31,32] or not to affect the

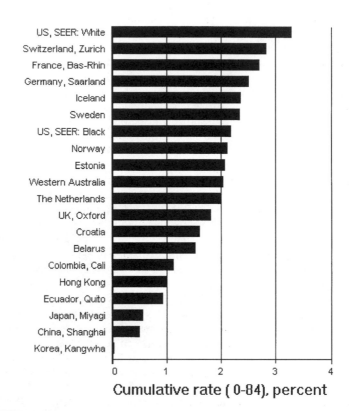

FIGURE 1. Cumulative rates of endometrial cancer in selected countries, 1988–1992. Data from Parkin *et al.*[7]

risk.[33,34] Exposures that have been associated with a protective effect also include parity,[16,23,35,36] smoking,[37,38] and physical activity.[39,40]

Unopposed Estrogen Hypothesis

Most of the risk and protective factors for endometrial adenocarcinoma can be effectively explained within the framework of the unopposed estrogen hypothesis.[41–43] This theory postulates that exposure to endogenous or exogenous estrogens not opposed by progesterone or synthetic progestins increases the mitotic activity of endometrial cells, resulting in increased DNA replication errors and somatic mutations, ultimately leading to endometrial hyperplasia and malignant phenotype.[44,45] The unopposed estrogen hypothesis is consistent with the known epidemiological features of the disease and provides plausible explanations for the mechanisms of action of various risk and protective factors for endometrial cancer, as summarized in TABLE 1.

Obesity

Obesity is a well-established risk factor for endometrial cancer among both premenopausal[21,44,46] and postmenopausal[16,21,27,44,45] women. Various indices of

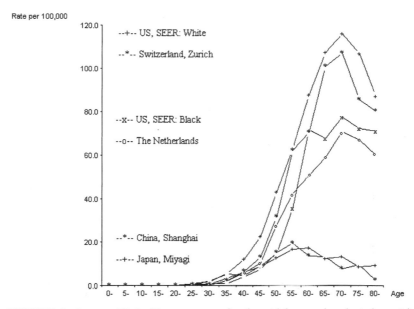

FIGURE 2. Age-specific incidence curves of endometrial cancer in selected countries, 1988–1922. Data from Parkin *et al.*[7]

obesity, including percentage of excess weight, body mass index (BMI = weight/height^2), waist-to-thigh ratio, and waist-to-hip ratio, were shown to be associated with increased risk.[46–48] The lifetime risk of being diagnosed with endometrial cancer in the U.S. is about 3%, whereas the cumulative risk increases to 9–10% in obese women.[6] Based on the prevalence of obesity and estimates of relative risk in U.S. women, excessive weight and a central pattern of fat distribution may account for 17–46% of endometrial cancer incidence in postmenopausal women.[6]

A substantial portion of the international variation in the incidence of endometrial cancer could be explained by differences in the prevalence of obesity. Comparisons of cumulative rates (ages 0–84) of endometrial cancer[7] with reported data on the prevalence of obesity (defined as BMI ≥ 30 kg/m^2) among women in developed[49] and developing[50] countries suggest that obesity may account for about 40% of worldwide variation in cumulative rates of endometrial cancer (FIG. 3).

Obesity in postmenopausal women leads to increased peripheral production of estrogens, mainly through the aromatization of androstenedione to estrone in adipose cells, which are rich in the aromatase enzyme necessary for this conversion.[51] This mechanism could be particularly important, because obesity also increases adrenal secretion of androgens, including androstenedione, a major precursor of estrogens in postmenopausal women.[51] Thus, elevated circulating estrogens in obese postmenopausal women may result from an enhanced production of androgen precursor by the adrenal glands as well as an increased rate of aromatization in adipose tissue. It has been shown that plasma concentrations of androstenedione and of the major estrogens (estradiol and estrone) are positively correlated with body weight in

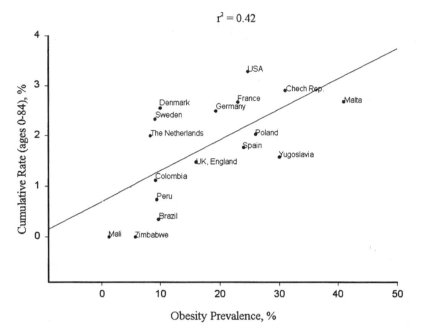

FIGURE 3. Association between obesity and endometrial cancer cumulative rate in selected countries.

postmenopausal women.[52,53] In addition, obesity is associated with decreased sex hormone binding globulin (SHBG) production in the liver and with increased proportions of bioavailable (free and albumin-bound) fractions of estradiol.[54,55] Key and Pike[44] estimated that doubling the body weight of postmenopausal woman from 54 kg to 109 kg would reduce SHBG concentration by 85% and increase total, free, and non-SHBG–bound estradiol levels by 60%. The increase in bioavailable estradiol was proposed as a cause of increased endometrial cancer risk in postmenopausal women.[42]

Among premenopausal women, obesity is thought to increase the risk of endometrial cancer because of the increased frequency of anovulatory cycles, amenorrhea,[56] and irregular menstrual periods,[57] which are associated with progesterone deficiency during the luteal phase of the cycle. Progesterone deficiency results in higher proliferation and lesser degree of desquamation of the endometrium, including endometrial transformed cells, and is considered a major risk factor of endometrial cancer in premenopausal women.[44]

Postmenopausal Hormone Replacement

An extensive search of the literature revealed that after the first two reports published in 1975 by Smith *et al.*[4] and Ziel *et al.*,[5] at least 130 studies have examined the association between postmenopausal hormone replacement and the risk of endometrial cancer. Overall, the use of unopposed estrogens for 1 year or more appears

TABLE 1. Established risk and protective factors for endometrial cancer in relation to unopposed estrogen exposure

Increased unopposed estrogen/risk factor	Proposed mechanism(s)
Exogenous	
Estrogen therapy for ovarian dysgenesis	Estrogenic effect on the endometrium.
Postmenopausal estrogen replacement	Unopposed effect on the endometrium.
Sequential estrogen–progestin replacement	Mimicking follicular phase endometrial mitotic rate during estrogen replacement stage.
Tamoxifen use	Binding to estrogen receptor, estrogenic effect on the endometrium.
Endogenous	
Obesity	*Adipose tissue*: Increased aromatization of androstenedione to estrone.
	Adrenal glands: Increased secretion of androgens (androstenedione, testosterone, dehydroepi androsterone) in postmenopausal women.
	Liver: Decreased SHBG production, increased proportion of bioavailable (free and albumin-bound) fractions of estradiol.
	Decreased 2-hydroxlation of estradiol.
	Ovary: Increased frequency of anovulation in obese premenopausal women, progesterone deficiency, unopposed estrogen exposure.
Ovarian dysfunction:	
Anovulation	Unopposed endometrial estrogen exposure.
Ovarian granulosa-cell and theca-cell tumors	Increased estrogen and androgen secretion.
Polycystic ovary syndrome	Increased androstenedione secretion and aromatization of androstenedione to estrone.
Early menarche/late menopause	Increased duration of estrogen exposure.
Nulliparity/infertility	Increased cumulative endometrial estrogen exposure/progesterone deficiency.
Diabetes mellitus, noninsulin dependent	Hyperinsulinemia, elevated estrogen levels.

Decreased unopposed estrogen/protective factor	Proposed mechanism(s)
Exogenous	
Continuous estrogen–progestin replacement	Opposed effect of synthetic progestin leading to reduced endometrial mitotic rate.
Smoking	Anti-estrogenic effect due to increased metabolic clearance of estrogens.
	Increased 2-hydroxylation of estradiol.
Physical activity	Maintenance of low body fat, moderation of extraglandular estrogen;
	Reduction of number of ovulatory cycles;
	Decreased cumulative endometrial estrogen exposure.
Endogenous	
Pregnancy	Decreased cumulative number of ovulations and subsequent endometrial estrogen exposure;
	During delivery, shedding of cells that have undergone malignant transformation.

to be associated with relative risks ranging from 1.5–10.0, depending on the control group. Risk estimates were usually higher in studies that used controls with non-gynecologic diseases and lower in studies that used controls with gynecologic diseases other than cancer. A meta-analysis of 30 studies yielded a summary relative risk (RR) of 2.3 for ever-users of estrogens compared to non-users (95% confidence interval [CI], 2.1–2.5).[15] Relative risk associated with prolonged duration of use was much higher (RR, 9.5 for 10 or more years).[15] The summary RR of endometrial cancer remained elevated 5 years or more after discontinuation of unopposed estrogen therapy (RR, 2.3).[15] Estrogen-induced endometrial tumors usually have favorable prognostic characteristics, such as low grade of differentiation and superficial invasion into the myometrium.[58]

Progestins antagonize the effects of estrogens on the endometrium and prevent the development of endometrial hyperplasia when added to estrogens.[59,60] Endometrial hyperplasia that develops in women taking unopposed estrogens is effectively treated with progestins.[61,62] Thus, since the 1980s, progestins have been added to estrogen replacement regimens to prevent the increased risk of endometrial cancer associated with unopposed estrogen therapy. Initially, estrogen replacement therapy was followed by the addition of progestins, usually for 7 or 10 days per month (sequential estrogen-progestin replacement therapy, SEPRT). SEPRT causes bleeding in many women and is associated with other side effects. Consequently, a continuous combined estrogen-progestin replacement therapy (CEPRT) regimen was developed in which estrogen and progestin are taken together.[33,34]

Among sequential estrogen-progestin users, four cohort studies[63–66] showed a decreased risk of endometrial cancer (RR, 0.4), whereas case control studies[67–69] reported an increase in risk (RR, 1.8).[15] The increased risk observed in some studies could be related to inadequate progestin dose or duration, use of less effective progestins, prior use of unopposed estrogen, and poor patient compliance.

Combined estrogen-progestin therapy has generally been associated with a reduced risk of endometrial cancer[23,27,31,32,46] or with no risk changes.[33,34] A recent study of different hormone replacement regimens by Pike and Ross[34] showed that the risk of endometrial cancer was strongly affected by the number of days of progestin administration. In a typical 28-day cycle of SEPRT, progestin use can be divided into short-progestin (SEPRT-SP, <10 days per cycle) and long-progestin (SEPRT-LP, ≥10 days per cycle) regimens. The risk of endometrial cancer was significantly increased among subjects on the SEPRT-SP regimen, whereas women on SEPRT-LP and CEPRT showed no evidence of significantly increased risk.[34] Pike and Ross[34] proposed that the increased risk of endometrial cancer among women on SEPRT-SP could be related to the lower degree of desquamation of the functional layer of the endometrium, where initial tumors often arise.

Tamoxifen Use

Tamoxifen is the most widely prescribed antineoplastic agent for the adjuvant treatment of breast cancer. It is a synthetic compound, which acts by blocking the binding of estrogen to the estrogen receptor. Animal studies suggest that tamoxifen may have contrasting effects in breast and endometrial tissues. Tamoxifen blocks the growth of breast tumors and stimulates the growth of endometrial carcinomas in athymic mice.[70] Experimental evidence suggest that tamoxifen exerts an estrogenic effect on the endometrium,[71] and several reports have documented the increased incidence of endometrial hyperplasia and polyps in women treated with tamoxifen.[72,73]

Since the first case report in 1985,[29] numerous cases of tamoxifen-associated uterine cancers have been documented in the literature.[74–78] The first large study, which assessed the association between tamoxifen and the risk of endometrial cancer in a group of postmenopausal women with early breast cancer who were treated in a randomized clinical trial of adjuvant tamoxifen, came from Sweden in 1989.[79] Compared to the control group, the relative risk of endometrial cancer in the tamoxifen-treated group was 6.4, with the greatest risk occurring after 5 years of use. In a Danish randomized clinical trial,[80] the cumulative incidence of endometrial cancer 10 years after treatment with radiation therapy plus tamoxifen was 1.0%, as compared to 0.3% in patients treated with radiation alone. In two other trials no increase was found in the incidence of endometrial cancer after tamoxifen therapy.[81,82] Magriples *et al.*,[83] analyzing data from the Yale Tumor Registry, reported that women treated with tamoxifen were more likely to develop high-grade endometrial cancers and have a worse prognosis. In two subsequent studies no apparent difference was found between the types of endometrial cancer diagnosed in tamoxifen-treated women and those found in their controls.[84,85] However, recent nationwide case-control study in the Netherlands found that long-term (at least 2 years) tamoxifen users have a worse prognosis for endometrial cancers, which seems to be due to less favorable histologic characteristics and a higher stage of tumor.[86]

A randomized clinical trial from the National Surgical Adjuvant Breast and Bowel Project reported on disease outcome for 2,843 patients with invasive, node-negative, estrogen-receptor positive breast cancer who were randomly assigned to receive a placebo or tamoxifen (20 mg/day).[30,87] Compared to the placebo group, the relative risk of endometrial cancer was significantly higher in the tamoxifen-treated group (risk ratio, 2.53; 95% confidence interval, 1.35–4.97).[87] Most tumors in the trial had favorable prognostic features, such as low stage and low grade. Jordan and Morrow[88] estimated that two to three women would develop endometrial cancer per 1,000 women treated with tamoxifen per year. This estimate should be balanced against the potential benefits of tamoxifen in women with breast cancer, and all women who take tamoxifen should have a routine annual gynecologic evaluation.[89]

Endogenous Estrogens in Postmenopausal Women

Whereas the role of exogenous estrogens in endometrial cancer has been extensively studied, epidemiologic evidence regarding the role of endogenous estrogens is limited. Key and Pike[44] suggested that there is an upper limit beyond which unopposed estrogen does not induce a further increase in mitotic rate and estimated this limit to be 50 pg/ml, the upper limit of estradiol during the follicular phase of the menstrual cycle. Postmenopausal women, whose estradiol levels are substantially lower, in the range of 5–20 pg/ml, may be particularly sensitive to even modest elevations in estrogen levels, which may enhance endometrial mitotic rate and subsequently increase the risk of endometrial cancer.[44] Although estradiol is the most biologically active estrogen, other steroids, such as estrone and estrone sulfate, become important after menopause, when levels of estradiol are low.

Using a MEDLINE search from January 1965 through December 2000, we identified 30 studies that have examined associations between endogenous levels of estrogens and endometrial cancer in postmenopausal women. Most of these studies were hospital-based case-control studies with a limited number of cases and with controls often selected among subjects with other gynecologic conditions. The earliest studies examined the conversion of androstenedione to estrone, the major estrogen after menopause. Hausknecht and Gusberg,[90] Rizkallah et al.,[91] and Calanog et al.[92] reported that the conversion of androstenedione to estrone was significantly greater in patients with endometrial cancer than in matched controls. These observation, however, were not confirmed in a similar, but larger study by MacDonald et al.[52] Strong correlations between androstenedione-to-estrone conversion and body weight have been reported, with the highest conversion occurring in obese postmenopausal women.[52,91] Subsequent hospital-based studies directly compared circulating estrogen concentrations between endometrial cancer cases and controls. These studies were based on the acceptance of several fundamental assumptions: (1) that measurements at a single point in time provide an accurate reflection of the true average circulating estrogen levels; (2) that the presence of tumor does not affect estrogen levels among the cases; (3) that circulating estrogens are predictive of tissue concentrations in the endometrium; and (4) that changes in endogenous estrogen levels translate into corresponding changes in endometrial mitotic rate. It is possible that some of these assumptions may be less than accurate, or even untrue, which would considerably affect the interpretation of study results.

Thirteen of 26 published hospital-based case-control studies reported a statistically significant increase in circulating estrogen levels in endometrial cancer cases compared to controls.[93–105] The most commonly reported elevated estrogens in postmenopausal endometrial cancer cases were estrone[94,95,98,99,101,104,105] and total estradiol.[93,94,97,101–105] Significant increases in estrone sulfate,[98,100,105] free estradiol,[96,104,105] and albumin-bound estradiol[105] were also reported. However, several other studies found no differences in circulating estrogen levels between endometrial cancer cases and controls.[53,92,106–116] It is noteworthy that most of the negative studies had matched cases and controls by weight. Because obesity is thought to increase risk by elevating estrogen levels, it is plausible that matching on weight would result in overmatching and, thus, would tend to attenuate the association between circulating estrogens and endometrial cancer. Moreover, small sample size, use of hospital controls, and lack of clearly defined selection criteria for both patient and control groups may explain the absence of hormonal differences between patients with endometrial cancer and non-cancer controls in some of the hospital-based case-control studies.

To date, the association between circulating estrogen levels and the risk of endometrial cancer in postmenopausal women has been assessed in three large epidemiologic studies[117–119] (TABLE 2). All three studies observed an evident increased risk of endometrial cancer with increasing circulating levels of estrone after adjustment for BMI and other possible confounders. In addition, two studies have reported an increased risk with increasing bioavailable (free and albumin-bound) fractions of estradiol and a trend of reduced risk with increasing SHBG.[118,119]

TABLE 2. Endogenous estrogens and risk of endometrial cancer in postmenopausal women

Reference	Cases		Controls		Measure	OR (95% CI)	Comments
	Source	n	Source	n			
Austin *et al.*[117] (1991)	Hospital	67	Optometry clinic	142	Estrone Quartiles (pg/ml): 1–2 (≤24) 4 (≥32) Total estradiol Quartiles (pg/ml): 1–2 (≤7) 4 (≥10)	1.0 (referent) 3.8 (1.7–8.4) 1.0 (referent) 2.9 (1.3–6.5)	Adjusted for BMI, age, race, and education.
Potischman *et al.*[118] (1996)	Hospital	208	Population	209	Estrone Tertiles (pg/ml): 1 (<26) 2 (26–40) 3 (≥41) Total estradiol Tertiles (pg/ml): 1 (<6) 2 (6–9.9) 3 (≥10) Free estradiol Tertiles (pg/ml): 1 (<0.08) 2 (0.08–0.13) 3 (≥0.14)	1.0 (referent) 2.2 (1.2–4.3) 2.2 (1.2–4.4) 1.0 (referent) 0.8 (0.4–1.5) 1.3 (0.7–2.5) 1.0 (referent) 0.6 (0.3–1.2) 1.7 (0.9–3.3)	Adjusted for BMI, waist-to-thigh ratio, age, study site, race, education, parity, current smoking, use of oral contraceptives, diabetes, exogenous estrogen use, serum cholesterol level, alcohol intake, saturated fat, and carbohydrate calories.
Zeleniuch-Jacquotte *et al.*[119] (2001)	Prospective cohort	57	Prospective cohort	222	Estrone Tertiles (pg/ml): 1 (<20) 2 (20–28) 3 (>28) Total estradiol Tertiles (pg/ml): 1 (<6) 2 (6–8) 3 (>8) Free estradiol Tertiles (%): 1 (<1.10) 2 (1.10–1.28) 3 (>1.28)	1.0 (referent) 2.0 (0.9–4.7) 3.2 (1.3–7.8) 1.0 (referent) 1.0 (0.5–2.3) 1.8 (0.8–4.2) 1.0 (referent) 0.9 (0.4–2.2) 2.8 (1.3–6.4)	Adjusted for BMI and height. Matched by age, menopausal status at enrollment, and number of blood donations.

Dualistic Model of Endometrial Carcinogenesis

There is growing evidence that estrogens may be associated with certain histologic types of endometrial cancer, such as endometrioid carcinoma, also known as type 1 endometrial carcinoma. Type 1 carcinoma is the most common, is believed to develop from endometrial hyperplasia induced by estrogen excess exposure, and tends to have a favorable prognosis.[120] Type 2 carcinoma is represented by serous carcinoma, which does not seem to be related to estrogenic exposure, develops from atrophic rather than hyperplastic epithelium, and has a less favorable clinical course than does endometrioid carcinoma.

Molecular evidence supports the existence of a dualistic model of endometrial carcinogenesis. Endometrioid carcinomas (type 1) are commonly associated with mutations in *ras* oncogene, *PTEN* tumor suppressor gene, and microsatellite instability, whereas serous (type 2) carcinomas are associated with *p53* mutations.[120] Sherman *et al.*[105] demonstrated that patients with endometrioid carcinoma have significantly higher circulating estrogen levels than do patients with serous carcinoma, who have hormone levels similar to community controls. The investigators conclude that sex hormone levels and molecular mechanisms differ between patients with endometrioid and serous carcinoma, suggesting at least two different pathways of endometrial carcinogenesis.[105,120]

Other Endogenous Hormones

Progesterone

Whereas the role of estrogens in endometrial cancer is well established, the significance of other hormones is less clear. Gambrell[121] and other investigators[44,122] have presented a case for progesterone deficiency as a key hormonal factor in patients with endometrial cancer. Key and Pike[44] proposed that the risk of endometrial cancer positively correlates with the endometrial mitotic rate, which is increased by estrogens and reduced by progesterone. Therefore, progesterone deficiency, as a result of anovulation, unopposed estrogen exposure, or progesterone receptor downregulation, could be a risk factor for endometrial cancer.

Epidemiologic evidence provides indirect support for this hypothesis. Women taking unopposed estrogen replacement therapy have an increased risk of endometrial cancer, wheres women taking combined estrogen-progesterone replacement therapy experience risk reduction[23,27,31,32,46] or no increase in risk.[33,34] In addition, miscarriage late in reproductive life, which is a marker of progesterone deficiency, is associated with increased risk of endometrial cancer.[123]

Studies directly examining the levels of progesterone in women with and without endometrial cancer are limited. Two small hospital-based studies found no significant differences in circulating progesterone levels between postmenopausal endometrial cancer cases and controls.[99,116] A larger case-control study from Bulgaria involving 62 women with endometrial cancer found marked hypoprogesteronemia in premenopausal and postmenopausal women with endometrial cancer and atypical hyperplasia.[124] Modan *et al.*[125] reported that infertile women with clinical criteria of progesterone deficiency had a significant excess of endometrial cancer (standardized incidence rate, 9.4; 95% confidence interval, 5.0–16.0).[125] Future epidemiologic studies should determine whether serum levels of progesterone could be used as a biomarker of endometrial cancer risk.

Adrenal Hormones

In postmenopausal women, the adrenal cortex is the main source of steroid hormones.[126] Lucas[127] suggested that patients with endometrial cancer have an increased "adrenal drive." Significantly elevated levels of adrenal hormones, such as cortisol,[103] androstenedione,[92,101,105,117,118] dehydroepiandrosterone,[95] and dehydroepiandrosterone sulfate,[103] were reported in women with endometrial cancer compared to control subjects. Other studies, however, failed to support such evidence.[97,102,104,108,110,112,114]

Two large epidemiologic studies[117,118] showed a positive association between serum androstenedione levels and endometrial cancer risk. Potischman *et al.*[118] reported that a strong association of endometrial cancer with circulating androstenedione remained after control for estrone and hypothesized that abnormal endometrial cells could produce estrone locally from the plasma pool of androstenedione and thus gain advantage independent of circulating estrogen levels. Studies of the estrogen biosynthesis by human endometrial cells *in vitro* seem to support this hypothesis.[128,129]

Ovarian Androgens

In postmenopausal women, the adrenal glands are the major source of androgens, but the ovaries still contribute substantial amounts of testosterone and androstenedione.[130] Among postmenopausal women with endometrial cancer, two studies reported a significant increase in the ovarian venous levels of androstenedione and testosterone, as compared to controls.[111,113] In the same studies, androgen levels in peripheral blood were not significantly different between cases and controls.[111,113] The existence of such an ovarian-peripheral gradient suggests that the ovaries of postmenopausal women with endometrial cancer may secrete more androgens than do the ovaries of women without cancer. Consequently, Nagamani *et al.*[113] proposed that the increase in ovarian androgen secretion could play a role in the pathogenesis of endometrial cancer.

Pituitary Hormones

Hormones secreted by the pituitary gland (follicle-stimulating hormone, FSH; luteinizing hormone, LH; and prolactin) have been studied in relation to endometrial cancer. Several investigators reported that FSH levels were significantly lower among postmenopausal women with endometrial cancer than among control subjects.[94,97,102,111] Although the direct effect of FSH cannot be excluded, FSH is regulated by estrogens through a negative feedback, and, thus, it is possible that reduced circulating FSH in endometrial cancer patients could result from increased peripheral estrogen levels. In postmenopausal women, who are physiologically characterized by low estrogen and elevated FSH and LH levels, no substantial case-control differences in immunoactive LH levels have been documented.[94,101,102,106,111,112] However, elevated bioactive LH levels in postmenopausal women with endometrial cancer[131] and increased expression of LH receptors have been reported in endometrial hyperplasia and carcinoma occurring among anovulatory women with polycystic ovarian syndrome.[132] These data suggest that elevated bioactive LH may increase ovarian steroid production and contribute to the pathogenesis of endometrial carcinoma in anovulatory women.

Prolactin is produced not only by the anterior pituitary gland but also by human endometrium.[133,134] Endometrial prolactin is biologically and immunologically equipotent with pituitary prolactin. Synthesis of prolactin in human endometrial stromal cells extends from the late luteal phase in the nonpregnant cycle and throughout the pregnancy. Endometrial prolactin is a marker of stromal cell differentiation (decidualization) and is thought to play a role in implantation, placentation, and regulation of amniotic fluid volume and electrolytes.[135] Progesterone induces the expression of prolactin and prolactin receptor by the stromal cells of the human endometrium[135–137] and suppresses proliferation of the endometrium induced by epidermal growth factor.[136] In addition, prolactin markedly inhibits the mitogenic activity of human endometrial fibroblasts.[138] These observations indicate that prolactin could serve as a local modulator of stromal endometrial cell growth and differentiation. Several studies have compared circulating prolactin levels between endometrial cancer cases and controls. Benjamin and Deutsch[94] reported that women with endometrial cancer have significantly higher levels of serum prolactin than do controls, but other studies found no significant differences.[103,106]

Insulin and Insulin-Like Growth Factor Family

Several studies reported an increased risk of endometrial cancer with a history of diabetes.[16–18,22] Parazzini et al.[18] reported that the association between endometrial cancer risk and diabetes is limited to a non-insulin dependent type of diabetes mellitus, which is characterized by insulin resistance and hyperinsulinemia. Hyperinsulinemia and higher levels of insulin-like growth factor I (IGF-I) are proposed to play a role in hormone-dependent neoplasia.[139] Hyperinsulinemia increases ovarian steroid hormone production,[140] stimulates aromatization of androgens to estrogens,[141] and suppresses circulating levels of SHBG.[142] Several studies demonstrated that serum estradiol concentrations correlate with IGF-I.[143,144] In addition, adrenal androgens may also affect circulating IGF-I levels in postmenopausal women.[145]

Experimental studies have shown that steroid hormones are involved in the regulation of the insulin and IGF-1 receptors in human endometrium.[146] Both insulin and IGF-I substantially increase the mitogenic activity of the human endometrial adenocarcinoma cell lines.[147,148] The insulin-IGF system is thought to function as a mediator of steroid hormone action in the endometrium. Rutanen et al.[149] have shown that imbalance between insulin-like growth factors and IGF binding proteins could trigger an uncontrolled endometrial cell proliferation and hypothesized that, like unopposed estrogen, IGF-I unopposed by IGF binding proteins may increase the risk of endometrial cancer.[150]

FUTURE DIRECTIONS

The critical role of hormones in endometrial cancer has long been recognized. The unopposed estrogen hypothesis successfully explains endometrial cancer risk associated with exposure to exogenous and endogenous estrogens. Future investigations should clarify the role of other hormonal factors, including estrogen metabolites, progesterone, androgens, gonadotropins, prolactin, insulin, and insulin-like growth factors, as well as the significance of genetic polymorphisms of the respective genes, in the pathogenesis of different types of endometrial cancer. In conclusion, understanding hormonal functions in endometrial cancer may result in the development of more successful strategies for primary prevention, early detection, and effective treatment of the disease.

REFERENCES

1. AMERICAN CANCER SOCIETY. 2000. Cancer Facts & Figures. American Cancer Society, Inc. Atlanta, GA.
2. RIES, L.A.G., M.P. EISNER, C.L. KOSARY, *et al.*, Eds. 2000. SEER Cancer Statistics Review, 1973-1997. National Cancer Institute. NIH Pub. No. 00-2789: 171–181. NIH. Bethesda, MD.
3. WEISS, N.S., D.R. SZEKELY & D.F. AUSTIN. 1976. Increasing incidence of endometrial cancer in the United States. N. Engl. J. Med. **294:** 1259–1262.
4. SMITH, D.C., R. PRENTICE, D.J. THOMPSON, *et al.* 1975. Association of exogenous estrogen and endometrial carcinoma. N. Engl. J. Med. **293:** 1164–1167.
5. ZIEL, H.K. & W.D. FINKLE. 1975. Increased risk of endometrial carcinoma among users of conjugated estrogens. N. Engl. J. Med. **293:** 1167–1170.
6. SCHOTTENFELD, D. 1995. Epidemiology of endometrial neoplasia. 1995. J. Cell. Biochem. Suppl. **23:** 151–159.
7. PARKIN, D.M., S.L. WHELAN, J. FERLAY, *et al.*, Eds. 1997. Cancer incidence in five continents. Vol. VII. IARC Sci. Pub. No. 143. IARC. Lyon.
8. MACMAHON, B. 1974. Risk factors for endometrial cancer. Gynecol. Oncol. **2:** 122–129.
9. CRAMER, D.W., S.J. CUTLER & B. CHRISTINE. 1974. Trends in the incidence of endometrial cancer in the United States. Gynecol. Oncol. **2:** 130–143.
10. JAVERT, C.T. & E.L. RENNING. 1963. Endometrial cancer – survey of 610 cases treated at Women's Hospital (1919–1960). Cancer **16:** 1057–1064.
11. WYNDER, E.L., G.C. ESCHER & N. MANTEL. 1966. An epidemiological investigation of cancer of the endometrium. Cancer **19:** 489–520.
12. GANGEMI, M., G. MENEGHETTI, O. PREDEBON, *et al.* 1987. Obesity as a risk factor for endometrial cancer. Clin. Exp. Obstet. Gynecol. **14:** 119–122.
13. DOWSETT, J.H. 1963. Corpus carcinoma developing in a patient with Turner's syndrome treated with estrogen. Am. J. Obstet. Gynecol. **86:** 622–625.
14. CLEMENT, P.B. & R.II. YOUNG. 1987. Atypical polypoid adenomyoma of the uterus associated with Turner's syndrome. A report of three cases, including a review of "estrogen-associated" endometrial neoplasms and neoplasms associated with Turner's syndrome. Int. J. Gynecol. Pathol. **6:** 104–113.
15. GRADY, D., T. GEBRETSADIK, K. KERLIKOWSKE, *et al.* 1995. Hormone replacement therapy and endometrial cancer risk: a meta-analysis. Obstet. Gynecol. **85:** 304–313.
16. ELWOOD, J.M., P. COLE, K.J. ROTHMAN, *et al.* 1977. Epidemiology of endometrial cancer. J. Natl. Cancer Inst. **59:** 1055–1060.
17. O'MARA, B.A., T. BYERS & E. SCHOENFELD. 1985. Diabetes mellitus and cancer risk: a multisite case-control study. J. Chronic Dis. **38:** 435–441.
18. PARAZZINI, F., C. LA VECCHIA, E. NEGRI, *et al.* 1999. Diabetes and endometrial cancer: an Italian case-control study. Int. J. Cancer **81:** 539–542.
19. MCDONALD, T.W., G.D. MALKASIAN & T.A. GAFFEY. 1977. Endometrial cancer associated with feminizing ovarian tumor and polycystic ovarian disease. Obstet. Gynecol. **49:** 654–658.
20. DAHLGREN, E., L.G. FRIBERG, S. JOHANSSON, *et al.* 1991. Endometrial carcinoma: ovarian dysfunction–a risk factor in young women. Eur. J. Obstet. Gynecol. Reprod. Biol. **41:** 143–150.

21. LA VECCHIA, C., S. FRANCESCHI, A. DECARLI, *et al.* 1984. Risk factors for endometrial cancer at different ages. J. Natl. Cancer Inst. **73:** 667–671.
22. BRINTON, L.A., M.L. BERMAN, R. MORTEL, *et al.* 1992. Reproductive, menstrual, and medical risk factors for endometrial cancer: results from a case-control study. Am. J. Obstet. Gynecol. **167:** 1317–1325.
23. PETTERSSON, B., H.O. ADAMI, R. BERGSTROM, *et al.* 1986. Menstruation span – a time-limited risk factor for endometrial carcinoma. Acta Obstet. Gynecol. Scand. **65:** 247–255.
24. KALANDIDI, A., A. TZONOU, L. LIPWORTH, *et al.* 1996. A case-control study of endometrial cancer in relation to reproductive, somatometric, and life-style variables. Oncology **53:** 354–359.
25. RON, E., B. LUNENFELD, J. MENCZER, *et al.* 1987. Cancer incidence in a cohort of infertile women. Am. J. Epidemiol. **125:** 780–790.
26. ESCOBEDO, L.G., N.C. LEE, H.B. PETERSON, *et al.* 1991. Infertility-associated endometrial cancer risk may be limited to specific subgroups of infertile women. Obstet. Gynecol. **77:** 124–128.
27. KELSEY, J.L., V.A. LIVOLSI, T.R. HOLFORD, *et al.* 1982. A case-control study of cancer of the endometrium. Am. J. Epidemiol. **116:** 333–342.
28. ALBREKTSEN, G., I. HEUCH, S. TRETLI, *et al.* 1995. Is the risk of cancer of the corpus uteri reduced by a recent pregnancy? A prospective study of 765,756 Norwegian women. Int. J. Cancer **61:** 485–490.
29. KILLACKEY, M.A., T.B. HAKES & V.K. PIERCE. 1985. Endometrial adenocarcinoma in breast cancer patients receiving antiestrogens. Cancer Treat. Rep. **69:** 237–238.
30. FISHER, B., J.P. COSTANTINO, C.K. REDMOND, *et al.* 1994. Endometrial cancer in tamoxifen-treated breast cancer patients: findings from the National Surgical Adjuvant Breast and Bowel Project (NSABP) B-14. J. Natl. Cancer Inst. **86:** 527–537.
31. SCHLESSELMAN, J.J. 1997. Risk of endometrial cancer in relation to use of combined oral contraceptives. A practitioner's guide to meta-analysis. Hum. Reprod. **12:** 1851–1863.
32. WEIDERPASS, E., H.O. ADAMI, J.A. BARON, *et al.* 1999. Risk of endometrial cancer following estrogen replacement with and without progestins. J. Natl. Cancer Inst. **91:** 1131–1137.
33. PIKE, M.C., R.K. PETERS, W. COZEN, *et al.* 1997. Estrogen-progestin replacement therapy and endometrial cancer. J. Natl. Cancer Inst. **89:** 1110–1116.
34. PIKE, M.C. & R.K. ROSS. 2000. Progestins and menopause: epidemiological studies of risks of endometrial and breast cancer. Steroids **65:** 659–664.
35. KVALE, G., I. HEUCH & G. URSIN. 1988. Reproductive factors and risk of cancer of the uterine corpus: a prospective study. Cancer Res. **48:** 6217–6221.
36. LAMBE, M., J. WUU, E. WEIDERPASS, *et al.* 1999. Childbearing at older age and endometrial cancer risk (Sweden). Cancer Causes Control **10:** 43–49.
37. LESKO, S.M., L. ROSENBERG, D.W. KAUFMAN, *et al.* 1985. Cigarette smoking and the risk of endometrial cancer. N. Engl. J. Med. **313:** 593–596.
38. BRINTON, L.A., R.J. BARRETT, M.L. BERMAN, *et al.* 1993. Cigarette smoking and the risk of endometrial cancer. Am. J. Epidemiol. **137:** 281–291.
39. LEVI, F., C. LA VECCHIA, E. NEGRI, *et al.* 1993. Selected physical activities and the risk of endometrial cancer. Br. J. Cancer **67:** 846–851.
40. MORADI, T., E. WEIDERPASS, L.B. SIGNORELLO, *et al.* 2000. Physical activity and post-menopausal endometrial cancer risk. Cancer Causes Control **11:** 829–837.
41. SIITERI, P.K., B.E. SCHWARZ & P.C. MACDONALD. 1974. Estrogen receptors and the estrone hypothesis in relation to endometrial and breast cancer. Gynecol. Oncol. **2:** 228–238.
42. SIITERI, P.K. 1978. Steroid hormones and endometrial cancer. Cancer Res. **38:** 4360–4366.
43. HENDERSON, B.E., R.K. ROSS, M.C. PIKE, *et al.* 1982. Endogenous hormones as a major factor in human cancer. Cancer Res. **42:** 3232–3239.
44. KEY, T.J.A. & M.C. PIKE. 1988. The dose-effect relationship between 'unopposed' oestrogens and endometrial mitotic rate: its central role in explaining and predicting endometrial cancer risk. Br. J. Cancer **57:** 205–212.

45. HENDERSON, B.E. & H.S. FEIGELSON. 2000. Hormonal carcinogenesis. Carcinogenesis **21:** 427–433.
46. FOLSOM, A.R., S.A. KAYE, J.D. POTTER, *et al.* 1989. Association of incident carcinoma of the endometrium with body weight and fat distribution in older women: early findings of the Iowa Women's Health Study. Cancer Res. **49:** 6828–6831.
47. SCHAPIRA, D.V., N.B. KUMAR, G.H. LYMAN, *et al.* 1991. Upper-body fat distribution and endometrial cancer risk. JAMA **266:** 1808–1811.
48. SWANSON, C.A., N. POTISCHMAN, G.D. WILBANKS, *et al.* 1993. Relation of endometrial cancer risk to past and contemporary body size and body fat distribution. Cancer Epidemiol. Biomarkers Prev. **2:** 321–327.
49. SEIDELL, J.C. & K.M. FLEGAL. 1997. Assessing obesity: classification and epidemiology. Br. Med. Bull. **53:** 238–252.
50. MARTORELL, R., L.K. KHAN, M.L. HUGHES, *et al.* 2000. Obesity in women from developing countries. Eur. J. Clin. Nutr. **54:** 247–252.
51. GRODIN, J.M., P.K. SIITERI & P.C. MACDONALD. 1973. Source of estrogen production in postmenopausal women. J. Clin. Endocrinol. Metab. **36:** 207–214.
52. MACDONALD, P.C., C.D. EDMAN, D.L. HEMSELL, *et al.* 1978. Effect of obesity on conversion of plasma androstenedione to estrone in postmenopausal women with and without endometrial cancer. Am. J. Obstet. Gynecol. **130:** 448–455.
53. JUDD, H.L., W.E. LUCAS & S.S. YEN. 1976. Serum 17 beta-estradiol and estrone levels in postmenopausal women with and without endometrial cancer. J. Clin. Endocrinol. Metab. **43:** 272–278.
54. ANDERSON, DC. 1974. Sex-hormone-binding globulin. Clin. Endocrinol. (Oxf.) **3:** 69–96.
55. MOORE, J.W., T.J.A. KEY, R.D. BULBROOK, *et al.* 1987. Sex hormone binding globulin and risk factors for breast cancer in a population of normal women who had never used exogenous sex hormones. Br. J. Cancer **56:** 661–666.
56. ROGERS, J. & G.W. MITCHELL. 1952. The relation of obesity to menstrual disturbances. N. Engl. J. Med. **247:** 53–55.
57. HARTZ, A.J., D.C. RUPLEY & A.A. RIMM. 1984. The association of girth measurements with disease in 32,856 women. Am. J. Epidemiol. **119:** 71–80.
58. CHU, J., A.I. SCHWEID & N.S. WEISS. 1982. Survival among women with endometrial cancer: a comparison of estrogen users and nonusers. Am. J. Obstet. Gynecol. **143:** 569–573.
59. WHITEHEAD, M.I. & D. FRASER. 1987. The effects of estrogens and progestogens on the endometrium. Modern approach to treatment. Obstet. Gynecol. Clin. North. Am. **14:** 299–320.
60. GELFAND, M.M. & A. FERENCZY. 1989. A prospective 1-year study of estrogen and progestin in postmenopausal women: effects on the endometrium. Obstet. Gynecol. **74:** 398–402.
61. GAMBRELL, R.D., JR. 1978. The prevention of endometrial cancer in postmenopausal women with progestogens. Maturitas **1:** 107–112.
62. THOM, M.H., P.J. WHITE, R.M. WILLIAMS, *et al.* 1979. Prevention and treatment of endometrial disease in climacteric women receiving oestrogen therapy. Lancet **2:** 455–457.
63. HAMMOND, C.B., F.R. JELOVSEK, K.L. LEE, *et al.* 1979. Effects of long-term estrogen replacement therapy. II. Neoplasia. Am. J. Obstet. Gynecol. **133:** 537–547.
64. PERSSON, I., H.O. ADAMI, L. BERGKVIST, *et al.* 1989. Risk of endometrial cancer after treatment with oestrogens alone or in conjunction with progestogens: results of a prospective study. Br. Med. J. **298:** 147–151.
65. NACHTIGALL, L.E., R.H. NACHTIGALL, R.D. NACHTIGALL, *et al.* 1979. Estrogen replacement therapy II: a prospective study in the relationship to carcinoma and cardiovascular and metabolic problems. Obstet. Gynecol. **54:** 74–79.
66. GAMBRELL, R.D., JR., F.M. MASSEY, T.A. CASTANEDA, *et al.* 1980. Use of the progestogen challenge test to reduce the risk of endometrial cancer. Obstet. Gynecol. **55:** 732–738.
67. VOIGT, L.F., N.S. WEISS, J. CHU, *et al.* 1991. Progestagen supplementation of exogenous oestrogens and risk of endometrial cancer. Lancet **338:** 274–277.

68. JICK, S.S., A.M. WALKER & H. JICK. 1993. Estrogens, progesterone, and endometrial cancer. Epidemiology **4:** 20–24.
69. BRINTON, L.A. & R.N. HOOVER. 1993. Estrogen replacement therapy and endometrial cancer risk: unresolved issues. The Endometrial Cancer Collaborative Group. Obstet. Gynecol. **81:** 265–271.
70. GOTTARDIS, M.M., S.P. ROBINSON, P.G. SATYASWAROOP, et al. 1988. Contrasting actions of tamoxifen on endometrial and breast tumor growth in the athymic mouse. Cancer Res. **48:** 812–815.
71. SATYASWAROOP, P.G., R.J. ZAINO & R. MORTEL. 1984. Estrogen-like effects of tamoxifen on human endometrial carcinoma transplanted into nude mice. Cancer Res. **44:** 4006–4010.
72. GAL, D., S. KOPEL, M. BASHEVKIN, et al. 1991. Oncogenic potential of tamoxifen on endometria of postmenopausal women with breast cancer – preliminary report. Gynecol. Oncol. **42:** 120–123.
73. COHEN, I., E. PEREL, D. FLEX, et al. 1999. Endometrial pathology in postmenopausal tamoxifen treatment: comparison between gynaecologically symptomatic and asymptomatic breast cancer patients. J. Clin. Pathol. **52:** 278–282.
74. ATLANTE, G., M. POZZI, C. VINCENZONI, et al. 1990. Four case reports presenting new acquisitions on the association between breast and endometrial carcinoma. Gynecol. Oncol. **37:** 378–380.
75. ALTARAS, M.M., R. AVIRAM, I. COHEN, et al. 1993. Role of prolonged stimulation of tamoxifen therapy in the etiology of endometrial sarcomas. Gynecol. Oncol. **49:** 255–258.
76. LANZA, A., E. ALBA, A. RE, et al. 1994. Endometrial carcinoma in breast cancer patients treated with tamoxifen. Two case report and review of the literature. Eur. J Gynaecol. Oncol. **15:** 455–459.
77. BERLIERE, M., C. GALANT & J. DONNEZ. 1999. The potential oncogenic effect of tamoxifen on the endometrium. Hum. Reprod. **14:** 1381–1383.
78. TREILLEUX, T., H. MIGNOTTE, C. CLEMENT-CHASSAGNE, et al. 1999. Tamoxifen and malignant epithelial-nonepithelial tumours of the endometrium: report of six cases and review of the literature. Eur. J. Surg. Oncol. **25:** 477–482.
79. FORNANDER, T., B. CEDERMARK, A. MATTSSON, et al. 1989. Adjuvant tamoxifen in early breast cancer: occurrence of new primary cancers. Lancet **1:** 117–120.
80. ANDERSSON, M., H.H. STORM & H.T. MOURIDSEN. 1992. Carcinogenic effects of adjuvant tamoxifen treatment and radiotherapy for early breast cancer. Acta Oncol. **31:** 259–263.
81. STEWART, H.J. 1992. The Scottish trial of adjuvant tamoxifen in node-negative breast cancer. Scottish Cancer Trials Breast Group. J. Natl. Cancer Inst. Monogr. **11:** 117–120.
82. RIBEIRO, G. & R. SWINDELL. 1992. The Christie Hospital adjuvant tamoxifen trial. J. Natl. Cancer Inst. Monogr. **11:** 121–125.
83. MAGRIPLES, U., F. NAFTOLIN, P.E. SCHWARTZ, et al. 1993. High-grade endometrial carcinoma in tamoxifen-treated breast cancer patients. J. Clin. Oncol. **11:** 485–490.
84. VAN LEEUWEN, F.E., J. BENRAADT, J.W.W. COEBERGH, et al. 1994. Risk of endometrial cancer after tamoxifen treatment of breast cancer. Lancet **343:** 448–452.
85. BARAKAT, R.R., G. WONG, J.P. CURTIN, et al. 1994. Tamoxifen use in breast cancer patients who subsequently develop corpus cancer is not associated with a higher incidence of adverse histologic features. Gynecol. Oncol. **55:** 164–168.
86. BERGMAN, L., M.L. BEELEN, M.P. GALLEE, et al. 2000. Risk and prognosis of endometrial cancer after tamoxifen for breast cancer. Comprehensive Cancer Centres' ALERT Group. Assessment of liver and endometrial cancer risk following tamoxifen. Lancet **356:** 881–887.
87. FISHER, B., J.P. COSTANTINO, D.L. WICKERHAM, et al. 1998. Tamoxifen for prevention of breast cancer: report of the National Surgical Adjuvant Breast and Bowel Project P-1 Study. J. Natl. Cancer Inst. **90:** 1371–1388.
88. JORDAN, V.C. & M. MORROW. 1994. Should clinicians be concerned about the carcinogenic potential of tamoxifen? Eur. J. Cancer **30A:** 1714–1721.
89. GREVEN, K.M. & B.W. CORN. 1997. Endometrial cancer. Curr. Probl. Cancer **21:** 65–127.

90. HAUSKNECHT, R.U. & S.B. GUSBERG. 1973. Estrogen metabolism in patients at high risk for endometrial carcinoma. II. The role of androstenedione as an estrogen precursor in postmenopausal women with endometrial carcinoma. Am. J. Obstet. Gynecol. **116:** 981–984.

91. RIZKALLAH, T.H., H.M. TOVELL & W.G. KELLY. 1975. Production of estrone and fractional conversion of circulating androstenedione to estrone in women with endometrial carcinoma. J. Clin. Endocrinol. Metab. **40:** 1045–1056.

92. CALANOG, A., S. SALL, G.G. GORDON, *et al.* 1977. Androstenedione metabolism in patients with endometrial cancer. Am. J. Obstet. Gynecol. **129:** 553–556.

93. ALEEM, F.A., M.A. MOUKHTAR, H.C. HUNG, *et al.* 1976. Plasma estrogen in patients with endometrial hyperplasia and carcinoma. Cancer **38:** 2101–2104.

94. BENJAMIN, F. & S. DEUTSCH. 1976. Plasma levels of fractionated estrogens and pituitary hormones in endometrial carcinoma. Am. J. Obstet. Gynecol. **126:** 638–647.

95. CARLSTROM, K., M.G. DAMBER, M. FURUHJELM, *et al.* 1979. Serum levels of total dehydroepiandrosterone and total estrone in postmenopausal women with special regard to carcinoma of the uterine corpus. Acta Obstet. Gynecol. Scand. **58:** 179–181.

96. NISKER, J.A., G.L. HAMMOND, B.J. DAVIDSON, *et al.* 1980. Serum sex hormone-binding globulin capacity and the percentage of free estradiol in postmenopausal women with and without endometrial carcinoma. A new biochemical basis for the association between obesity and endometrial carcinoma. Am. J. Obstet. Gynecol. **138:** 637–642.

97. VON HOLST, T., K. KLINGA & B. RUNNEBAUM. 1981. Hormone levels in healthy post–menopausal women and in women with post-menopausal bleeding with or without endometrial carcinoma. Maturitas **3:** 315–320.

98. JASONNI, V.M., C. BULLETTI, F. FRANCESCHETTI, *et al.* 1982. Analysis of estrone sulphate levels in post-menopausal women with and without endometrial cancer. Eur. J. Gynaecol. Oncol. **3:** 206–209.

99. OETTINGER, M., I. SAMBERG, Z. LEVITAN, *et al.* 1984. Hormonal profile of endometrial cancer. Gynecol. Obstet. Invest. **17:** 225–235.

100. JASONNI, V.M., C. BULLETTI, F. FRANCESCHETTI, *et al.* 1984. Estrone sulphate plasma levels in postmenopausal women with and without endometrial cancer. Cancer **53:** 2698–2700.

101. GIMES, G., Z. SZARVAS & G. SIKLOSI. 1986. Endocrine factors in the etiology of endometrial carcinoma. Neoplasma **33:** 393–397.

102. PETTERSSON, B., R. BERGSTROM & E.D. JOHANSSON. 1986. Serum estrogens and androgens in women with endometrial carcinoma. Gynecol. Oncol. **25:** 223–233.

103. MOLLERSTROM, G., K. CARLSTROM, A. LAGRELIUS, *et al.* 1993. Is there an altered steroid profile in patients with endometrial carcinoma? Cancer **72:** 173–181.

104. NYHOLM, H.C., A.L. NIELSEN, J. LYNDRUP, *et al.* 1993. Plasma oestrogens in postmenopausal women with endometrial cancer. Br. J. Obstet. Gynaecol. **100:** 1115–1119.

105. SHERMAN, M.E., S. STURGEON, L.A. BRINTON, *et al.* 1997. Risk factors and hormone levels in patients with serous and endometrioid uterine carcinomas. Mod. Pathol. **10:** 963–968.

106. LUCAS, W.E. & S.S. YEN. 1979. A study of endocrine and metabolic variables in postmenopausal women with endometrial carcinoma. Am. J. Obstet. Gynecol. **134:** 180–186.

107. SCHENKER, J.G., D. WEINSTEIN & E. OKON. 1979. Estradiol and testosterone levels in the peripheral and ovarian circulations in patients with endometrial cancer. Cancer **44:** 1809–1812.

108. JUDD, H.L., B.J. DAVIDSON, A.M. FRUMAR, *et al.* 1980. Serum androgens and estrogens in postmenopausal women with and without endometrial cancer. Am. J. Obstet. Gynecol. **136:** 859–871.

109. DAVIDSON, B.J., J.C. GAMBONE, L.D. LAGASSE, *et al.* 1981. Free estradiol in postmenopausal women with and without endometrial cancer. J. Clin. Endocrinol. Metab. **52:** 404–408.

110. SCIRPA, P., D. MANGO, F. BATTAGLIA, *et al.* 1982. Plasma androstenedione and oestrone levels before and after the menopause. I. Glandular hyperplasia and adenocarcinoma of the endometrium. Maturitas **4:** 33–42.

111. BREMOND, A.G., B. CLAUSTRAT, R.C. RUDIGOZ, *et al.* 1982. Estradiol, androstenedione, testosterone, and dehydroepiandrosterone sulfate in the ovarian and peripheral blood of postmenopausal patients with and without endometrial cancer. Gynecol. Oncol. **14:** 119–124.
112. FALSETTI, L., U. OMODEI, D. DORDONI, *et al.* 1983. Profiles and endocrine correlations in endometrial carcinoma. Eur. J. Gynaecol. Oncol. **4:** 30–34.
113. NAGAMANI, M., E.V. HANNIGAN, E.A. DILLARD, JR., *et al.* 1986. Ovarian steroid secretion in postmenopausal women with and without endometrial cancer. J. Clin. Endocrinol. Metab. **62:** 508–512.
114. BONNEY, R.C., M.J. SCANLON, D.L. JONES, *et al.* 1986. The relationship between oestradiol metabolism and adrenal steroids in the endometrium of postmenopausal women with and without endometrial cancer. Eur. J. Cancer Clin. Oncol. **22:** 953–961.
115. REED, M.J., P.A. BERANEK, M.W. GHILCHIK, *et al.* 1986. Estrogen production and metabolism in normal postmenopausal women and postmenopausal women with breast or endometrial cancer. Eur. J. Cancer Clin. Oncol. **22:** 1395–1400.
116. BOND, A.P., M.J. DIVER & J.C. DAVIS. 1987. Plasma progesterone concentration in women with and without adenocarcinoma of the endometrium. Am. J. Obstet. Gynecol. **156:** 437–440.
117. AUSTIN, H., J.M. AUSTIN, JR., E.E. PARTRIDGE, *et al.* 1991. Endometrial cancer, obesity, and body fat distribution. Cancer Res. **51:** 568–572.
118. POTISCHMAN, N., R.N. HOOVER, L.A. BRINTON, *et al.* 1996. Case-control study of endogenous steroid hormones and endometrial cancer. J. Natl. Cancer Inst. **88:** 1127–1135.
119. ZELENIUCH-JACQUOTTE, A., A. AKHMEDKHANOV, I. KATO, *et al.* 2001. Postmenopausal endogenous estrogens and risk of endometrial cancer: results of a prospective study. Br. J. Cancer. **84:** 975–981.
120. SHERMAN, M.E. 2000. Theories of endometrial carcinogenesis: a multidisciplinary approach. Mod. Pathol. **13:** 295–308.
121. GAMBRELL, R.D. 1979. The role of hormones in the etiology of breast and endometrial cancer. Acta Obstet. Gynecol. Scand. Suppl. **88:** 73–81.
122. GREENBLATT, R.B., R.D. GAMBRELL, JR. & L.D. STODDARD. 1982. The protective role of progesterone in the prevention of endometrial cancer. Pathol. Res. Pract. **174:** 297–318.
123. MCPHERSON, C.P., T.A. SELLERS, J.D. POTTER, *et al.* 1996. Reproductive factors and risk of endometrial cancer. The Iowa Women's Health Study. Am. J. Epidemiol. **143:** 1195–1202.
124. GORCHEV, G. & A. MALEEVA. 1993. Serum E2 and progesterone levels in patients with atypical hyperplasia and endometrial carcinoma [Bulgarian]. Akush. Ginekol. (Sofiia) **32:** 23–24.
125. MODAN, B., E. RON, L. LERNER-GEVA, *et al.* 1998. Cancer incidence in a cohort of infertile women. Am. J. Epidemiol. **147:** 1038–1042.
126. VERMEULEN, A. 1976. The hormonal activity of the postmenopausal ovary. J. Clin. Endocrinol. Metab. **42:** 247–253.
127. LUCAS, W.E. 1974. Causal relationships between endocrine–metabolic variables in patients with endometrial carcinoma. Obstet. Gynecol. Surv. **29:** 507–528.
128. TSENG, L., J. MAZELLA, W.J. MANN, *et al.* 1982. Estrogen synthesis in normal and malignant human endometrium. J. Clin. Endocrinol. Metab. **55:** 1029–1031.
129. TSENG, L., J. MAZELLA, M.I. FUNT, *et al.* 1984. Preliminary studies of aromatase in human neoplastic endometrium. Obstet. Gynecol. **63:** 150–154.
130. LUCISANO, A., M.G. ACAMPORA, N. RUSSO, *et al.* 1984. Ovarian and peripheral plasma levels of progestogens, androgens and oestrogens in post-menopausal women. Maturitas **6:** 45–53.
131. NAGAMANI, M., M.G. DOHERTY, E.R. SMITH, *et al.* 1992. Increased bioactive luteinizing hormone levels in postmenopausal women with endometrial cancer. Am. J. Obstet. Gynecol. **167:** 1825–1830.
132. KONISHI, I., M. KOSHIYAMA, M. MANDAI, *et al.* 1997. Increased expression of LH/hCG receptors in endometrial hyperplasia and carcinoma in anovulatory women. Gynecol. Oncol. **65:** 273–280.

133. RIDDICK, D.H. & W.F. KUSMIK. 1977. Decidua: a possible source of amniotic fluid prolactin. Am. J. Obstet. Gynecol. **127:** 187–190.
134. GOLANDER, A., T. HURLEY, J. BARRETT, *et al.* 1978. Prolactin synthesis by human chorion-decidual tissue: a possible source of prolactin in the amniotic fluid. Science **202:** 311–313.
135. TSENG, L. & J. MAZELLA. 1999. Prolactin and its receptor in human endometrium. Semin. Reprod. Endocrinol. **17:** 23–27.
136. SAJI, M., M. TAGA & H. MINAGUCHI. 1990. Epidermal growth factor stimulate cell proliferation and inhibits prolactin secretion of the human decidual cells in culture. Endocrinol. Jpn. **37:** 177–182.
137. SCHATZ, F., C. PAPP, S. AIGNER, *et al.* 1997. Biological mechanisms underlying the clinical effects of RU 486: modulation of cultured endometrial stromal cell stromelysin-1 and prolactin expression. J. Clin. Endocrinol. Metab. **82:** 188–193.
138. IMAI, A., T. FURUI, T. OHNO, *et al.* 1993. Prolactin binds to human endometrial fibroblasts and inhibits mitogenicity of an endometrial carcinoma extract. Proc. Soc. Exp. Biol. Med. **203:** 117–122.
139. KAZER, R.R. 1995. Insulin resistance, insulin-like growth factor I and breast cancer: a hypothesis. Int. J. Cancer **62:** 403–406.
140. PORETSKY, L. & M.F. KALIN. 1987. The gonadotropic function of insulin. Endocr. Rev. **8:** 132–141.
141. GARZO, V.G. & J.H. DORRINGTON. 1984. Aromatase activity in human granulosa cells during follicular development and the modulation by follicle-stimulating hormone and insulin. Am. J. Obstet. Gynecol. **148:** 657–662.
142. NESTLER, J.E., L.P. POWERS, D.W. MATT, *et al.* 1991. A direct effect of hyperinsulinemia on serum sex hormone-binding globulin levels in obese women with the polycystic ovary syndrome. J. Clin. Endocrinol. Metab. **72:** 83–89.
143. GREENDALE, G.A., S. EDELSTEIN & E. BARRETT-CONNOR. 1997. Endogenous sex steroids and bone mineral density in older women and men: the Rancho Bernardo Study. J. Bone Miner. Res. **12:** 1833–1843.
144. POEHLMAN, E.T., M.J. TOTH, P.A. ADES, *et al.* 1997. Menopause-associated changes in plasma lipids, insulin-like growth factor I and blood pressure: a longitudinal study. Eur. J. Clin. Invest. **27:** 322–326.
145. DE PERGOLA, G., M.R. COSPITE, V.A. GIAGULLI, *et al.* 1993. Insulin-like growth factor-1 (IGF-1) and dehydroepiandrosterone sulphate in obese women. Int. J. Obes. Relat. Metab. Disord. **17:** 481–483.
146. REYNOLDS, R.K., F. TALAVERA, J.A. ROBERTS, *et al.* 1990. Regulation of epidermal growth factor and insulin-like growth factor I receptors by estradiol and progesterone in normal and neoplastic endometrial cell cultures. Gynecol. Oncol. **38:** 396–406.
147. NAGAMANI, M. & C.A. STUART. 1998. Specific binding and growth-promoting activity of insulin in endometrial cancer cells in culture. Am. J. Obstet. Gynecol. **179:** 6–12.
148. PEARL, M.L., F. TALAVERA, H.F. GRETZ, 3RD, *et al.* 1993. Mitogenic activity of growth factors in the human endometrial adenocarcinoma cell lines HEC-1-A and KLE. Gynecol. Oncol. **49:** 325–332.
149. RUTANEN, E.M., T. NYMAN, P. LEHTOVIRTA, *et al.* 1994. Suppressed expression of insulin-like growth factor binding protein-1 mRNA in the endometrium: a molecular mechanism associating endometrial cancer with its risk factors. Int. J. Cancer **59:** 307–312.
150. RUTANEN, E.M. 1998. Insulin-like growth factors in endometrial function. Gynecol. Endocrinol. **12:** 399–406.

Doppler Investigation in Intrauterine Growth Restriction—From Qualitative Indices to Flow Measurements

A Review of the Experience of a Collaborative Group

ENRICO FERRAZZI,[a] MARIA BELLOTTI,[a] HENRY GALAN,[b]
GIANCARLO PENNATI,[c] MADDALENA BOZZO,[a] SERENA RIGANO,[a]
AND FREDERICK C. BATTAGLIA[b]

[a]Department of Obstetrics and Gynecology, ISBM L. Sacco and DMCO San Paolo,
University of Milan, 20157 Milan, Italy

[b]Division of Perinatal Medicine, Departments of Obstetrics and Gynecology and
Pediatrics, University of Colorado, Denver, Colorado, USA

[c]Department of Bioengineering, Polithecnics of Milan, Milan, Italy

ABSTRACT: In 1997 we started a collaboration among three groups, combining
our experience with Doppler examination of the human fetus, blood flow studies on fetal lamb, and mathematical modeling of human circulation. In preliminary investigations on fetal lambs, the same Doppler method designed for the
human fetus was used to measure venous blood flow in the umbilical veins of
seven fetal lambs. Doppler measurements and diffusion technique groups for
umbilical venous flow were 210.8 ± 18.8 and 205.7 ± 38.5 ml/min/kg, respectively ($p = 0.881$). In human pregnancy the interobserver variabilities for the vein
diameter, mean velocity, and absolute umbilical venous blood were 2.9%,
7.9%, and 12.7%, respectively. A cross-sectional study allowed us to establish
normal reference values. Venous blood flow/kg of estimated fetal weight
showed a nonsignificant linear reduction with gestational age, from 128.7 ml/
min/kg at 20 weeks to 104.2 ml/min/kg at 38 weeks. In a series of 37 growth-
restricted fetuses, the UV flow per kilogram was significantly lower in the more
severe growth-restricted fetuses (abdominal circumference below the second
percentile and abnormal umbilical arterial p.i.) than in normal comparable fetuses ($p < 0.001$). In a series of 140 normal fetuses, we calculated that the absolute blood flow rate in the ductus venosus (DV) increases significantly with
advancing gestational age from 20 to 38 weeks of gestation (from 23.2 ± 9.6 ml/
min to 43.5 ± 21.5 ml/min). This means that the percentage of umbilical blood
flow shunted through the DV decreases significantly during gestation (from
50% at midgestation to 20% at 38 weeks). In a series of 45 growthrestricted fetuses, delivered because of nonreactive fetal heart rate (group 2) and for other
reasons but still with a normal heart rate pattern (group 1), we measured the
ductal inlet diameter. In these fetuses, the diameters at the ductal isthmus, normalized for the dimension of the abdominal circumference (inlet diameter/
abdominal circumference), were significantly larger (group 1 = 6.8 ± 2.3;

Address for correspondence: Enrico Ferrazzi, Direttore, Clinica Ostetrica e Ginecologica, Isti-
tuto di Sceinze Biomediche L. Sacco, Università di Milano, Via G.B. Grassi, 74, 20157 Milano,
Italy. Voice: 39-02-3904-2264; fax: 39-02-356-5061.
ferrazzi@tin.it

group 29.4 ± 2.8) than in the control group (6.1 ± 0.3). This means that in this subset of fetuses the amount of blood shunted can be increased as a compensatory mechanism.

KEYWORDS: fetal growth restriction; umbilical venous flow; ductus venosus; Doppler ultrasound

INTRODUCTION

Many publications have greatly strengthened the associations between intrauterine growth retardation (IUGR) pregnancies and long-term health hazards in those IUGR infants when they reach adulthood. The recent works clarified the associations by including good gestational age information.[1–6] Thus, it is now well established that the link between hypertension, heart disease, and diabetes and being born as an IUGR infant is not due to prematurity but to true intrauterine growth restriction. This is a major contribution, since earlier work had used birth weight without gestational age information.

Fetal growth restriction is a relevant disease that can complicate up to 7–15% of pregnancies. This percentage depends on the population studied and on the definition of the disease. As far as the definition is concerned, the first criterion to acknowledge is that growth restriction not a synonymous for small for gestational age at birth. Under this stricter definition, the percentage of births involving fetal growth restriction remains high (5–7%). It is likely that these are, in fact, the cases that should be identified prenatally and on which we should invest time and resources.

A number of recent studies have attempted to link specific fetal surveillance data of growth-restricted fetuses with clinical outcomes.[7–10] Umbilical Doppler velocimetry has helped to identify prenatally, among growth-restricted fetuses, those with the worst placental damage[11,12] and the worst perinatal outcome.[8,9,13]

Although qualitative waveform analyses have been feasible and used extensively with the above-quoted results, quantitative flow studies have always been neglected because of the relative inaccuracy of the measurement of vessel diameters, flow velocities, and fetal weight, all associated with time-consuming, cumbersome procedures. It is blood flow, however, not velocimetry, that determines O_2 delivery to the fetal tissues, hence its potential importance. High-tech sonographic imaging, color Doppler imaging, and pulsed-wave Doppler imaging are a big challenge for this new area of investigation of fetal circulation. In 1997 we started a collaboration among three groups, combining our experience with Doppler examination of the human fetus with blood flow studies on fetal lamb and with mathematical modeling of human circulation.

ACCURACY AND FEASIBILITY OF DOPPLER MEASUREMENT OF UMBILICAL VENOUS BLOOD FLOW

Doppler Methodology and Preliminary Investigations on Fetal Lambs

A preliminary step was taken to validate Doppler technology with more traditional methods to assess flow in the human fetus.[14] The same Doppler method designed for the human fetus was used to measure venous blood flow in the umbilical veins of seven fetal lambs from 125 to 133 days of gestation (comparable to 235–250 days of human gestation). A 2.0–5.0 MHz convex probe was used on an ultrasound unit with triplex operative mode (ATL; Seattle, WA). The umbilical vein (UV) was sampled at three different free loops along the cord to allow for any minor differences in diameter along the cord. The internal diameter of the UV was measured by obtaining perpendicular views of the cord at maximum magnification followed by caliper placement at the inner edge of the vessel. The average of three consecutive diameters was reported in millimeters. The UV mean velocity was calculated by the formula time-averaged peak velocity multiplied by 0.5.[15]

The velocity range of the color imaging was set between 10 and 14 cm/sec, and the Doppler sample volume was positioned so that it covered the entire lumen of the vessel with the Doppler beam angle closest to zero. The wall filter was set at 25 Hz. Velocity values were reported as the mean of three different measurements. Umbilical vein blood flow was calculated and expressed as an absolute value, and as per kilogram of fetal weight:

$$\text{UV flow } (\text{ml}^2\text{min}^{-1}) = \text{vessel cross-sectional area} \times \text{mean velocity} \times 60 \ [/\text{kg}]$$

For the ovine fetus, the results obtained were multiplied by two. This study proved that no significant differences were detected between the Doppler measurements and diffusion technique groups for umbilical venous flow (210.8 ± 18.8 and 205.7 ± 38.5 ml/min/kg, $p = 0.881$). Both gestational age and fetal weights did not differ between the animals studied by Doppler technique (129.6 ± 2.8 days; 2.75 ± 0.26 kg, respectively) and steady-state data derived from historical data from 34 ewes (131.6 ± 4.1 days; 2.94 ± 0.68, respectively).[16] Nevertheless, one of the assumptions of this work, that is, that the difference between the two veins is negligible, was questionable and a possible source of unexplained variability.

Advanced Investigations in the Fetal Lamb

In a second series of ovine pregnancies, Doppler measurements and diffusional techniques were performed on the same fetuses.[17] In addition, we took into account in this further study the possible differences of flow in the two veins. Following a five-day recovery period, umbilical venous flow measurements were determined by triplex mode ultrasound and followed by transplacental steady-state diffusion technique (SST). In fact, SST has become a "gold standard" by which other blood-flow techniques have been compared.[18–20] It has the clear advantage over all other techniques of providing both uterine and umbilical flow measurements. At completion of the blood flow studies, the animals were euthanized, in order to obtain the fetal weights, to obtain the number and weights of cotyledons serving each umbilical vein, and to verify catheter locations. The mean umbilical flow in this study was $602.8 \text{ ml} \cdot \text{min}^{-1}$ or $208.1 \text{ ml} \cdot \text{kg}_{\text{fetus}}^{-1} \cdot \text{min}^{-1}$, which is consistent with studies reported previously.[21] Blood flow was assessed also per vein because Rudolph and Heymann,[22] using electromagnetic flow meters, provided perhaps the first evidence that blood flow is frequently different in each of a given pair of umbilical veins. In the seven sheep studied,[17] the ratio of flows between a given vein pair was nearly identical to the ratio of microsphere distribution in the cotyledons serving the veins for each pregnant sheep. Applying these criteria, although the smaller veins had a significantly lower mean umbilical blood flow than the larger veins, when normalized for either the weight or number of cotyledons serving the umbilical veins, there were no differences in blood flow between large and small umbilical veins. This suggests that blood flow per gram of placenta is similar.

Reproducibility and Feasibility in Human Pregnancy

The intra- and interobserver reproducibility of UV blood flow measurements was tested in 10 human fetuses.[14] The intraobserver coefficients of variation for the vein diameter, mean velocity, and absolute umbilical venous blood were 3.3%, 9.7%, and 10.9%, respectively. The interobserver variabilities for the same parameters were 2.9%, 7.9%, and 12.7%, respectively. The mean length (± SD) of all 70 examinations was 3 ± 1 minutes. These findings showed that the high-resolution digital imaging system currently available can play an innovative role in obtaining, within 3 minutes, reproducible measurements of the internal venous diameter and of the umbilical vein mean velocity. In summary, two operators studying these endpoints can be expected to achieve less than 13% variability.

The accuracy of umbilical blood flow measurements per kilogram fetal weight using Doppler ultrasound was reported by Rasmussen[23] in 1987. He reported an intraoperator mean coefficient of variance of 6.8%. The feasibility in each fetus and length of examination were not described, but in our experience these were far from 100% of the cases and 3 minutes' duration, as is obtainable with present ultrasound units. More recently, Lees, using modern technology, has confirmed our values both in reproducibility and feasibility.[24]

NORMAL VALUES OF UMBILICAL BLOOD FLOW IN HUMAN PREGNANCY

A cross-sectional study was performed from 20 weeks' gestation to term in 70 normal fetuses.[14] Venous blood flow per kilogram of estimated fetal weight showed a nonsignificant linear reduction with gestational age, from 128.7 ml/min/kg at 20 weeks to 104.2 ml/min/kg at 38 weeks, consistent with the results of Gerson,[25] Gill,[26] and Sutton.[27] It is interesting to observe that in ovine pregnancy UV flow is much greater. Bell *et al.*[28] reported an umbilical blood flow of 468 ± 57 ml/min/kg fetus at midgestation in sheep which is approximately four times the flow for human pregnancies at midgestation. Moreover, there is a much steeper decline in umbilical blood flow per kilogram until term, falling more than 50% during gestation. At midgestation the higher ovine flow is largely explained by differences in the rate of placental growth: sheep placenta is already near its maximal weight (486 g), whereas the human placenta (126 g) is approximately 25% of its maximal weight. Throughout gestation, the human fetus manifests a much lower umbilical blood flow (ml/min/kg) than the sheep fetus. One potential advantage is that a greater fraction of the human fetal cardiac output can be diverted for perfusion of the much larger fetal brain throughout gestation.

Knowledge of the umbilical flow per kilogram is of great physiological interest. For clinical purposes, however, there are limitations to the accuracy of the weight determination because fetal weight in the human is derived from linear measurements of the head, abdomen, and femur. In general, the estimation of fetal weight has a possible error of approximately 10% in 68% of cases. The use of direct linear measurements has obvious potential advantages. The abdominal circumference as measured by ultrasound has been shown in many studies to serve as an early and sensitive biometric indicator of fetal growth restriction. On the contrary, head growth is less influenced by restricted or accelerated growth. For clinical purposes, this latter measurement can serve as an indicator of fetal body development.

DOPPLER MEASUREMENT OF UMBILICAL VENOUS BLOOD FLOW IN GROWTH-RESTRICTED FETUSES

Evidence of a severe reduction in umbilical venous flow in the most severely growth-restricted fetuses had already been shown by Laurin *et al.* in 1987,[29] using the technology available at that time. In that work, fetuses weighing 32% less than normal mean weight had an umbilical vein flow as low as of 67.7 ± 36.7 ml/min/kg. We examined 37 growth-restricted fetuses by Doppler ultrasound within four hours of the last nonstress test before delivery.[30] This population was divided into two groups of different clinical severities: group 1, IUGR fetuses with normal umbilical Doppler arterial velocities, and group 2, with abnormal umbilical arterial Doppler velocities. Overall, UV flow per kilogram was significantly lower in the more severely growth-restricted fetuses (abdominal circumference below the second percentile and abnormal umbilical arterial p.i.) than in comparable normal fetuses ($p < 0.001$). UV flow per unit head circumference was also significantly lower in less severely growth-restricted fetuses (abdominal circumference below the second percen-

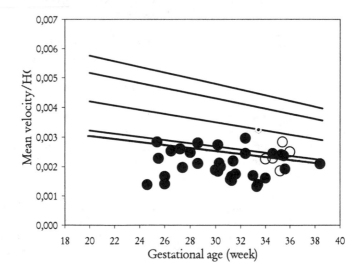

FIGURE 1. Umbilical vein velocity (cm/sec) per unit head circumference versus gestational age in growth-restricted fetuses: group 1 ○ and group 2 ●. Continuous lines represent the 5th, 10th, 50th, 90th, and 95th percentile of 70 normal cases.

tile only) than in the control population. The UV diameter/HC was normal, whereas UV velocity/HC was significantly lower in IUGR fetuses than in comparable controls (FIG. 1). Limitations of this study were the relatively small number of cases with a normal umbilical p.i. and the cross-sectional design.

However, it is possible to conclude from our data that normalization of flow for head circumference, rather than estimated weight, provides the most sensitive parameter in sorting out differences in umbilical vein flow between normal and IUGR fetuses of different severities. Reduction in venous blood velocity is the principal component in determining flow decrease in growth-restricted fetuses.

DOPPLER MEASUREMENT OF VENOUS BLOOD FLOW IN THE DUCTUS VENOSUS

Another area of study focused on determining whether blood flow could also be measured in the fetal ductus venosus (DV). This is a far more difficult vessel to study, but crucial to an understanding of the fetal circulation. Its importance stems from the fact that the ductus venosus shunts blood from the umbilical vein to the inferior vena cava, thus bypassing the fetal liver. The umbilical vein carries O_2 and nutrients obtained from the placenta to the fetus. Shunting through the ductus venosus increases the supply of nutrient-rich and O_2-rich blood to the brain. In animal studies, the magnitude of the shunt changes with fetal hypoxia. The difficulties arise from the complex architecture of this part of the fetal circulation in human pregnancies.

Methodological Problems and Accuracy

Many difficulties arise from the complex architecture of this part of the fetal circulation in human pregnancies. FIGURE 2 presents a drawing of the circulation in this small, trumpet-shaped vessel. The conical nature of the vessel sets an absolute condition that velocity wave forms will change along the course of the vessel. Many clinical studies are attempting to use velocimetry measurements alone in assessing the perfusion through this vessel. We have completed several papers examining the modeling in the circulation of the ductus in terms of the predictable changes in velocity waveforms.[31,32] From these studies we were able to model the calculation of the mean velocity within the vessel from the usual velocity measurements along its course. With the mean velocity and measurements of inlet/outlet diameter and length of the vessel, we are able to calculate blood flow in the ductus. This method has been validated by comparing the blood flow calculated at the inlet of the vessel with that at the outlet of the vessel (the two values should be identical within the limits of measurement). In 26 normal fetuses the time-averaged blood flow rates at the isthmus and at the outlet were not significantly different (36.3 ± 22.1 vs. 39.4 ± 24.0 ml/min) (correlation coefficient = 0.87). The mean percent difference between the results obtained by inlet and outlet measurements on the same ductus was 7.1% ($p < 0.001$).

Blood Flow Changes in the Ductus Venosus during Normal Pregnancy

In a series of 140 normal fetuses, we calculated that the absolute blood flow rate in the ductus venosus increases significantly with advancing gestational age from 20 to 38 weeks of gestation from 23.2 ± 9.6 ml/min to 43.5 ± 21.5 ml/min.[33] However,

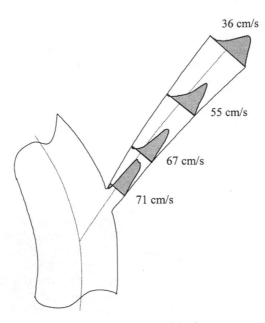

FIGURE 2. Velocity profile at different levels of the ductus venous, according to its co-nicity. These velocity profiles are the experimental basis for the calculation of the mean blood velocity in this vessel.

the flow per unit body weight significantly decreases with advancing gestation from 41.7 ± 17.2 ml/min to 17.9 ± 9.1 ml/min. Moreover, because the blood flow per unit body weight in the umbilical vein does not decrease significantly through gestation,[14] the percentage of umbilical blood flow rate shunted through the DV decreases significantly during gestation (from 50% at midgestation to 20% at 38 weeks). Our data, in agreement with those in animal models, suggest a minor role of the human ductus venosus in the third trimester of gestation in shunting the oxygenated blood flow to the brain and myocardium, with a higher proportion of blood flow to the liver and splancnic organs.

DUCTAL CHANGES OF THE DUCTUS VENOSUS IN IUGR FETUSES

Experimental animal data suggested that the volume of blood shunted through the DV increased during hypovolemia and hypoxia and could reach as much as 70% of the umbilical blood flow.[34,35] Similarly, in the human fetus during hypoxia or reduced umbilical flow, a compensatory mechanism is supposed to increase the oxygenated blood flow through the ductus venosus. We reported for the first time in 1998 on Doppler flow measurements at the isthmus, both in dilated and steady conditions. Our findings showed that the mean blood flow through the DV increases substantially (>70%) for high dilatation[32] compared with steady conditions. At the same time the waveform of the venous flow showed a steep decrease of the a-wave.

TABLE 1. Ductus venosus (DV) diameter normalized for abdominal circumference in IUGR fetuses

	Control (n = 37)	Group 1[b] (n = 22)	Group 2[c] (n = 23)
Mean DV diameter[a]	6.1 ± 0.3	6.8 ± 2.3	9.4 ± 2.8[d]
Mean weight ±SD	1540 ± 460	1300 ± 208	961 ± 315
Mean gestational age ±SD	30 ± 3	32.1 ± 2.1	29.6 ± 2.6

[a](DV diameter/abdominal circumference)1000.
[b]Group 1 IUGR—normal heart pattern: delivered for reasons unrelated to fetal heart rate challenge test.
[c]Group 2 IUGR—delivered because of nonreactive fetal heart rate.
[d]$p < 0.05$.

The mathematical modeling of this phenomenon (i.e., dilatation of the isthmus and increased blood flow) showed that, in parallel with dilatation, there occurs a significant decrease of the a-wave. Therefore, this steep decrease is not determined by increased atrial pressure, but is a consequence of hemodynamic changes in the velocity profile of this vessel.

TABLE 1 shows recent, unreported data from our center on the ductal diameter normalized for the abdominal circumference in 45 growth-restricted fetuses delivered because of nonreactive fetal heart rate (group 2) and for other reasons but still with a normal heart rate pattern (group 1). In these fetuses, the diameters at the ductal isthmus, normalized for the dimension of the abdominal circumference, were larger than in the control group. The ductal dilatation and the increase of blood flow rate were related to the severity of the IUGR condition as evidenced by an abnormal heart rate pattern. Since the umbilical blood flow per kilogram is decreased in the IUGR fetuses compared with the normal fetuses, the percentage of umbilical vein blood flow shunted through the ductus is higher in this condition. These observations supported the hypothesis that, in human fetuses under reduced oxygen conditions, the isthmic sphincter mechanism could determine a fetal circulatory adaptation that is likely to be the most distressing form of adaptation before intrauterine demise.

ACKNOWLEDGMENTS

These studies were supported by National Institutes of Health Program Project Grants PO1 HD20761 and 1RO1 HD34837 and March of Dimes Grant #6-F497-0174.

REFERENCES

1. CURHAN, G.C., W.C. WILLETT, E.B. RIMM & M.J. STAMPFER. 1996. Birthweight and adult hypertension and diabetes in US men. Am. J. Hyperten. **9:** 11A.
2. MARTYN, C.N., D.J.P. BARKER & C. OSMOND. 1996. Mothers pelvic size, fetal growth and death from stroke in men. Lancet **348:** 1264–1268.
3. FRANKEL, S., P. ELWOOD, P. SWEETNAM, *et al.* 1996. Birthweight, body mass index in middle age, and incident coronary heart disease. Lancet **348:** 1478–1480.

4. LAW, C.M. & A.W. SHIELL. 1996. Is blood pressure inversely related to birthweight? The strength of evidence from a systematic review of the literature. J. Hypertens. **14:** 935–941.
5. COOPER, C., C. FALL, P. EGGER, et al. 1997. Growth in infancy and bone mass in later life. Ann. Rheum. **56:** 17–21.
6. PHILLIPS, D.I.W. & D.J.P. BARKER. 1997. Association between low birthweight and high resting pulse in adult life: is the sympathetic nervous system involved in programming the insulin resistance syndrome. Diabet. Med. **14:** 673–577.
7. BAHADO-SINGH, R.O., E. KOVANCI, A. JEFFRIES, et al. 1999. The Doppler cerebrosplacental ratio and perinatal outcome in intrauterine growth restriction. Am. J. Obstet. Gynecol. **180:** 750–756.
8. FERRAZZI, E., C. VEGNI, M. BELLOTTI, et al. 1991. Role of umbilical Doppler velocimetry in the biophysical assessment of the growth-retarded fetus: answers from neonatal morbidity and mortality. J. Ultrasound Med. **10:** 309–315.
9. KARLSDORP, V.H.M., J.M.G. VAN VUGT, H.P. VAN GEIJN, et al. 1994. Clinical significance of absent or reversed end diastolic velocity waveforms in umbilical artery. Lancet **344:** 1664–1668.
10. DIVON, M.Y. 1996. Umbilical artery Doppler velocimetry: clinical utility in high-risk pregnancies. Am. J. Obstet. Gynecol. **174:** 10–14.
11. FERRAZZI, E., G. BULFAMANTE, R. MEZZOPANE, et al. 1999. Uterine Doppler velocimetry and placental hypoxic-ischemic lesion in pregnancies with fetal intrauterine growth restriction. Placenta **20(5-6):** 389–394.
12. LAURINI, R., J. LAURIN & K. MARSAL. 1994. Placental histology and fetal blood flow in intrauterine growth retardation. Acta. Obstet. Gynecol. Scand. **73(7):** 529–534.
13. PARDI, G., I. CETIN, A.M. MARCONI, et al. 1993. Diagnostic value of blood sampling in fetuses with growth retardation. N. Engl. J. Med. **328:** 692–696.
14. BARBERA, A., H.L. GALAN, E. FERRAZZI, et al. 1999. Relationship of umbilical vein blood flow to growth parameters in the human fetus. Am. J. Obstet. Gynecol. **181(1):** 174–179.
15. KISERUD, T., H. EIK-NES, H.G. BLAAS, et al. 1994. Ductus venosus blood velocity and the umbilical circulation in the seriously growth-retarded fetuses. Ultrasound. Obstet. Gynecol. **4:** 109–114.
16. WILKENING, R.B., S. ANDERSON, L. MARTENSSON & G. MESCHIA. 1982. Placental transfer as a function of uterine blood flow. Am. J. Physiol. **242:** H429–436.
17. GALAN, H.L., M. JOZWIK, S. RIGANO, et al. 1999. Umbilical vein blood flow determination in the ovine fetus: comparison of Doppler ultrasonographic and steady-state diffusion techniques. Am. J. Obstet. Gynecol. **181(5, Pt. 1):** 1149–1153.
18. RUDOLPH, A.M. & M.A. HEYMANN. 1967. Validation of the antipyrine method for measuring fetal umbilical blood flow. Circ. Res. **21:** 185–190.
19. MAKOWSKI, E.L., G. MESCHIA, W. DROEGEMUELLER & F.C. BATTAGLIA. 1968. Measurement of umbilical arterial blood flow to the sheep placenta and fetus in utero. Circ. Res. **23:** 539–547.
20. SCHMIDT, K.G., M. DI TOMMASO, N.H. SILVERMAN & A.M. RUDOLPH. 1991. Doppler echocardiographic assessment of fetal descending aortic and umbilical blood flows. Validation studies in fetal lambs. Circulation **83:** 1731–1737.
21. THUREEN, P.J., K.A. TREMBLER, G. MESCHIA, et al. 1992. Placental glucose transport in heat-induced fetal growth retardation. Am. J. Physiol. **263:** R578–585.
22. RUDOLPH, A.M. & M.A. HEYMANN. 1967. The circulation of the fetus in utero. Methods for studying distribution of blood flow, cardiac output and organ blood flow. Circ. Res. **21:** 163–184.
23. RASMUSSEN, K. 1987. Precision and accuracy of Doppler flow measurements: in vitro and in vivo study of the applicability of the method in human fetuses. Scand. J. Clin. Lab. Invest. **47:** 311–318.
24. LEES, C., G. ALBAIGES, C. DEANE, et al. 1999. Assessment of umbilical arterial and venous flow using color Doppler. Ultrasound Obstet. Gynecol. **14(4):** 250–255.
25. GERSON, A., D. WALLACE, R. STILLER, et al. 1987. Doppler evaluation of umbilical venous and arterial blood flow in the second and in the third trimesters of normal pregnancy. Obstet. Gynecol. **70(4):** 622–626.

26. GILL, R.W., B.J. TRUDINGER, W.J. GARRETT, *et al.* 1981. Fetal umbilical venous flow measured in utero by pulsed Doppler and B-mode ultrasound. I. Normal pregnancies. Am. J. Obstet. Gynecol. **139**: 720–725.
27. SUTTON, M.S., M.A. THEARD, S.J. BHATIA, *et al.* 1990. Changes in placental blood flow in the normal human fetus with gestational age. Pediatr. Res. **28(4)**: 383–387.
28. BELL, A.W., J.M. KENNAUGH, F.C. BATTAGLIA, *et al.* 1986. Metabolic and circulatory studies of the fetal lamb at mid gestation. Am. J. Physiol. **250**: E538–544.
29. LAURIN, J., G. LINGMAN, K. MARSAL & P.K. PERSSON. 1987. Fetal blood flow in pregnancies complicated by intrauterine growth retardation. Obstet Gynecol. **69(6)**: 895–902.
30. FERRAZZI, E., S. RIGANO, M. BOZZO, *et al.* 2000. Umbilical vein blood flow in growth restricted fetuses. Ultrasound Obstet. Gynecol. **16(5)**: 432–438.
31. PENNATI, G., M. BELLOTTI, E. FERRAZZI, *et al.* 1998. Blood flow through the ductus venosus in human fetus: calculation using Doppler velocimetry and computational findings. Ultrasound Med. Biol. **24**: 477–487.
32. BELLOTTI, M., G. PENNATI, G. PARDI & R. RUMERO. 1998. Dilation of the ductus venosus in human fetuses: ultrasonographic evidences and mathematical modeling. Am. J. Physiol. **275**: H1759–H1767.
33. BELLOTTI, M., G. PENNATI, C. DE GASPERI, *et al.* 2000. Role of the ductus venosus in the distribution of umbilical blood flow in human fetuses during the second half of pregnancy. Am. J. Physiol. Heart Circ. Physiol. **279(3)**: H1256–1263.
34. BEHRMAN, R.E., R.N. LEES, E.N. PETERSON, *et al.* 1970. Distribution of the circulation in the normal and asphyxiated primate. Am. J. Obstet. Gynecol. **108**: 956–969.
35. EDELSTONE, D.I., A.M. RUDOLPH & M.A. HEYMANN. 1980. Effects of hypoxemia and decreasing umbilical flow on liver and ductus venosus blood flow in fetal lambs. Am. J. Physiol. **238**: H656–663.

A Critical Birth Weight and Other Determinants of Survival for Infants with Severe Intrauterine Growth Restriction

MEN-JEAN LEE,[a] ELLEN L. CONNER,[a] LAMA CHARAFEDDINE,[b]
JAMES R. WOODS, JR.,[b] AND GIUSEPPE DEL PRIORE[a]

[a]Department of Obstetrics and Gynecology, New York University School of Medicine, New York, New York 10016, USA

[b]University of Rochester School of Medicine, Departments of Obstetrics and Gynecology and Pediatrics, Rochester, New York 14627, USA

ABSTRACT: OUR objective was to assess the perinatal management and neonatal outcomes of premature, severely intrauterine growth-restricted (IUGR) neonates. A cohort of neonates <1000 grams, ≤ first percentile for weight, and <37 weeks' gestation was identified and matched 2:1 to two control sets of premature, appropriate-for-gestational age (AGA) infants—one with similar gestational age (AGA-GA group) and the other with similar birth weight (AGA-BW group) to determine the effect of IUGR on the outcome of the premature infant. The IUGR group was then examined in detail for descriptive statistics. Data were analyzed by t-tests and Chi-square analyses where appropriate. The IUGR infants had worse outcomes than AGA-GA controls but had somewhat better results than the AGA-BW controls. In the IUGR group, a birth weight less than 550 grams was significantly associated with neonatal death ($p < 0.001$). However, increasing gestational age was not associated with neonatal survival ($p = 0.661$) if birthweight remained below 550 grams. Classical cesarean delivery was associated with neonatal death ($p = 0.003$). Neonatal variables associated with poor outcome included patent ductus arteriosus ($p = 0.034$), feeding intolerance ($p = 0.046$), and failure to thrive ($p = 0.05$). Overall, neonatal survival was 73%. Of the surviving neonates, 69% had evidence of neurodevelopmental delay when tested at 6 and 12 months. Premature, growth-restricted neonates with birth weights of <550 grams versus those of >550 grams have dismal outcomes despite a gestational age that is compatible with survival.

KEYWORDS: intrauterine growth restriction; premature infant; very low birth weight infant; pregnancy outcome; infant mortality

INTRODUCTION

During the past decade, innovations in antepartum fetal surveillance and neonatal intensive care have markedly improved the survival of premature infants, and low-

Address for correspondence: Men-Jean Lee, M.D., Department of Obstetrics and Gynecology, New York University Medical Center, 550 First Avenue, Room 9E2, New York, NY 10016. Voice: 212-263-8687; fax: 212-263-8887.

mjl5@nyu.edu

ered the threshold of viability of normal fetuses to 24 weeks' gestation where survival is approximately 50%.[1] Furthermore, when evaluating birth weight as a criterion for survival in appropriately grown infants, those weighing 1250 grams or less at birth had survival rates of 62.1% to a high of 85.2%[2] and a weight limit of viability that has been suggested by other authors to be about 600 g.[3] During this same time period, there have been a number of reports in the medical literature of the remarkable survival of premature, extremely low-birthweight (ELBW) infants (birth weight less than 1000 g) with severe intrauterine growth restriction (IUGR), weighing as little as 280 to 390 g at 25 to 26 weeks' gestation,[4,5,6] which push the limits of viability even further. A significant percentage of IUGR fetuses die before birth.[7] However, traditionally, those "stressed" IUGR fetuses that survive until after delivery are thought to have better neonatal outcomes because of a theoretical increase in organ maturity compared with their appropriately grown,"nonstressed" counterparts of the same gestational age.[8] This commonly held opinion, the recent advances in medical care, and these impressive case reports may altogether sway healthcare providers to be overly optimistic in counseling concerned parents. Survival rates and long-term outcomes of ELBW neonates that have severe IUGR have not been realistically evaluated to assess the efficacy of obstetrical and neonatal interventions. Furthermore, recent reports of long-term outcomes of premature neonates following discharge from the neonatal intensive care unit (NICU) during the first six years of life have revealed neurodevelopmental delay and impairment.[9,10]

The purpose of this study was to examine perinatal risk factors associated with survival of preterm ELBW infants with severe IUGR. The obstetrical and neonatal management of these infants was also described, as well as survival rates and long-term outcomes. The impact of IUGR was then determined by comparing these infants to appropriate for gestational age (AGA) controls that had either similar gestational age or birth weight.

MATERIALS AND METHODS

A cohort of neonates born between January 1, 1991, and March 31, 1994, at Strong Memorial Hospital, University of Rochester, Rochester, New York, was identified by the hospital-based birth certificate computer database that met the following criteria: preterm (gestational age less than 37 weeks' gestation at delivery), ELBW (birth weight less than 1000 g), and severe IUGR (birth weight less than 3 standard deviations or the first percentile for the mean birth weight as determined by the standard growth curves of Usher and McLean[11]). Multiple gestations were not excluded. Twenty-two neonates met the inclusion criteria for the study out of a total of 13,608 live births recorded in the established time period (FIG. 1). The assigned gestational age for each infant obtained from the birth certificate database was based on maternal last menstrual period and confirmed by physical examination, which included ultrasound in the majority of the cases. Neonatal gestational age was determined by a modified Dubowitz examination. If both obstetric and neonatal estimates were within two weeks, the obstetric estimate was used as the final gestational age; otherwise the neonatal estimate was used for analysis.

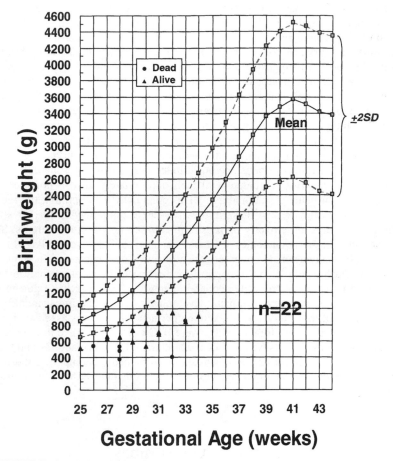

FIGURE 1. Birth weight and gestational age of IUGR cohort. (Normal curves adapted from Usher and McLean.[11])

To assess the overall impact of growth restriction on survival, the IUGR infants were matched to two sets of AGA controls using the same institutional computer birth certificate database: one group matched for gestational age (AGA-GA group), the other group matched for birth weight (AGA-BW group) (TABLE 1). The controls were matched 2:1 with each index IUGR infant and were identified by selection of the two next-born infants of similar gestational age (±2 weeks) and the two next-born infants of similar birth weight (±75 grams). Pertinent data were abstracted from the University of Rochester Division of Neonatology Neonatal Database.

Maternal and neonatal medical records were retrieved for detailed study of IUGR maternal and infant data including tobacco and illicit drug use, elevated maternal serum α-fetoprotein (MSAFP), severe preeclampsia, abnormal umbilical artery Doppler flow studies, and oligohydramnios. Sonographic assessments of estimated fetal

TABLE 1. Selection of AGA controls

	IUGR cases ($n = 22$)	AGA-GA controls ($n = 44$)	AGA-BW controls ($n = 44$)
Mean EGA (wks)	30 ± 2.4	30 ± 2.6	24 ± 2.3
Mean BW (g)	689 ± 181	1462 ± 384	707 ± 179

ABBREVIATIONS: AGA, approriate for gestational age; AGA-GA, appropriate for gestational age matched for gestational age; AGA-BW, appropriate for gestational age matched for birth weight; EGA, estimated gestational age; BW, birth weight.

weight (EFW) obtained within one week before delivery were also retrieved. Obstetrical management data, such as the administration of prophylactic maternal steroids and the method of delivery (vaginal or low-transverse cesarean section or classical cesarean section), were also recorded.

Neonatal data abstracted from each infant's medical record included gestational age, birth weight, sex, umbilical cord blood gas values, surfactant therapy, antibiotic use, presence of congenital anomalies or infection, abnormal karyotype, days on hyperalimentation, duration of ventilatory support, and length of hospitalization in the NICU. Common neonatal morbidities were identified, including respiratory distress syndrome (RDS), bronchopulmonary dysplasia (BPD), patent ductus arteriosus (PDA), intraventricular hemorrhage (IVH), necrotizing enterocolitis (NEC), and retinopathy of prematurity (ROP). Feeding intolerance was defined by a gastric residual obtained at two hours postinfusion that was greater than 20% of the volume of feeds, making it difficult to meet calculated nutritional requirements. Failure to thrive was defined as a lack of consistent weight gain of 15 grams per day over a three-week period. Information on each neonate's condition upon discharge (alive or dead) and disposition (home or alternate-care facility) from the NICU was obtained. Data from the neonatal medical record were corroborated for accuracy with the institutional Neonatology Database. Hospitalization costs were obtained from the billing office at Strong Memorial Hospital. Neonatology physician charges were not available for analysis.

The infants surviving NICU admission were followed prospectively in the Neonatal Continuing Care Clinic (NCCC) for long-term outcomes at 6 and 12 months of corrected age. A thorough neurological examination by a pediatric neurologist and a developmental assessment, using the Bayley Scales for Infant Development and administered by a pediatric psychologist or a certified nurse practitioner, were determined at each interval visit. A Mental Development Index (MDI) of >85 points was considered normal. Infants with MDI scores of less than 70 points were referred to early interventional programs. An infant with a score between 70 and 85 was referred to an interventional program at the pediatrician's discretion, depending on the neurological examination and the patient's home environment. Infant growth measurements were also assessed at these visits for catch-up growth, denoted when the patient was no longer below the third percentile for growth in head circumference, length, and weight. Any interval death of a neonate following NICU discharge was confirmed by the NCCC.

TABLE 2. Comparison of IUGR infants to control infants — neonatal complications

	IUGR (%)	AGA-GA control (%)	AGA-BW control (%)	p value
Mortality	27.3	2.3	47.7	$p < 0.01$
RDS	68.2	59.5	96.6	$p < 0.01$
PDA	40.9	28.6	69.0	$p < 0.01$
NEC	4.5	0	9.1	$p < 0.01$
IVH	22.7	14.6	27.6	$p = NS$
ROP	59.1	10.0	55.5	$p < 0.01$

NOTE: Chi-square test.
ABBREVIATIONS: RDS, respiratory distress syndrome; PDA, patent ductus arteriosus; NEC, necrotizing enterocolitis; IVH, intraventricular hemorrhage; ROP, retinopathy of prematurity.

TABLE 3. Comparison of IUGR infants to control infants—days of NICU requirements

	IUGR	AGA-GA control	AGA-BW control	p value
VENT	24	10	27	$p < 0.05$
ABX	17	11	27	$p < 0.05$
HAL	24	10	27	$p < 0.05$
NICU	74	31	80	$p < 0.05$

NOTE: Chi-square test
ABBREVIATIONS: VENT, ventilator; ABX, antibiotics; HAL, hyperalimentation; NICU, neonatal intensive care unit.

Paired t-tests were used to analyze continuous variables. Statistical analysis of categorical data included either the chi-square test or Fisher's exact test, where appropriate. A p value of less than or equal to 0.05 was considered significant.

RESULTS

The IUGR infants were appropriately matched with gestational age- and birth-weight-matched controls (TABLE 1). Intuitively, when focusing on the entire cohort including controls, both estimated gestational age and birth weight are significantly associated with neonatal survival (Mann-Whitney U, $p < 0.01$ for both); that is, survival increases as birth weight and/or gestational age increases. Nevertheless, the IUGR infants suffered more complications than AGA-GA controls, but fared better than infants of similar weights that were correspondingly younger (AGA-BW) (TABLE 2). The IUGR infants also required more specialized care than AGA controls (TABLE 3). When compared to gestational age-matched controls, significantly more IUGR infants died (27% versus 2%, Fishers, $p = 0.004$). When the IUGR infants

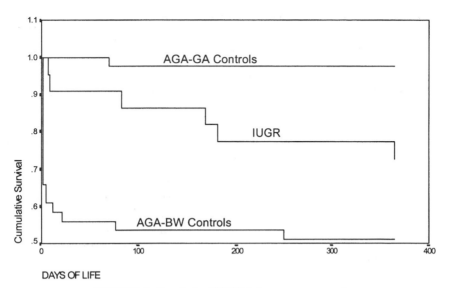

FIGURE 2. Survival of IUGR infants versus controls.

were compared to birthweight-matched controls, more of the latter died (48% versus 27%), but the difference in survival was not significant (Fishers, $p = 0.091$). Although the median survival was not achieved using the Kaplan and Meier product-limit method, it was estimated to exceed 365 days in all three groups. Survival curves were significantly different among the three groups (FIG. 2) using the Log Rank Test Statistic for Equality of Survival Distribution, with $p < 0.01$. The AGA-BW infants tended to expire within the first day of life, whereas the IUGR infants died after a longer time interval, and the AGA-GA controls did well.

Survival of IUGR neonates from the NICU was 77% (17/22), but the overall survival of IUGR offspring at the 12-month corrected age assessment was 73% (16/22). Of the 22 neonates that met the strict criteria for inclusion into our study, 17 (77%) were discharged alive from the NICU, with one more infant dying 10 months after NICU discharge because of respiratory failure and failure to thrive, resulting in a total survival rate of 73%. The IUGR infants of focus in the study were, by definition, less than the first percentile for birth weight (FIG. 1), but were also all less than the third percentile for length and head circumference at birth for their respective gestational ages. Of the 16 surviving infants, 15 complied with NCCC assessment at 6 months, but only 8 patients were compliant with the 12-month follow-up visits.

The mean maternal age was 26.2 ± 5.7 years. The severely IUGR babies in our study were relatively evenly distributed among white and black populations, single and married women, and Medicaid versus patients with private insurance. None of the mothers had insulin-dependent diabetes mellitus (IDDM); diet-controlled gestational diabetes was diagnosed in only one woman. Other medical problems in the study group included chronic hypertension, hypothyroidism, asthma, idiopathic thrombocytopenic purpura (ITP), and psychiatric illness. Tobacco and cocaine use

TABLE 4. Obstetrical management in IUGR pregnancies

Variable[a]	Entire group	Alive (n = 16)	Dead (n = 6)	p value
EGA at delivery (weeks)[b]	29.7 ± 2.4	29.9 ± 2.4	29.2 ± 2.7	NS
Birth weight (grams)[b]	689 ± 180	750 ± 149	530 ± 170	0.008
Sex				
Female	15 (68%)	9 (56%)	6 (100%)	0.05
Male	7 (32%)	7 (44%)	0 (0%)	NS
Delivery route				
Vaginal	1 (5%)	1 (6%)	0 (0%)	NS
Low transverse C/S	12 (54%)	12 (75%)	0 (0%)	NS
Classical C/S	9 (41%)	3 (19%)	6 (100%)	0.003
Maternal steroids	12 (55%)	11 (69%)	1 (17%)	0.09

NOTE: Student's t-test
[a]Percent value is for column data.
[b]Mean ± standard deviation.

was uncommon in the IUGR cohort. Only five women (23%) reported a history of cigarette smoking and another five women admitted to cocaine use. There were no significant differences in infant survival based on any of these pertinent maternal characteristics.

Preeclampsia was diagnosed in 15 women (68%) with IUGR gestations. Abnormal placental pathology results (increased syncytial knots, infarction) were found in 19 pregnancies (86%). Of the 12 women that consented to prenatal MSAFP screening, 9 (75%) had abnormally elevated levels that warranted further investigation that predated the diagnosis of IUGR. Oligohydramnios was noted in 19 (86%) of patients. Of the 21 fetuses with antenatal umbilical cord Doppler studies, 19 had abnormal ratios. Although 4 had elevated S/D ratios, 12 had no diastolic flow, and 3 had reverse flow, none were predictive of neonatal survival or outcome. The only antenatal predictor of neonatal death was mean antepartum ultrasound EFW (t-test, $p = 0.05$).

Several obstetrical management variables were compared between surviving and nonsurviving IUGR infants (TABLE 4). The most significant difference in the birth data and obstetrical management variables associated with improved outcome was birth weight. The mean birth weight of infants who survived was significantly higher than that for those who died. Furthermore, when birth weight was stratified into groups greater or less than 550 grams, those neonates with birth weights less than 550 grams were at significantly increased risk of neonatal death (FIG. 3).

Although more female IUGR infants were delivered alive, they were at a significantly higher risk for death than males. In fact, all the infants that died in the IUGR group were female in comparison to the equal proportions of male and female deaths in both control groups (AGA-GA: 0/20 female vs. 1/24 male, AGA-BW: 10/20 vs. 11/24, respectively).

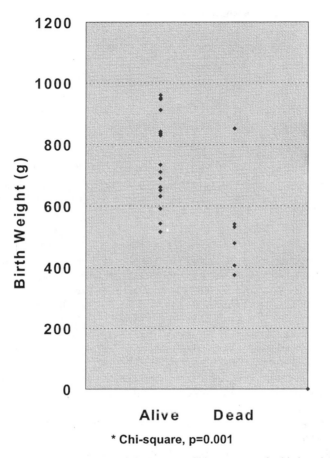

FIGURE 3. Survival by birth weight (grams). Chi-square test for birth weight <550 g, *p* < 0.001.

Decisions regarding the timing and route of delivery were based on maternal and fetal status and were made by the managing attending obstetrician for each IUGR pregnancy. Cesarean sections were performed primarily for fetal heart-rate abnormalities, deteriorating maternal status, and/or breech presentations. Classical cesarean delivery was associated with higher neonatal mortality when compared with other modes of delivery. Urgency of delivery precluded the administration of prophylactic steroids in several patients. The use of antenatal maternal steroid prophylaxis against RDS was associated with increased neonatal survival, but was not statistically significant.

Neonatal management variables were also analyzed in the IUGR infants (TABLE 5). Although the duration of ventilator and hyperalimentation support was higher in nonsurvivors, these factors were not statistically significant when compared with infants that survived. There was great variation in the length of NICU hospitalization at Strong Memorial Hospital; dying infants had a tendency toward longer NICU

TABLE 5. Neonatal management in IUGR cohort

Characteristics[a]	Entire group	Alive ($n = 16$)	Dead ($n = 6$)	p value
Surfactant use	8 (36%)	6 (38%)	2 (33%)	NS
Cord pH ($n = 18$)	7.22	7.20 ± 0.1	7.20 ± 0.1	NS
Antibiotics (days)[b]	11 (0–74)	9 (0–40)	9 (2–74)	NS
Ventilator (days)[b]	10 (0–154)	1 (0–70)	47 (0–154)	0.09
Hyperalimentation (days)[b]	12 (1–157)	8 (2–55)	25 (1–157)	NS
NICU stay (days)[b]	65 (5–180)	43 (5–142)	98 (6–180)	NS
Hospital charges	$149,180	$129,679	$201,182	NS

[a]Percent value is for column data.
[b]Median (range).

stays. One surviving infant was transferred to a level II nursery at a hospital closer to home at 5 days after birth, and two infants expired within a week of birth. Otherwise, all patients were hospitalized at least 28 days before death or discharge from the NICU. The hospital charges for caring for infants that ultimately died were almost double of those that survived; however, the difference was not significant.

Rates for neonatal morbidity in the IUGR cohort were evaluated systematically (TABLE 6). Generally, there were low rates of IVH, neonatal seizures, congenital anomalies, and congenital infections. Of the 15 patients that had karyotype analysis by either amniocentesis or neonatal blood, two had partial chromosome duplications (both of these infants survived). Minor congenital anomalies were identified such as ambiguous genitalia ($n = 2$), ventricular septal defect ($n = 1$), atrial septal defect ($n = 1$), and extrahepatic biliary atresia ($n = 1$). Two infants were prophylactically treated for asymptomatic congenital syphilis. Complications associated with neonatal death included patent ductus arteriosus, feeding intolerance, and failure to thrive. All of the neonates that died were diagnosed with feeding intolerance and met the criteria for failure to thrive. Causes of death for the six neonates included respiratory failure from viral pneumonitis ($n = 1$), BPD ($n = 3$), sepsis ($n = 1$), and NEC with pulmonary hemorrhage ($n = 1$), all of which are known complications of prematurity.

When growth measurements were determined for the 16 surviving infants at the 6- and 12-month-interval NCCC visits, 44% (7/16) of them exhibited catch-up growth and were no longer below the third percentile for weight, height, and head circumference. At 6 months, results of neurological examinations were available for 15 patients, and 13 of them had complete developmental assessments. The one infant that was lost to follow-up (the same patient that was transferred out of the NICU at 5 days of age at parental request) was reportedly "doing well, without any problems," according to his mother at a new obstetrical visit. At 12 months, 8 patients were available for neurological examinations, and 7 had complete developmental assessments. Altogether, 11 of the 15 tested patients (73%) had evidence of moderate to severe neurological impairment and/or developmental delay at either 6 and 12 month evaluations. These children have since been referred to early interventional programs. The infant that died at 11 months of age was also severely neurologically

TABLE 6. Comparison of neonatal complications

Characteristics[a]	Entire group	Alive (n = 16)	Dead (n = 6)	p value
RDS	15 (68%)	10 (63%)	5 (83%)	NS
IVH	5 (23%)	3 (19%)	2 (33%)	NS
Seizures	1 (5%)	0 (0%)	1 (17%)	NS
NEC	1 (5%)	0 (0%)	1 (17%)	NS
Feeding intolerance	3 (59%)	7 (44%)	16 (100%	0.046
Failure to thrive	9 (41%)	3 (19%)	6 (100%)	0.05
ROP	13 (59%)	6 (38%)	3 (75%)*	NS
BPD	9 (41%)	5 (31%)	4 (100%)*	NS
PDA	2 (9%)	4 (25%)	5 (83%)	0.034
Congenital anomalies	6 (27%)	4 (25%)	2 (33%)	NS
Congenital infection	2 (9%)	1 (6%)	1 (16%)	NS

NOTE: Student's *t*-test.
ABBREVIATIONS: RDS, respiratory distress syndrome; IVH, intraventricular hemorrhage; NEC, necrotizing enterocolitis; ROP, retinopathy of prematurity; BPD, bronchopulmonary dysplasia; PDA. patent ductus arteriosus.
[a]n = 4.

and developmentally impaired based on multiple hospitalization admission examinations, but was too ill to comply with formal neurodevelopmental testing.

DISCUSSION

Over the past decade, collaborative efforts on the part of obstetricians and neonatologists at tertiary care institutions have become increasingly sophisticated in the resuscitation and care of the very low birthweight infant. The gestational age limit of viability has progressively been lowered from 26 weeks in the 1970–80s[12] to 24 weeks in the 1990s.[1] Survival of infants below 750 grams has also increased from 21% to over 50% from 1981 to 1987,[13] with a lower birthweight limit of 700 grams in the 1970s,[14] decreasing further to 600 grams in the 1980s.[3] Obstetricians have traditionally placed more emphasis on gestational age of a fetus in directing aggressive management for salvaging a pregnancy, as compared to their counterparts, the pediatricians, who have been more interested in birth weight as a predictor of survival.[2] Because the limits of viability have been set at 24 weeks and with a corresponding birthweight of 500 to 750 g, some practitioners have attempted to push the limit further by attempting to save IUGR fetuses at these early gestational ages that would weigh even less. However, survival data in the case of the premature, very severely growth-restricted fetus have been limited and not critically studied because so few of these pregnancies reach viability. Despite the infrequency of pregnancies with this degree of growth restriction presenting this early in gestation, they represent a major challenge for patient counseling by obstetricians and pediatricians because of the paucity of useful outcome data.

As expected, when looking at the entire cohort, both estimated gestational age and birth weight are significantly associated with neonatal survival. It is a well-known fact that, in general, survival increases as birth weight and/or gestational age increases. The IUGR neonates evaluated in this study, however, were in the first percentile of birth weight between 25 and 33 weeks' gestation and, therefore, are the most severely growth-restricted infants that have ever been described in the literature. (The fact that this condition is so rare accounts for the small sample size and also makes prospective analysis impractical.) Although only 22 out of 13,608 live births during this time period met the strict criteria (<37 weeks, BW <1000 g, ≤ first percentile for BW) for the study, they border on the lower limits of survival in both birth weight and gestational age. Survival of premature, extremely IUGR neonates with birth weights less than 550 grams rarely occurred (1 out of 16) in our series. This is consistent with the findings of Hack and Fanaroff[3] that the probability of survival is very poor for newborns with birth weights less than 600 grams even in an AGA population. We found this weight cutoff to hold true for every given gestational age in our IUGR population, including a 32-week infant weighing 405 grams. There was one 25-week survivor that weighed 514 grams at birth that met the criteria for severe IUGR, but she was proportionally larger than some of her more mature counterparts. There was no obvious gestational age cutoff or gestational age trend towards increased survival in these IUGR patients, except for the observation that there were no viable growth-restricted neonates at 24-weeks' gestation and only two IUGR fetuses delivered between 25 and 26 weeks' gestation. The lower birthweight babies in this series died, regardless of gestational age. To examine the contribution if IUGR to survival, gestational age- and birthweight-matched controls were derived from the computerized database. Although more AGA-BW controls died in comparison to IUGR infants, the difference was not significant. These statistics are obviously affected by exclusion of other AGA pregnancies of similar extremely low birth weights that were considered abortions and therefore not resuscitated. AGA-GA controls had a significantly higher survival rate in comparison to IUGR infants. This suggests that when gestational age is controlled, birth weight makes the difference—a lower birth weight has a negative effect on survival.

It is interesting to note that such severe degrees of IUGR are occurring in women with essentially no predisposing medical risk factors such as IDDM, tobacco smoking, or cocaine use. This extreme IUGR also crosses all racial barriers, as well as socioeconomic statuses. However, abnormal placental pathology results, abnormally elevated MSAFP, abnormal Doppler flow studies, and severe preeclampsia were common manifestations for many of these patients. Abnormally high MSAFP values were found in 75% of patients who had this test performed. This was consistent with the finding of Katz et al.,[15] who noted that "unexplained" elevations of MSAFP levels were associated with a high incidence of subsequent fetal growth restriction. However, in the present study, elevation MSAFP values were not predictive of neonatal survival.

A preponderance of female infants (14 vs. 6) is found in this IUGR population as compared to a slightly higher number of live-born males in AGA populations (48 vs. 40). One might speculate that more female IUGR babies are born alive because more male IUGR fetuses are stillborn. However, despite the increased ratio of female to male live births in the setting of IUGR, the female neonates were at higher risk for neonatal death. However, sex had no effect on survival in AGA-GA and AGA-BW controls, where the overall proportion of females who died was similar to males, confirming the lack of systemic bias in our study design. It seems that the difference found in the IUGR population may be a result of a predisposition for female fetuses, especially those that died, to be lower in birth weight and thus at higher risk of neonatal death when compared to viable males of the same gestation. These results are in contrast with the findings of Phelps and colleagues, in which premature female infants fared better than males in weight-matched and gestational age–matched controls.[2]

The obstetrician's best tool in predicting survival outcome of these fetuses may be ultrasound EFW, despite its limitations. An accurate determination of EFW is often difficult to obtain in the setting of oligohydramnios that usually accompanies IUGR, but it may be the only prenatal assessment that can be used to direct obstetrical and neonatal interventions. Measurements of fetal umbilical cord Doppler flow studies may predict impending intrauterine fetal demise if the fetus is left undelivered[16] but were not useful in our study for determining postnatal survival. However, Craigo *et al.* found that absent or reversed diastolic end flow was associated with adverse neonatal outcome in infants with fetal weights less than the 10th percentile, specifically with neonatal death, BPD, and NEC.[17] The administration of maternal steroids demonstrated a trend toward improved neonatal survival, but because of limited use of steroids during the study period, our data were not sufficient to make definitive recommendations. However, this recommendation is supported by the National Institues of Health, who found evidence that antenatal steroids do in fact increase survival, as well as decrease pulmonary and cerebral morbidity, among infants of less than a 1500-gram birth weight.[18]

There was an increased tendency to deliver these ELBW babies by cesarean section; only one fetus was delivered vaginally in our series. Bottoms *et al.* found that the willingness to perform a cesarean delivery was associated with increased likelihood of survival independent of actually performing cesarean delivery.[19] Despite the aggressive measures to deliver the babies by cesarean section, particularly classical cesarean sections, almost all neonates less than 550 grams at birth still did not survive. Because our study is retrospective, it is possible that selection bias has confounded this result. Rates of IVH were similar in both surviving and dead infants, despite the higher rate of classical cesarean section in an attempt to provide a less traumatic delivery. Nevertheless, the neonatology team should be consulted far in advance to discuss intensity of resuscitative efforts with the patient. This counseling should also include mode of delivery and realistic descriptions of neonatal morbidity and mortality.

Many days of expensive and highly specialized treatment in the NICU were required for the care of these ELBW infants, such as prolonged intravenous antibiotic infusions, ventilator support, and hyperalimentation. Despite the time, money, and effort expended on behalf of these neonates, half of the nonsurviving babies died following more than 100 days of NICU care. This contradicts the finding of Meadow *et al.*, who noted that from 1989 to 1991, 80% of deaths of ELBW infants (<1000 g) occurred in the first three days of life.[20] However, it supports the finding of Hack *et al.*, who noted that from 1982 to 1988 until 1990 to 1992, fewer infants of 500–750-

gram birth weight died at <24 hours of life and more died at more than 28 days of life, most likely reflecting the improvements in neonatal intensive care, such as surfactant and postnatal dexamethasone.[21] Moreover, in our study, it appears that many of these infants have a protracted neonatal course complicated by feeding intolerance, with failure to thrive, and ultimately succumb to these consequences. In contrast, as depicted in the survival curves, AGA-BW controls that are destined to die, expire within the first few days of life, and AGA-EGA controls essentially all fared well to NICU discharge.

The allocation of resources to infants with such poor chances of survival deserves a thorough evaluation of cost efficacy. Although the hospitalization costs for infants that did not survive were greater than the costs for those that lived, the long-term costs of health care and interventional programs for the survivors have yet to be determined. Some provocative data now suggest that IUGR infants may be predisposed to developing certain chronic medical diseases in adulthood, such as coronary artery disease, hypertension, and diabetes, which may incur additional health-care expenditures.[22,23] It has been well documented in the literature that ELBW neonates develop behavioral and educational problems in childhood.[9,10,24] Although the birth weights in this series are much lower than those reported in previous studies and the examinations of these patients at 6 and 12 months of corrected age may be too early for accurate assessments, more than half of them already have exhibited neurological abnormalities and developmental delay. These difficult neurodevelopmental problems may respond well to early interventional regimens, as well as dedicated parental participation in care. Follow-up of the 16 survivors into the grade school years will need to be assessed by the NCCC.

In summary, premature, severely IUGR neonates weighing less than 550 grams at birth have a very poor prognosis for survival despite a gestational age at which survival is highly likely. Aggressive measures to save these very small fetuses appear to be futile and may be unnecessarily prolonging their ultimate demise. In this setting, classical cesarean sections that have such detrimental implications for a woman's future reproductive care may not improve neonatal outcome and, therefore, should not be encouraged. However, aggressive management of severely IUGR neonates weighing greater than 550 grams at birth may be considered because of improved morbidity and mortality rates in the modern NICU. Neonates developing PDA, feeding intolerance, and failure to thrive have a poor prognosis for survival. The quality of life for the surviving infants and costs of long-term health care into adulthood remain an important area for study. In the meantime, we echo the recommendation by Muraskas *et al.* for responsible counseling of parents before delivery of extremely IUGR fetuses and for realistically weighing the medical, ethical, financial, and emotional costs of caring for this unique subgroup of patients by all involved.[25]

REFERENCES

1. ALLEN, M.C., P.K. DONOHUE & A.E. DUSMAN. 1993. The limit of viability—neonatal outcome of infants born at 22 to 25 weeks' gestation. N. Engl. J. Med. **329:** 1597–1601.
2. PHELPS, D.L., *et al.* 1991. 28-day survival rates of 6676 neonates with birth weights of 1250 grams or less. Pediatrics **87:** 7–17.

3. HACK, M. & A.A. FANAROFF. 1989. Outcomes of extremely-low-birth-weight infants between 1982 and 1988. N. Engl. J. Med. **321:** 1642–1647.
4. MURASKAS, J.K., *et al.* 1991. Survival of a 280-g infant. N. Engl. J. Med. **324:** 1598–1599.
5. SHERER, D.M., *et al.* 1992. Case report: survival of an infant with a birth weight of 345 grams. Birth **19:** 151–153.
6. AMATO, M. & H. Schneider. 1991. Survival of a 390-gram Swiss infant. J. Perinat. Med. **19:** 313–315.
7. LEVENO, K.J., *et al.* 1983. Perinatal outcome in the absence of antepartum fetal heart rate acceleration. Obstet. Gynecol. **61(3):** 347–355.
8. GLUCK, L. & M.V. KULOVICH. 1973. Lecithin/sphingomyelin ratios in amniotic fluid in normal and abnormal pregnancy. Am. J. Obstet. Gynecol. **115:** 539–546.
9. HALSEY, C.L., M.F. COLLIN & C.L. ANDERSON. 1993. Extremely low birth weight children and their peers: a comparison of preschool performance. Pediatrics **91:** 807–811.
10. SUNG, I.K., B. VOHR & W. OH. 1993. Growth and neurodevelopmental outcome of very low birth weight infants with intrauterine growth retardation: comparison with control subjects matched by birth weight and gestational age. J. Pediatr. **123:** 618–624.
11. USHER, R. & F. MCLEAN. 1969. Intrauterine growth of live-born Caucasian infants at sea level: standards obtained from measurements in 7 dimensions of infants born between 25–44 weeks of gestation. J. Pediatr. **74:** 901–910.
12. HERSCHEL, M., *et al.* 1982. Survival of infants born at 24 to 28 weeks' gestation. Obstet. Gynecol. **60:** 154–158.
13. FERRARA, T.B., *et al.* 1989. Changing outcome of extremely premature infants (26 weeks' gestation and 750 gm): survival and follow-up at a tertiary center. Am. J. Obstet. Gynecol. **161:** 1114–1118.
14. BRITTON, S.B., P.M. FITZHARDINGE & S. ASHBY. 1981. Is intensive care justified for infants weighing less than 801 gm at birth? J. Pediatr. **99:** 937–943.
15. KATZ, V., N.C. CHESCHIER & R. CEFALO. 1990. Unexplained elevations of maternal serum alpha-fetoprotein. Obstet. Gynecol. Surv. **45:** 719–726.
16. REED, K.L., C.F. ANDERSON & L. SHENKER. 1987. Changes in intracardiac Doppler blood flow velocities in fetuses with absent umbilical artery diastolic flow. Am. J. Obstet. Gynecol. **157:** 774–779.
17. CRAIGO, S.D., *et al.* 1996. Ultrasound predictors of neonatal outcome in intrauterine growth restriction. Am. J. Perinatol. **13:** 465–471.
18. NATIONAL INSTITUTES OF HEALTH. 1994. Effect of corticosteroids for fetal maturation on perinatal outcomes: NIH consensus statement. Natl. Inst. Health **12:** 1–24.
19. BOTTOMS, S., *et al.* and the NATIONAL INSTITUTE OF CHILD HEALTH AND HUMAN DEVELOPMENT NETWORK OF MATERNAL–FETAL MEDICINE UNITS. 1997. Obstetric determinants of neonatal survival: influence of willingness to perform cesarean delivery on survival of extremely low-birth-weight infants. Am. J. Obstet. Gynecol. **176:** 960–966.
20. MEADOW, W., T. REIMSHISEL & J. LANTOS. 1996. Birth weight-specific mortality for extremely low birth weight infants vanishes by four days of life: epidemiology and ethics in the neonatal intensive care unit. Pediatrics **97:** 636–643.
21. HACK, M., H. FRIEDMAN & A.A. FANAROFF. 1996. Outcomes of extremely low birth weight infants. Pediatrics **98:** 931–937.
22. BARKER, D.J., *et al.* 1993. The relation of small head circumference and thinness at birth to death from cardiovascular disease in adult life. Br. Med. J. **306:** 422–426.
23. PHIPPS, K., *et al.* 1993. Fetal growth and impaired glucose tolerance in men and women. Diabetalogia **36:** 225–228.
24. SMEDLER, A.C., *et al.* 1992. Psychological development in children born with very low birth weight after severe intrauterine growth retardation: a 10-year follow-up study. Acta Paediatr. **81:** 197–203.
25. MURASKAS, JONATHAN, MONIKA BHOLA, PAUL TOMICH & DAVID THOMASMA. 1998. Neonatal viability: pushing the envelope. Pediatrics **101(6):** 1095–1096.

Role of the Proteasome in the Regulation of Fetal Fibronectin Secretion in Human Placenta

YUEHONG MA, DONATO D'ANTONA, LINDA LaCHAPELLE, JAE SHIN RYU, AND SETH GULLER

Department of Obstetrics and Gynecology, New York University School of Medicine, New York, New York 10016, USA

ABSTRACT: The goal of the current study was to examine the role of the ubiquitin-proteasome system (UPS), a pathway of intracellular degradation, in the regulation of fetal fibronectin (FFN) expression in human placenta. Primary cultures of cytotrophoblasts (CTs) and placental mesenchymal cells (PMCs) were isolated from human term placentas and were maintained in serum-free medium (SFM) in the presence of inhibitors of proteasome-mediated degradation (e.g., MG132) as well as inhibitors of other proteases. Levels of secreted FFN and interleukin (IL)-8 in culture media were quantitated by enzyme-linked immunosorbent assay (ELISA), and cell viability was assessed by trypan blue exclusion. Intracellular levels of FFN and ubiquinated proteins were measured by Western blotting, and levels of fibronectin mRNA were determined following Northern blotting. We found that proteasome inhibitors (MG132, MG262, and PSI) potently suppressed levels of secreted FFN in cultures of CTs, but they not did affect levels of IL-8. Lysosomal, calpain, and serine protease inhibitors as well as the anti-inflammatory compound sulfasalazine did not markedly affect levels of secreted FFN in CT cultures. Proteasome inhibitors did not compromise cell viability during the initial 16–18 hours of treatment and did not affect intracellular levels of FFN protein or fibronectin mRNA. The efficacy of suppression of FFN in CT culture media by proteasome inhibitors reflected their effects on intracellular accumulation of ubiquinated proteins. By contrast, the presence of proteasome inhibitors did not alter levels of secreted FFN in cultures of PMCs. We conclude that inhibitors of proteasome-mediated degradation potently and specifically suppressed extracellular expression of FFN in CTs through a cell type-specific pathway that did not involve alterations in FFN synthesis. This suggests that accumulation of ubiquinated proteins in the presence of proteasome inhibitors blocks FFN secretion or promotes the extracellular degradation of FFN. This experimental paradigm will be useful for dissecting the role of the UPS in regulating CT function.

KEYWORDS: proteasome; fibronectin; placenta; fetal fibronectin; cytotrophoblasts; placental mesenchymal cells; serum-free medium

Address for correspondence: Dr. Seth Guller, Department of OB/GYN, NYU School of Medicine, 550 First Ave., New York, NY 10016. Voice: 212-263-8594; fax: 212-263-5742.
gulles01@med.nyu.edu

INTRODUCTION

Eukaryotic cells contain two major pathways for intracellular protein degradation. The first to be described was the lysosomal system involving acid proteases (cathepsins) that degrade proteins in membrane-enclosed vacuoles.[1] Over the last several years it has become evident that most intracellular proteins are degraded by the ubiquitin-proteasome system (UPS) in a process requiring ATP. Protein degradation by this pathway involves the covalent attachment of ubiquitin to target proteins and subsequent degradation of the ubiquinated protein by the 26S proteasome complex.[2,3] The addition of ubiquitin to a protein determines the specificity of the UPS and occurs sequentially through the actions of the ubiquitin-activating enzyme (E1), one of several ubiquitin-conjugating enzymes (E2), and one of several ubiquitin ligases (E3) that ultimately covalently attach ubiquitin to a lysine residue of the target protein.[2,3] The use of synthetic pharmacologic proteasome inhibitors (e.g., MG132) have enabled investigators to assess the importance of the UPS in the turnover of specific proteins.[3] For *in vitro* studies, if the presence of proteasome inhibitors increases the level of a protein or slows its turnover, the UPS is generally implicated in protein degradation.[2,3] This approach demonstrated a role for the UPS in the rapid degradation of transcription regulators including activating transcription factor-2 (ATF-2),[4] IκB,[5] inducible cAMP early repressor,[6] hypoxia-inducible factor (HIF)-1,[7] and p53.[8] Other roles of the UPS include presentation of peptide fragments as MHC antigens[9] and removal of mutated or post-translationally damaged proteins through endoplasmic reticulum-associated degradation.[10,11] It was initially believed that UPS function was limited to the degradation of cytosolic and nuclear proteins, but recent results suggest that membrane-anchored and secretory proteins are also degraded by this system.[12] The clinical utility of proteasome inhibitors is based on their anti-inflammatory properties.[3]

Oncofetal fibronectin (FFN) is a uniquely glycosylated fibronectin produced by the placenta that plays a critical role in placental development. FFN in placenta and certain tumors is recognized by the monoclonal antibody FDC-6.[13,14] Immunohistochemistry revealed high levels of FFN at uterine-placental and decidual-fetal membrane interfaces, suggesting that it mediates adherence at these sites.[15,16] Its specific localization to the ECM connecting extravillous anchoring cytotrophoblasts (CTs) and CT cell columns to the uterus suggested that FFN functions as a "trophoblast glue."[16] Recent *in vitro* studies using trophoblast explants and function-perturbing antibodies suggest that FFN and the α5β1 integrin (i.e., the FN receptor) play an important role in anchoring extravillous CTs to the uterus.[17] We have shown that all fibronectin expressed and released by CTs isolated from term placentas contains the oncofetal epitope,[18] reflecting its pattern of expression *in vivo*.[15,16]

Previous work in our laboratory has shown that glucocorticoids (GCs) regulate FFN expression in human and non-human primate placenta and fetal membranes.[19] Our *in vitro* studies demonstrate that GCs downregulate FFN expression in epithelial cells of placenta and amnion, whereas GCs stimulate FFN expression in mesenchymal cells isolated from these tissues.[19] Therefore, we suggested that the periparturitional rise in GCs remodels extracellular matrices at maternal-fetal junctions prior to expulsion of the fetus.

To date, there is no information on the role of proteolytic systems in the regulation of FFN secretion by human placenta. Therefore, the goal of the current study was to assess the contribution of proteasome-mediated degradation in the regulation of placental FFN expression using CTs isolated from human term placentas as a model.

MATERIALS AND METHODS

Materials

Tissue culture media were obtained from Sigma (St. Louis, MO). Bovine sera were purchased from Gemini Bio-Products (Calabasas, CA). Laboratory plasticware was obtained from Falcon, Becton-Dickinson Labware (Lincoln Park, NJ). ITS+, a mixture containing insulin, transferrin, and selenium, was purchased from Collaborative Research-Becton-Dickinson (Bedford, MA). MG132 was purchased from CALBIOCHEM (San Diego, CA). MG262, PSI, and lactacystin/β-lactone were obtained from Affiniti Research Products (Exeter, UK). Calpain inhibitor-1 was purchased from Boehringer Mannheim (Indianapolis, IN). Leupeptin, antipain, and sulfasalazine were obtained from Sigma (St. Louis, MO). Calpeptin inhibitor was obtained from a previously described source.[20] Ultraspec used for RNA isolation was purchased from BIOTECX Laboratories, Inc. (Houston, TX). ^{32}P-dCTP was from New England Nuclear (Boston, MA). Plasmids containing cDNAs to fibronectin and glyceraldehyde-3-phosphate dehydrogenase (GAPDH) were obtained from the American Type Culture Collection (Rockville, MD). Other reagents used in tissue culture and Northern blotting and Western blotting were from previously described sources.[21,22]

Methods

Cell Culture

Human placental tissue ($n = 9$) was obtained from pregnancies with normally grown, singleton fetus delivered at term (37–42 weeks of gestation) by cesarean section. For the isolation of cytotrophoblasts (CTs), approximately 45 g of villous tissue was dissected from the placental disc, and digestions with trypsin were carried out as described.[21,23] Tissue digests were separated on continuous percoll gradients in which CTs sedimented as a ring of cells at a density of approximately 1.05 g/ml.[21,23] Using these procedures we obtain CTs with purities of ≥95% as judged by immunocytochemistry.[18]

Placental mesenchymal cells (PMCs) were isolated based on a modification of our previous method.[22] Briefly, washed villi were digested for 45 minutes in a 1:1 mixture of phenol red-free Ham's F12-Dulbecco's Modified Eagle's medium (basal medium) containing 0.1% collagenase and 0.01% DNase. Dispersed cells were filtered through a 160-μm stainless steel sieve, and the eluate was collected. To obtain a more homogeneous preparation of PMCs, cells were then resuspended in basal medium and centrifuged ($2000 \times g$, 15 min) on a discontinuous gradient containing 40 and 60% percoll. Cells were collected from the interface of the two gradients and were washed and resuspended in basal medium. Using this procedure, we obtained preparations of PMCs with ≥95% of the cell population showing positive staining for vimentin by immunocytochemistry.

Following isolation, CTs and PMCs were plated at a density of 1–4 x 10^5 cells/ 24-well dish for ELISA studies and 2–10 x 10^6 cells per 10-cm dish for Northern and Western blot analyses in culture medium containing basal medium with 10% charcoal-stripped calf serum and ITS$^+$ (a supplement used to achieve a final concentration of insulin of 6.25 µg/ml, transferrin 6.25 µg/ml, selenous acid 6.25 ng/ml, bovine serum albumin 1.25 mg/ml, and linoleic acid 5.35 µg/ml).[21,22] After 24 hours, the monolayers were washed twice with HBSS and serum-free medium (SFM), consisting of the aforementioned media formulation without serum,[24] was added. After the indicated time in culture, conditioned media were saved for ELISA, and protein and RNA were extracted from adherent cells.

Cells were maintained at 37°C in a humidified atmosphere of 5% CO_2/95% air.

ELISA

Levels of FFN in culture media were measured by an ELISA using FDC-6 monoclonal antibody, according to information provided by the manufacturer (Adeza Biomedical, Sunnyvale, CA), as we previously described.[18] Levels of IL-8 were determined with a kit obtained from R & D Systems (Minneapolis, MN), as described.[25] The concentration of FFN in culture media was determined in triplicate wells and was normalized to cell protein using the D_C Protein Assay from Bio-Rad Laboratories (Hercules, CA).

Northern and Western blotting

For Northern blotting, RNA was extracted from CTs and PMCs using UltraSpec RNA (Biotecx, Houston, TX) as reported.[22] Approximately 20 µg total RNA were separated on a 1% agarose gel containing formaldehyde. Following transfer, fibronectin and GAPDH mRNAs were detected using ^{32}P-labeled cDNA probes.[22] Autoradiographic signals were quantitated using the Electrophoresis Documentation and Analysis System 120 and Digital Science 1D Image Software (Eastman Kodak, Rochester, NY). For Western blotting, proteins were separated on 7% (w/v) polyacrylamide gels under reducing conditions. Following transfer of proteins to nitrocellulose filters, immunodetection of FFN with FDC-6 antibody was carried out using ECL detection as reported.[26] FDC-6 antibody and the secondary antibody/ peroxidase conjugate were diluted 1:1000 and 1:8000, respectively.

Statistics

Unless stated otherwise, FIGURES 1–5 show results from one experiment representing three to four identically conducted ones. Cumulative data showing the effect of MG132 treatment on FFN and IL-8 levels in CTs were performed by Student's *t* test using SigmaStat software (Jandel, San Rafael, CA). Results are expressed as mean ± SE.

Human Subjects and Animal Care

The study protocol was approved by the institutional review board committee at New York University School of Medicine. Placentas were obtained with the consent of the surgeon and the pathologist.

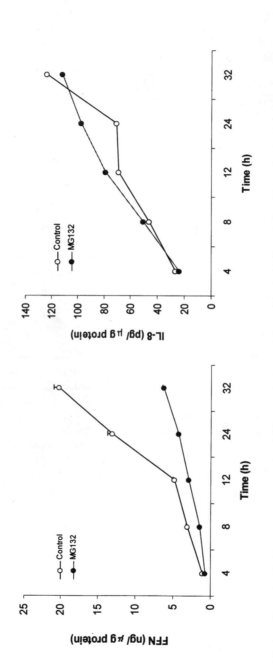

FIGURE 1. Effect of MG132 treatment on levels of FFN and IL-8 in culture media from CTs. Cells were maintained in SFM for the indicated time with and without 1 μM MG132 and levels of FFN (*left panel*) and IL-8 (*right panel*) in culture media were determined by ELISA. Each point represents the mean ± SE of determinations carried out in triplicate wells. SEs that fell within the symbol are not presented.

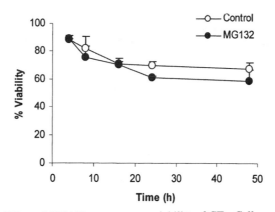

FIGURE 2. Effect of MG132 treatment on viability of CTs. Cells were maintained in SFM in the presence and absence of 1 µM MG132, and cell viability was assessed by trypan blue exclusion. Data are presented as mean ± SE of determinations performed in triplicate.

RESULTS

CTs isolated from human term placentas were maintained for 4–32 hours in SFM ± 1 µM MG132 (a peptide aldehyde proteasome inhibitor) and levels of immuno-detectable FFN (left panel) and IL-8 (right panel) in culture media were determined by ELISA. We observed that MG132 treatment suppressed levels of FFN in culture media to 15 to 60% of control levels, but it did not affect levels of secreted IL-8. Note that MG132 effects on FFN levels were rapid and occurred at the earliest time point of detectability (~4 h). Cumulative results from four different preparations of CTs revealed that treatment of CTs with 1 µM MG132 for 16–18 hours significantly reduced media levels of FFN to 37 ± 3% of control ($p < 0.01$). By contrast, media levels of IL-8 in three different preparations of MG132-treated cells was 142 ± 27% of control ($p = 0.19$). As shown in FIGURE 2, MG132 treatment did not markedly affect cell viability up to 16 hours of treatment as measured by trypan blue exclusion. Treatment of CTs with MG132 for 24 or 48 hours resulted in a 10–20% loss in viability relative to controls. These results suggest that the MG132-mediated reduction in secreted FFN levels was not associated with a general reduction in function of CTs.

We found that MG132 treatment inhibited FFN secretion in CTs with an IC_{50} of approximately 0.15 µM (TABLE 1). *N*-benzoylcarbonyl-ile-flu-(*O-t*-Bu)-ala-leucinal (PSI) and lactacystin/β-lactone, other proteasome inhibitors, reduced levels of secreted FFN secretion to 10–30% of control levels with IC_{50}s of 1 and 2 µM, respectively (TABLE 1). MG262, a boronic acid derivative proteasome inhibitor with 100-fold greater potency in inhibiting proteasome-mediated degradation compared to MG132,[26] inhibited FFN secretion with an IC_{50} of approximately 1 nM. Conversely, the lysosomal inhibitor calpeptin, the serine protease inhibitors leupeptin and anti-pain, as well as the anti-inflammatory agent sulfasalazine did not affect levels of secreted FFN at concentrations between 1 and 100 µM (TABLE 1). Calpain inhibitor-1, an inhibitor of calpains and a relatively weak inhibitor of proteasome activity,[3] had modest suppressive activity.

TABLE 1. Potency of protease inhibitors in reducing levels of fetal fibronectin (FFN) in cytotrophoblast culture media[a]

Compound	Specificity	IC_{50} (µM)
MG262	Proteasome	0.001
MG132	Proteasome	0.150
PSI	Proteasome	1.0
Lactacystin β-lactone	Proteasome	2.0
Calpain inhibitor-1	Calpains/proteasome	10
Sulfasalazine	Inflammatory pathways	>100
Calpeptin inhibitor	Lysosome	>100
Leupeptin	Serine proteases	>100
Antipain	Serine proteases	>100

[a]Cells were maintained in serum-free medium with the indicated protease inhibitor at concentrations ranging from 10 pM to 100 µM for 18 hours, and levels of FFN in culture media were determined by ELISA. The concentration of inhibitors that elicits a 50% reduction in FFN levels relative control (IC_{50}) is presented from a single experiment representing two or three identically conducted ones. The primary site of action is shown for each inhibitor.

We also observed that treatment of CTs with 1 µM MG132 for 18 hours did not affect levels of cell-associated FFN protein, as detected by Western blotting (FIG. 3, left panel). Similarly, an 8-hour treatment of CTs with 1 µM MG132 did not affect levels of fibronectin mRNA as detected by Northern blotting and normalization to levels of GAPDH mRNA (FIG. 3, right panel). We noted that longer treatments of CTs with MG132 (≥18 h) reduced levels of fibronectin and GAPDH mRNA to the same extent relative to control (not shown), suggesting a generalized transcriptional suppression at longer time points. These results indicate that the MG132-mediated reduction in secreted FFN in CTs was not due to suppression of FFN synthesis. Note

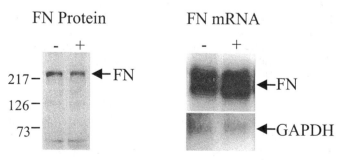

FIGURE 3. Levels of FFN protein and FN mRNA in control and MG132-treated CTs. Cells maintained for 18 hours in SFM with (+) and without (−) 1 µM MG132 were lysed and cell-associated FFN was determined following Western blotting (*left panel*). Molecular weights of protein standards are presented at the left of the panel. In addition, CTs were maintained for 8 hours in SFM in the presence or absence of 1 µM MG132 and levels of FN mRNA were determined following Northern blotting and hybridization with ^{32}P-labeled cDNA probes to FN and GAPDH (*right panel*).

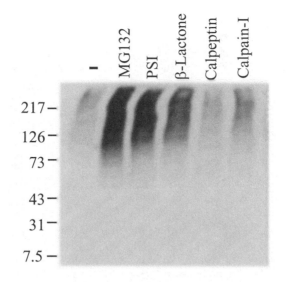

FIGURE 4. Effect of protease inhibitors on the expression of ubiquinated proteins in CTs. Cells were incubated in SFM without (-) or with the indicated protease inhibitor (1 μM), and levels of cell-associated ubiquinated proteins were determined by Western blotting and detection with anti-ubiquitin Ab. Ubiquinated proteins appear as a high molecular weight smear.

that in this study and in previous studies, [18,23] we observed that levels of FFN protein and fibronectin mRNA were similarly regulated in CTs. This is most likely due to the finding that virtually all fibronectin protein secreted by CTs contains the oncofetal epitope.[18]

Western blotting with anti-ubiquitin Ab (which detects both free and protein-conjugated ubiquitin) was carried out to assess the efficacy of inhibitors (1 μM) in blocking proteasome-mediated protein degradation in CTs. We observed that treatment with the proteasome inhibitors MG132, PSI, and lactacystin/β-lactone (denoted β-lactone) increased expression of ubiquinated proteins (as indicated by the appearance of a high molecular weight smear), whereas the lysosomal inhibitor, calpeptin inhibitor (denoted calpeptin), and calpain inhibitor-1 (denoted calpain-I) had little effect (FIG. 4). These results suggest that peptide aldehydes and other compounds that reduce FFN secretion by CTs do so by suppressing proteasome activity.

To determine whether MG132 effects on fibronectin secretion were cell type-specific, we tested the effect of MG132 treatment on FFN production by PMCs. We observed that the presence of 1 or 10 μM MG132 for 4–32 hours did not affect levels of FFN in culture media of PMCs (FIG. 5). This indicates that proteasome activity regulates levels of secreted FFN in CTs but not in PMCs.

Our results indicate that proteasome activity specifically controls levels of secreted FFN in CT cultures.

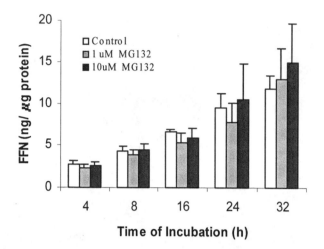

FIGURE 5. Levels of FFN in media of control and MG132-treated placental mesen-chymal cells (PMCs). Cells were maintained for 4-32 hours in SFM with 0.1 or 10 µM MG132 and levels of FFN in culture media were determined by ELISA. Results depict the mean and range of cumulative data from 2 independent experiments.

DISCUSSION

Our experiments link proteasome function with FFN expression in human placenta. We specifically show that levels of secreted FFN in cultures of CTs are markedly and specifically suppressed by the presence of inhibitors of proteasome-mediated degradation. Treatment of CTs with MG132, a well characterized peptide aldehyde proteasome inhibitor,[3] decreased levels of secreted FFN while suppressing proteasome function, as evidenced by the accumulation of polyubiquinated proteins on Western blots. It is of note that the IC_{50} for suppression of FFN by MG132 was 0.15 µM, approximately 20-fold lower than that reported for MG132-mediated inhibition of proteolysis in cell cultures.[3] Similarly, we noted that the presence of relatively low concentrations of MG132 (~0.1 µM) also markedly increased the expression of ubiquinated proteins (not shown). Moreover, the IC_{50} for FFN suppression by MG262, that is, a boronic acid derivative proteasome inhibitor,[27] was approximately 1 nM, suggesting that this compound will be particularly useful in future *in vitro* studies that examine the role of the UPS in placental function. We observed that the presence of 10% calf serum reduced the efficacy of MG132 in FFN suppression 10–20-fold (not shown). Therefore, it is likely that proteasome inhibitors were effective at low concentrations due to our use of serum-free culture medium. The enhanced potency of proteasome inhibitors under serum-free conditions allowed us to use these compounds at concentrations that did not reduce cell viability for the initial 16–18 hours of culture.

Our experiments indicate that proteasome activity indirectly regulates levels of secreted FFN in CTs, because the presence of MG132 treatment did not affect intra-cellular levels of FFN. If FFN was a proteasome substrate, its intracellular levels would be expected to increase in the presence of proteasome inhibitors, as has been observed for other proteins degraded by the proteasome including IκB[5] and HIF-1.[6] Although the proteasome was originally implicated in the degradation of short-lived transcriptional regulators,[28] secreted proteins including fibrinogen[29] as well as integral membrane proteins[30] were found to be substrates for ubiquitination and proteasome-mediated degradation. Fibronectin has been indirectly linked to the UPS through its interaction with the von Hippel-Lindau tumor suppressor protein (pVHL), a component of a ubiquitin E3 complex that binds fibronectin at the endoplasmic reticulum and is required for the extracellular assembly of fibronectin.[30] However, it is unlikely that pVHL is involved in the MG132-mediated effects observed in the present study, because pVHL was reported to be important in the extracellular organization of fibronectin in CHO cells but it did not regulate fibronectin secretion.[30]

Based on our results we suggest that two pathways may be involved in the MG132-mediated reduction in levels of secreted FFN in cultures of CTs. In both pathways it is assumed that the inhibition of proteasome function leads to the accumulation of ubiquinated proteasome substrates that alter extracellular levels of FFN without affecting its synthesis (i.e., intracellular levels of FFN protein and fibronectin mRNA were not altered by MG132 treatment). These accumulated proteins could bind FFN, leading to improper folding. FFNs, like other proteins, form dimers in the endoplasmic reticulum prior to glycosylation in the Golgi vesicles.[31] Misfolding could preclude dimer assembly, leading to intracellular accumulation and degradation of FFN.[12] Alternatively, inhibition of proteasome activity may lead to enhanced extracellular degradation of FFN by proteases secreted by CTs. Potential MG132-activated proteases include matrix metalloproteinases (72 and 92 kD gelatinases, stromelysin-1, and matrilysin), which catalyze the extracellular degradation of fibronectin.[32] In addition, MG132 treatment could also activate urokinase-type plasminogen activator (uPA), which is known to degrade fibronectin and is expressed at high levels by CTs.[33,34] Furthermore, most of the FFN-degrading activity in conditioned media from CT cultures was mediated by uPA.[35] It is also possible that MG132 treatment reveals latent autocatalytic activites in the fibronectin molecule, as has been observed following cleavage of purified fibronectin with cathepsin.[36] Significantly, it was recently demonstrated that a caspase-3 like protease responsible for bcl-2 cleavage is upregulated in leukemic cells by treatment with MG132.[37]

In conclusion, our results show that proteasome activity regulates extracellular levels of FFN in cultures of CTs. Since FFN expression is linked to changes in adhesion and differentiation and migration of CTs, it is likely that the UPS plays an important role in controlling placental development. Our studies provide a model with which to dissect the role of the UPS in placental function.

ACKNOWLEDGMENTS

These studies were supported in part through National Institutes of Health Grant HD 33909 (S.G.).

REFERENCES

1. WARD, C.L., S. OMURA, S & R.R. KOPITO 1995. Degradation of CFTR by the ubiquitin-proteasome pathway. Cell **83:** 121–127.
2. BIEDERER, T., C. VOLKWEIN & T. SOMMER. 1996. Degradation of subunits of the Sec61p complex, an integral component of the ER membrane, by the ubiquitin-proteasome pathway. EMBO J. **15:** 2069–2076.
3. PLEMPER, R.K. & D.H. WOLF. 1999. Retrograde protein translocation: ERADication of secretory proteins in health and disease. Trends Biochem. Sci. **24:** 266–270.
4. MATSUURA, H. & S.I. HAKOMORI. 1985. The oncofetal domain of fibronectin defined by the monoclonal antibody FDC-6:its presence in fibronectins from fetal and tumor tissues and its absence in those normal adult tissues and plasma. Proc. Natl. Acad. Sci. USA **82:** 6517–6521.
5. MATSUURA, H., K. TAKIO, K. TITANI, et al. 1988. The oncofetal structure of human fibronectin defined by monoclonal antibody FDC-6. J. Biol. Chem. **263:** 3314–3322.
6. LOCKWOOD, C.J., A.E. SENYEI, M.R. DISCHE, et al. 1991. Fetal fibronectin in cervical and vaginal secretions as a predictor of preterm delivery. N. Engl. J. Med. **325:** 669–674.
7. FEINBERG, R.F., H.J. KLIMAN & C.J. LOCKWOOD. 1991. Is oncofetal fibronectin a trophoblast glue for human implantation? Am. J. Pathol. **138:** 537–543.
8. APLIN, J.D., T. HAIGH, C.J.P. JONES, et al. 1999. Development of cytotrophoblast columns from explanted first-trimester human placental villi: role of fibronectin and integrin $\alpha_5\beta_1$. Biol. Reprod. **60:** 828–838.
9. GULLER, S., N. LACROIX, G. KRIKUN, et al. 1993. Steroid regulation of oncofetal fibronectin expression in human cytotrophoblasts. J. Steroid. Biochem. Molec. Biol. **46:** 1–10.
10. MA, Y., C.J. LOCKWOOD, A.L. BUNIM, et al. 2000. Cell type-specific regulation of fetal fibronectin expression in amnion: conservation of glucocorticoid responsiveness in human and nonhuman primates. Biol. Reprod. **62:** 1812–1817.
11. YANG, M.-X. & A.I. CEDERBAUM. 1997. Characterization of cytochrome P4502E1 turnover in transfected HepG2 cells expressing human CYP2E1. Arch. Biochem. Biophys. **341:** 25–33.
12. GULLER, S., L. MARKIEWICZ, R. WOZNIAK, et al. 1994. Developmental regulation of glucocorticoid-mediated effects on extracellular matrix protein expression in the human placenta. Endocrinology **134:** 2064–2071.
13. YOON, D.Y., Y. MA, G. KRIKUN, et al. 1998. Glucocorticoid effects in the human placenta: evidence that dexamethasone-mediated inhibition of fibronectin expression in cytotrophoblasts involves a protein intermediate. J. Clin. Endocrinol. Metab. **83:** 632–637.
14. GULLER, S., R. WOZNIAK, G. KRIKUN, et al. 1993. Glucocorticoid suppression of human placental fibronectin expression: implications in uterine-placental adherence. Endocrinology **133:** 1139–1146.
15. GULLER, S., R. WOZNIAK, L. KONG, et al. 1995. Opposing actions of transforming growth factor-β and glucocorticoids in the regulation of fibronectin expression in the human placenta. J. Clin. Endocrinol. Metab. **80:** 3273–3278.
16. ROSEN, T., G. KRIKUN, E.Y. WANG, et al. 1998. Chronic antagonism of nuclear factor κB activity in cytotrophoblasts by dexamethasone: a potential mechanism for antiinflammatory action of glucocorticoids in human placenta. J. Clin. Endocrinol. Metab. **83:** 3647–3652.
17. RUNIC, R., C.J LOCKWOOD, Y. MA, et al. 1996. Expression of Fas ligand by human cytotrophoblasts: implications in placentation and fetal survival. J. Clin. Endocrinol. Metab. **81:** 3119–3122.
18. MCCORMACK, T., W. BAUMEISTER, L. GRENIER, et al. 1997. Active site-directed inhibitors of the Rhodococcus 20S proteasome. Kinetics and mechanism. J. Biol. Chem. **272:** 26103–26109.
19. STANCOVSKI, I., H. GONEN, A. ORIAN, et al. 1995. Degradation of the proto-oncogene product c-Fos by the ubiquitin proteolytic system *in vivo* and *in vitro*: identification and characterization of the conjugating enzymes. Mol. Cell. Biol. **15:** 7106–7116.

20. XIA, H. & C. REDMAN. 1999. The degradation of nascent fibrinogen chains is mediated by the ubiquitin proteasome pathway. Biochem. Biophys. Res. Commun. **261:** 590–597.
21. OHH, M., R.L. YAUCH, K.M. LONERGAN, *et al.* 1998. The von Hippel-Lindau tumor suppressor protein is required for proper assembly of an extracellular fibronectin matrix. Mol. Cell. **1:** 959–968.
22. SCHWARZBAUER, J.E. 1991. Fibronectins: from gene to protein. Curr. Opin. Cell. Biol. **3:** 786–791.
23. BIRKEDAL-HANSEN, H. 1995. Proteolytic remodeling of extracellular matrix. Curr. Opin. Cell Biol. **7:** 728–735.
24. QUIGLEY, J.P., L.I. GOLD, R. SCHWIMMER, *et al.* 1987. Limited cleavage of cellular fibronectin by plasminogen activator purified from transformed cells. Proc. Natl. Acad. Sci. USA **84:** 2776–2780.
25. QUEENAN, J.T., JR., L.C. KAO, C.E. ARBOLEDA, *et al.* 1987. Regulation of urokinase-type plasminogen activator production by cultured human cytotrophoblasts. J. Biol. Chem. **262:** 10903–10906.
26. MONZON-BORDONABA, F., C.L. WANG & R.F. FEINBERG. 1997. Fibronectinase activity in cultured human trophoblasts is mediated by urokinase-type plasminogen activator. Am. J. Obstet. Gynecol. **176:** 58–65.
27. LAMBERT VIDMAR, S., F. LOTTSPEICH, I. EMOD, *et al.* 1991. Latent fibronectin-degrading serine proteinase activity in *N*-terminal heparin-binding domain of human plasma fibronectin. Eur. J. Biochem. **201:** 71–77.
28. ZHANG, X.M., H. LIN, C. CHEN, *et al.* 1999. Inhibition of ubiquitin–proteasome pathway activates a caspase-3-like protease and induces Bcl-2 cleavage in human M-07e leukaemic cells. Biochem. J. **340:** 127–133.

The Embryo Question

CARLO FLAMIGNI

First Institute of Obstetrics and Gynecology, Clinics of Obstetrics and Gynecology and Physiopathology of Reproduction, University of Bologna, Bologna, Italy

Policlinico S. Orsola, via Massarenti 13, 40138 Bologna, Italy

ABSTRACT: In Italy, the seat of the Vatican, the problem of the "rights of the embryo" has been particularly felt and has caused bitter debate between laymen and clergy. The disagreement has focused primarily on the definition of "person," "individual," and the "beginning of life." Catholics, for the most part, have contested the concept of the "pre-embryo" and have tried to have a law passed that would impede the production and freezing of supernumerary embryos (according to the hypothesis of the "simple case"). In the same way, Catholics have strongly opposed the possible manipulation of embryos, including pre-implant genetic investigations. In addition to Catholic teachings, the National Committee for Bioethics has also declared itself favorable to the protection of the "waking life." It published a special document on the theme in a period in which the Committee was composed only of strict Catholics, following action taken by the then Prime Minister, Berlusconi, who believed it necessary to exclude and remove all lay members from the Committee. The document of the National Committee for Bioethics, which distinguishes itself for having declared that "the embryo is one of us," has been the cause of a transversal political aggregation that has gathered Catholic parliamentarians from different political parties and that has begun a campaign to acknowledge the prerogatives and rights of the embryo which Italian law attributes only to the baby after its birth. An intense debate continues on all these themes, and in back of all this is the warning from the Church to re-examine the Italian law dealing with the voluntary interruption of pregnancy.

KEYWORDS: embryo; origins; bioethics

INTRODUCTION

From time immemorial, man has been fascinated with the mystery of his origins, and certainly, myths and legends on this subject are numerous. I remind you of Genesis and the story of Adam and Eve. It is certain that if the fact that God created man and woman with the same human nature could be scientifically proved and was not only a matter of faith, we could not do more than the author of Genesis in imagining and describing how those facts came about. The theory of evolution challenged science and the imagination when it tried to explain how the first men appeared on earth. An even greater challenge was presented to philosophers and theologians

Address for correspondence: Dr. Carlo Flamigni, First Institute of Obstetrics and Gynecology, Clinics of Obstetrics and Gynecology and Physiopathology of Reproduction, University of Bologna, Bologna, Italy. Voice: +30-051-342823; fax: +39-051-301994.

when they had to explain the transformation of animal life into human life, the incarnation.

Even if these discussions and questions regard seemingly remote events, which presumably took place millions of years ago, modern man confronts similar problems when he wants to understand when individual life began for each of us. One thing is certain; each of us began to exist, eventually becoming a human being, starting from something else, very different from what we are now. There was a time when we "were not," except perhaps for a glint in the eyes of our parents. And there was a time when we began to be. The mystery is placed between these two moments.

The beginning of man, our beginning, is certainly a mystery destined never to lose its fascination. The development of the biology of reproduction has added new interests, interests predominantly practical to the problem of the beginning of individual life. This points out the great importance that an answer to this question could have for a series of moral problems.

The probability of having the first phases of development of the zygote take place *in vitro* and the prospect of experimentation for therapeutic ends have put the problem of the "status" of the product of conception under different profiles — biological, moral, and legal — and of its safeguarding. In this regard, different conceptual positions exist which refer to the different stages of the prenatal period as the moment of the beginning of individual human life. The events considered critical for the recognition of this quality are distributed over the entire period of uterine life. According to the criteria used more or less extensively, they can vary from fecundation to the initial or complete implantation of the product of conception in the endometrium, to the completion of organogenesis, to the appearance of brain activity, and to the acquisition of capability of autonomous life (about 20 weeks of gestation) until birth.

The concept of individual human life correlates to that of the person. Nevertheless, biology cannot define the person for that which he is, but can only "circumstantiate" or give support to this reality with the notion of a specific individual. The progress of molecular biology and genetics has certainly contributed to consolidating the principle not only of biological identity, but also of individual identity that DNA permits us to almost certainly recognize an individual genome in a single cell beginning from the zygote. But genomic individuality does not necessarily coincide with the individuality of the subject, considered a real person or *in fieri*. Opinions about the moment in which individual life appears differ substantially on this point and are ascribable to two major schools of thought. According to the first, the beginning of human life is not separable from the reality of the person and is placed at the moment of the formation of the zygote. The reasons that sustain this theory are the following: fusion of the gametes leads to the formation of a genetic system that is characterized by its uniqueness and the completeness of the information necessary for the expression of all the individual characteristics in a sequential process without interruption. The genome of the zygote not only has the capacity to direct the synthesis of all the genetic products that determine the manifestation of the various characteristics, but also contains the indicators of regulation that, interacting in the sites and at the right moment with external indicators, permit the normal execution of the program of development. Both structural and regulatory information is expressed very early in the first phases of the division of the zygote. According to data obtained in laboratory animals (mice and rabbits) and, recently, also in humans, on products of *in vitro* fecundation, the synthesis of new molecules that carry genetic messages of the zygote itself already begins the second cellular division. This means that the dependence on the maternal messengers is limited to the first two divisions on the flow of genetic information directly from DNA of the new individual begins at the 4–8 blastomere stage, at about 80 hours after fecundation.

A second school of thought considers the beginning of individual human life as presupposed by the recognition of the quality of the person, not coinciding with fecundation, but delayed to a successive moment of development. Furthermore, the acquisition of this state would be progressive and would have a useful effect with the aim of protecting the product of conception in correspondence with a threshold by some fixed at the 6th and 7th day, but for most at the 14th day of gestation. The reasons used to sustain the postzygote theory of the origin of human individuality, also defined as gradualist, are based on a series of biological indices that refer to the structure of the embryo itself and to the connection with maternal tissue. For the earliest fixed limit, such structures correspond to the formation of the embryonic disk evident in the blastocysts at the moment of its implantation into the uterine wall. The limit fixed later, the structure index, is the primitive line that gives the coordinates of the embryo and traces the organizational plan. The appearance of the primitive line signals the completion of a unitary organized structure, no longer separable into individuality and totally communicating with the maternal organism.

Objections to the theory of the zygotic origin of individual human life indicate the absence of evidence of an integrated function of the cells that constitute the product of the first division of the zygote, so that the vitality of the conceived in these first phases can be measured only as survival of the cell taken singularly. The consideration that a program of complete development involves the entering into function, in a sequential and concerted way, of all the genes involved in the different morphologic processes is opposed to the aforementioned theory, namely, that the argument of genetic expression is already demonstrable in the early phases of development.

In the initial undifferentiated state of the cells derived from the first divisions of the zygote and in the progressive loss of this characteristic, with maintenance of the capacity of contributing to sharing in the generations of many individuals by successive division, a contrary indication to the determination of the individuality of the conceived is recognized.

As can be noted, the biologic datum analyzed under different profiles and with different accentuation of various phenomena can furnish objective references and explanatory/explicative elements useful in clearing up different positions of principle, essentially those of constitutivity and the gradual acquisition of human individuality. New knowledge of genetics and developmental biology have brought us to a convergence of the concept of genetic identity demonstrable from the moment of fecundation and of the continuity of the developmental process seen as differential genetic activation. Points of view diverge on the significance to attribute to the different events that happen during this process. Research on the molecular mechanism of development is continually progressing; the sequentiality of the human genome will certainly permit the individualization and localization of the genetic determinants responsible for the different functions that are integrated into the formation of the organism. The birth of the individual from the initial phases will be able to be reconstructed with greater approximation, through analysis of both experimental systems and virtual reality, thus allowing a comparison of the different interpretative models on an objective scientific basis.

Embryologists began to debate the problem of the embryo many years ago. Already in 1930, in some obstetrics textbooks published in the United States, the idea of considering the preembryo separately (that is, the product of conception that has not yet been implanted in the uterus, the preimplanted embryo) from the embryo (for which implantation has already begun) had been proposed. The Science and Technology Commission of the European Council in 1988 proposed the use of the term preembryo for the period of time from conception to the end of nesting, which lasts about 14 days. The Commission justified its proposal with the fact that in this period, besides a phase of cellular independence, which characterizes the initial stages of cellular division, there is no evidence of the embryonic stripe/streak, which is the first proof of the existence of an embryo inside this agglomerate/conglomeration of cells. Furthermore, and until the end of implantation, that is, in those 14 days that the geneticist Forabosco defined as the presomatic and preindividual period of the conceived, the preembryo does not have nerve cells or immunologic capacity; it is impossible to say if it will become one embryo or two (or if there will be two embryos in one chimera) or no embryo or if it will be transformed into tumoral tissue. On this basis and on the basis of the lack of unity and uniqueness in this, a kind of cellular colony, the Commission concluded that the moral evaluation in comparison to a preembryo cannot be the same, which will become obligatory successively, when the phase of implantation is concluded.

This definition of "preembryonal phase" was accepted by some and contested, also with a certain amount of violence, by others. Internationally, Spanish and English laws were favorable, whereas German law negated its agreement. In the United Kingdom, a commission was even instituted which has the task of evaluating the requests for experimental investigations to carry out on preembryos and to consent to them only in exceptional cases.

Even if it has been widely used by scientists, the term "preembryo" has raised a lot of suspicion. I would like to forget the most common objections (which sometimes take root in saying that this is only "antiscientific" and "pretextual" terminology) in order to remember that, certainly stronger but put in a polite manner, according to which that term would essentially represent an exercise of linguistic engineering useful for rendering acceptable to the public scientific research on embryos. However, R. McCormick, professor of Christian Ethics in the Theology Department of the University of Notre Dame, strongly maintains that the intentions of the American Fertility Society in choosing this definition did not have anything to do with moral and research problems, but bore in mind the fact that only the first stages of development of mammals concern the formation of the nonembryonal trophoblast and not that of the embryo. The biologist Clifford Grobstein, member of the same Committee, affirms exactly the same thing: "...It's a case of being more accurate in characterizing the initial phase of the development of mammals...."

Lay philosophical reflection recently reported analysis from the field of biology to that of philosophy and has posed new and different questions. It has asked, for example, if it is really important to know when life begins or if, instead, it is not essential to understand when to attribute importance to the beginning of life, if it is really important to know what an embryo is at different moments of its development or if it is more useful to understand when the embryo becomes a "person." If this last is the real key to the problem, then the answer cannot come from biology because the problem is no longer scientific. A person is characterized by rational capacity, and there is no discipline, either natural science or biology, that can define rational capacity. The discussion on the meaning of "person" will certainly last for a long time. Intuitively, one tends to say that a "person" is an individual in some way aware and rational, so that for some it is still necessary to return to the definition of Severino Boezio (*rationalis naturae individua substantia*). It is certain that if this definition is accepted, the first 14 days of development of the "conceived" seem to exclude the definition of "person," because the lack of nervous tissue excludes a rational mixture (and also because there is no individuality until the cells are completely independent).

The importance of being able to understand whether or not the embryo is a "person" has returned to the center of attention of bioethicists since the National Committee for Bioethics published its document on the statute of the embryo in June 1997. One is dealing with an argument that is not easily read (even the media did not understand the basic theory of the Committee) and that is promoted as a document which has found unanimity of consensus, where even a minimally attentive reading cannot but register a notable series of differences of opinion and distinctions.

More than half of the document is dedicated to the philosophical problem of whether or not the embryo is a person. This, despite the fact that some members of the Committee would have willingly avoided discussing the question, was not considered a "condition indispensable and crucial in order to confront bioethical problems." Not taking into account this position, the Committee dedicated in-depth reflection to the philosophical problem, holding that "the force of moral consideration with respect to and for the protection of the embryo varies considerably according to whether or not the characteristic of being a person is recognized and, because, actually, the debate on the rights of protection recognized for the human embryo is very often concentrated in the literature on the subject, on the question of whether or not it is a person." Furthermore, adds the document, this question, even if not crucial (or decisive), is certainly "very relevant with respect to ethical problems." It is even too evident that for the Committee, an affirmative answer to the question "Is an embryo a person?" would resolve all the various normative questions on the subject, making any further investigation superfluous. Instead, a negative answer would not involve, as a consequence, the decision not to protect the embryo because other reasons capable of justifying a precise duty in this regard may exist.

In effect, until this moment, the Committee seems to be interested in pointing out the importance of the philosophical question of whether or not the embryo is a person, but with particular attention to the difference between "absolute importance and nondecisive importance" of the answer to the question. So, we are surprised by the conclusion of the document which says, "the Committee has unanimously decided to recognize the moral right to treat human embryos, immediately from fecundation, according to the criteria of respect and protection that must be adopted in comparison with human individuals to whom the characteristics of a person are commonly attributed apart from the fact that the characteristic of a person in its technically philosophical sense is attributed with certainty to the embryo, right from the beginning." Maurizio Mori justly points out that, in this way, the document contradicts the initial assumption according to which the importance of putting the question of the embryo at the center of the investigation, the fact that the force of the duty of protection cannot but change according to the answers given "is seldom deniable." The conclusions are instead in favor of the absolute irrelevance of the problem.

The layout of the document brings us to believe that the ontological problem of the embryo is a problem of description and as such, it can receive an answer on the basis of rational considerations — cognitive, analogously to that which happens with other descriptive problems. Now instead, we have to recognize that, in reality, this is a descriptive problem whose solution depends on the attitude of he who interprets it considers it, that is, from a preceding moral choice. In other words, at first, it seemed that the problem under examination concerned the type of "being" (ontology) of the embryo itself, but now we discover that this problem concerns the type of "attitude" (of a moral option) which you have to have in comparison to the embryo, because it is the attitude assumed which determines the type of "being" of the embryo.

The conclusions that must be reached with this analysis, however, are of great importance. The Committee recognizes (unanimously!!) that rational-cognitive analysis cannot give an unequivocal answer to the question of whether or not the embryo is a person right from fecundation (because the answer depends on the attitude of the interpreter), accepting the fact that the total potentiality itself of the first embryonal cells creates an insurmountable difficulty to the affirmation of the theory that the embryo is a person from the moment of the first cellular divisions. This is, basically, the central idea of the celebrated Warnock report in which the importance of the preembryonal phase is described.

Regarding the application of the "golden rule," the fact that every specification of the criteria of similarity, which allows the identification of "our fellow man," damages the theory of the Committee. This is even more important, considering the fact that, in the case in point, the embryo is not yet considered a "person." The fact that the similarity in question is identified in a temporal antecedence leaves us very perplexed, because if it is true that before being a person we were embryos, it is also true that before being embryos, we were a strange cell (certainly not definable as "embryo") which contained two separate nuclei and a polar globule, and, before that, we were two cells that were partially united by a fusion of membranes, and before that we were two gametes, a spermatozoon and an oocyte. There is no doubt that we come from things very different from what we are, things that we cannot consider "our fellow man" and in comparison to which we do not feel we have to predispose rules of protection analogous to those that are due to people.

I cannot continue this critical analysis because the document is very long, the subjects are discussed in an articulate and complex manner, and the critical evaluations are verbose and difficult to summarize. Personally, I feel that the stages of the development of the embryo are gradual and that this graduality is the characteristic element of the appearance of new characteristics. In this sense, fecundation is an important stage, but it is not the decisive stage for the substantial change required to be a person, which can take place only when the process has reached an adequate organizational complexity, differentiating and specializing parts of itself so as to consent to the presence of rational functions and to make the properties that characterize the characteristic/distinctive type of being of a person.

In effect, the reproductive process is a special teleologic process, finalized to give birth to new organisms that, before reaching the final aim, go through various stages characterized by the specific teleologicity of the bodies involved. Because the gametes are also alive, human, and intrinsically directed to develop, one must recognize that reproduction begins when two people, freely deciding to have a sexual relationship, give origin to a new process of human life. In fact, after this act, not only is there already teleologically direct human life *in fieri* in the body of the woman (gametes), but there is also the chromosomal set of the eventual future person, even if still separate. This human life, nevertheless, is still in a very uncertain state (many gametes do not manage to reach their aim) and undetermined (various combinations of chromosomal sets are possible). Eventual fecundation signals an important stage, because the vital process already begun becomes more precise because the chromosomal set of the eventual future person is united under the same membrane (in which the genetic material of the second polar globule is also present for a brief but definite period of time), initiating a new level of organization of the vital process. This process, however, is even more uncertain (many fertilized ovules are lost naturally) and still rather undetermined (it is still completely independent, that is, capable of splitting into twins or fusing with another embryo). After a few days, human life is even more determined, losing total independence and assuming somatic individuality, and for a while, it has a level of organization analogous to that vegetative because only metabolic and growth functions are present. Then, the process is more determined, differentiating itself and specializing itself so that, with the appearance of cerebral structures, it passes to an even more complex level characterized by the acquisition of new functions such as sensitivity and the capacity of movement. Finally, when the cerebral structures are almost complete, the vital process is so complex as to cause the characteristics of the new level of existence typical of a person to merge, with the conclusion of the finalism of the reproductive process. I have indicated the principal stages of the reproductive process, showing that the substantial change required of a person can happen only in the more advanced stages of the process.

This perspective puts in its correct place the *graduality* intrinsic to biological development and takes into account some of the other aspects of the "biological way of thinking" (finalism, emergence, etc.) managing, in this way, to explain also in which sense that what is relative to the nature of the embryo is a *philosophical* problem (and not merely biological) of a descriptive character, which can be resolved starting from rational and cognitive considerations. In this way, it is possible both to put in order all the various aspects of the question, avoiding many of the difficulties that made the conclusions of the Committee so confused, and to resolve the problem of individuality in the first phases after fecundation.

Some brief conclusive comments. The Italian National Committee for Bioethics has, in practice, published a document affirming that "the embryo is one of us," because, let me say it brutally, it has a soul. An extraordinary scientific and cultural result! However, the damage of this document is immediate and considerable. Immediately after its publication, a group of Catholic parliamentarians constituted the umpteenth lobby (the so-called "embryo party" with which many Catholic intellectuals, including the President of the Italian National Committee for Bioethics, have lined up), which intends to propose to the Italian Parliament the approval of a law that would recognize the dignity of the fertilized egg and the right of human beings. It is not even necessary to comment on this initiative, already discussed in the newspapers, evidently directed, as a first intention, to again examine the law on voluntary abortion and to consider illegal some therapy for sterility.

Among other things, evidently a little clouded by enthusiasm, the drafters of the various documents that concern this new juridical statute of the embryo have continued to anticipate the moment in which a person is determined, when it is no longer that of the fusion of the two genomes, but even that of the penetration of the spermatozoon and the fusion of the membranes of the two gametes.

Hard and unpleasant opposition such as that which is taking place on the question of the embryo, work of some Catholic integralists, cannot but damage the growth and civil maturation of the country. The alternative is that of accepting widely shared mediation, such as that which considers the human embryo deserving of respect and of protection (due to its potentiality), but not to protection equal to that of a person, according to the principles expressed in 1979 by the Ethics Committee of the American Society of Fertility and Sterility. It is therefore, once again, the very vituperated proposal of Engelhardt, that of agreeing on themes apparently open to irremediable conflicts going to the *"island for moral foreigners,"* a not so imaginary place, which is always open to good-hearted people and always closed to dogmas — religious, philosophical, or scientific — that exist.

Ethical Issues in Selecting Embryos

ROSAMOND RHODES

Mount Sinai School of Medicine, New York, New York 10029, USA

ABSTRACT: People involved in assisted reproduction frequently make decisions about which of several embryos to implant or which of several embryos to reduce from a multiple pregnancy. Yet, others have raised questions about the ethical acceptability of using sex or genetic characteristics as selection criteria. This paper reviews arguments for rejecting embryo selection and discusses the subject of choosing offspring in terms of the centrality of liberty and autonomous choice in ethics. It also presents a position on the acceptable scope of embryo selection and the professional responsibilities of those who practice reproductive medicine.

Keywords: ethics; embryos; sex selection; reproductive choice; liberty; disabilities; discrimination

INTRODUCTION

People involved in assisted reproduction frequently make decisions about which of several embryos to implant or which of several embryos to reduce from a multiple pregnancy. Physicians involved in embryo transfers or pregnancy reductions have to choose which embryos will have a chance of developing into a baby and which will not. Currently, the embryos that look healthiest are most often the ones to be implanted and the ones that appear unhealthy or are conveniently positioned are the ones that are most commonly discarded or reduced.

Developing technology will enable doctors to know more about the embryos among which they are selecting. Embryos can already be selected because of their gender or because they do not have some specific genetic anomaly. But, being able to do something does not mean that it should be done. In the case of selecting embryos, people have already raised questions about the ethical acceptability of using sex as a selection criterion. Disabilities activists have challenged the morality of using criteria related to illness, disease, or disability. And fiction writers and others with vivid imaginations have raised questions about possible future uses of diagnostic technology in fashioning future human beings. They spark reflection about whether it is acceptable to select an embryo because its genes promise great intelligence, aggressiveness, physical prowess, and blue eyes. These issues also change significantly when we consider them from the perspective of different decision makers. Is the selection of embryos a choice for physicians to make or should it be left to government, to insurance providers, or to parents? If the choice is to be made by

Address for correspondence: Dr. Rosamond Rhodes, Mount Sinai School of Medicine, Box #1108, One Gustave Levy Place, New York, New York 10029. Voice: 212-241-3757; fax: 212-427-7862.

rosamond_rhodes@mssm.edu

persons other than the physician, when should a physician cooperate with their choice and when should a physician refuse to act on their grounds for embryo selection?

With the possibility of selecting against kinds of humans, people worry about the morality of using the new technology. They are anxious about the ethical borders that might be crossed, they are apprehensive about eugenics, concerned about reinforcing negative social attitudes about gender and disability, and uneasy about producing humans without intending to allow them to live and to develop. The religiously inclined are concerned about meddling with the "sanctity of life." As Paul Ramsey explained, "the value of human life is ultimately grounded in the value God is placing on it. . . . [The] essence [of human life] is [its] existence before God and to God, and it is from Him." For believers, selecting embryos sounds dangerously close to playing God, trespassing in His domain, or treading on the sanctity of life.

In response to such concerns from so many disparate perspectives, specialists in assisted reproduction have been hesitant in making their techniques available on request, because of uncertainty about making decisions on the ethical frontier and concerns about their moral reputation. Nevertheless, this paper will argue that, for the most part, we must resist the movement to proscribe or prohibit embryo selection. Our society's commitment to liberty requires that we allow individuals to make choices according to their own lights, and in the absence of actual substantial evidence that such practices cause serious harm or at least a demonstration of a significant likelihood of untoward repercussions, we are not justified in denying individuals the option.

In this presentation, I review some of the important considerations for allowing embryo selection and arguments that have been put forward for rejecting embryo selection criteria based on sex or genetic characteristics. I discuss the subject of choosing our offspring in terms of the centrality to ethics of liberty and autonomous choice and in terms of well accepted ideas about limiting liberty because of harm to others. In light of these remarks, I shall present a position on the acceptable scope of embryo selection, on who should be making the choices, and on the professional responsibilities of those who practice reproductive medicine.

LIBERTY

From its inception, our society has embraced the value of liberty. Freedom has been our creed and the foundation for building our government both because of its inherent value and because it is such a crucial component of happiness. In particular, reproductive freedom is a very important human value. Through reproductive choice people are allowed to act on their own values and to try to create their own image of happiness. For the most part, people want the liberty to choose their own reproductive partners, the timing of their reproduction, and their rate of reproduction.

While there has been a great deal of discussion about the concept of liberty, John Stuart Mill's account has been given significant weight in moral and political philosophy, and in this discussion, because of the strength of his arguments and their analytic power, I will follow his account. As Mill has explained, for people who extol liberty, "the sole end for which mankind are warranted, individually or collectively, in interfering with the liberty of action of any of their number is self-protection."

This principle for limiting legislative and policy intervention with liberty has become known as the "harm principle." It demands that no action be forbidden unless it can be shown to cause harm to others in the enjoyment of their rights. According to Mill,

> As soon as any part of a person's conduct affects prejudicially the interests of others, society has jurisdiction over it, and the question whether the general welfare will or will not be promoted by interfering with it becomes open to discussion. But there is no room for entertaining any such question when a person's conduct affects the interests of no person besides himself, or need not affect them unless they like.

Although anything one person does may give another affront, upset, or sadness and thereby cause some harm, only those actions that "violate a distinct and assignable obligation to any person or persons" may be proscribed by legislation. For example, my yard art and the landscaping around my home might offend the esthetic sensitivities of some people who pass by, but since I have no specific obligation to decorate in accordance with their taste, and since I have made no one any promise about the limitations on the decoration of my property, I have violated no one's right. Therefore, society has no grounds for limiting my freedom of self-expression through landscaping by legislating against my esthetic choices.

EMBRYO SELECTION, RIGHTS, AND HARMS

Rights. With respect to embryo selection, the question relevant to Mill's criterion is whether someone's use of the technology would violate anyone else's rights? To answer, we must consider all of those who we could anticipate might have rights violated. As far as I can foresee, those who might be harmed by the production of selected offspring would include the perspective children, their peers, and those in the community who would be upset by people overstepping the line into God's domain. Under any circumstances of implanting only a few of several embryos or reducing a pregnancy of one or more of several embryos, only some of the possible embryos will actually become children. Without invoking a theological argument about fertilized eggs having a right to life, it is hard to imagine that the destruction of a nonselected embryo would involve a violation of rights. None of the others who might claim some harm would suffer any violation of rights.

Devaluation and Discrimination. Some disabilities activists worry that by selecting against embryos with genetic abnormalities we would diminish our appreciation of people with disabilities. Similarly, some feminists worry that by allowing people to select against females we would encourage sexist attitudes and support gender discrimination. These concerns do not meet Mill's standard for prohibiting individual choice. First, it is not at all clear that the imagined untoward affects will actually occur, and if the attitudes did arise in a few instances, it is not clear that their limited social impact could justify limiting reproductive liberty. These are empirical matters, and a significant amount of evidence would have to be amassed before the concern reached the level of meriting a restrictive social policy. Second, it seems that no one has a right to prevent the existence of the selected others who might, in some way, be preferred or superior to themselves and, just by living, make the less desired or inferior feel unappreciated. That embryo selection technology might be the means to enable fewer females or fewer individuals with disabilities to be born does not, therefore, violate the rights of women, or people with disabilities, or anyone else.

Religious Concerns. The religious concern over interfering with the sanctity of life also fails to meet Mill's criterion for legislating against a practice. While liberty allows individuals the freedom to choose a religious perspective and the freedom to live according to the religious views they embrace, it limits individuals' infringement on the similar rights of others. In other words, no one may impose his own religious views on others. So while no one has the right to interfere with anyone else's religious practice, the others who he respects have no right to intervene in his living by his own religious or nonreligious standards. The religious liberty guaranteed by the harm principle does not extend rights to control the lives of others, and so those whose religious sensitivities are upset by the prospect of other people meddling with the creation of human life cannot claim that harm as grounds for limiting others' procreative practice.

Justification. Some people base their objections to embryo selection on the particular moral justification that people may offer for their choice. Yet, while we may consider some reasons better than others, efforts to constrain peoples' moral judgments are rejected by Mill as illegitimate "moral legalism." Many people consider the medical reason of wanting to avoid having a child with a serious genetic disease and the nonmedical reason of family balance as good reasons for embryo selection. Putting these "good" reasons aside, it is important to point out that we do not question the reasoning that motivates nontechnology-assisted reproduction. The ordinary desire to have biologically related offspring is not challenged even in the face of overpopulation and the large numbers of orphaned children around the world. Without aid and without society's interference people have children in order to pass along their genes, or to pressure a partner into marriage, or to get an apartment, or to keep a marriage together, or to get an inheritance, or to have a real live doll to play with, or to have some body to love. It is not even clear which reasons are "good" reasons and which are not. But it is clear that privacy and respect for autonomy require that people be allowed to follow their own reasons. So reasons for procreation should be irrelevant to policy makers. And, at least since Hobbes's writings in the seventeenth century, it has been understood that law could only govern action and not thought or belief.

FURTHER CONSIDERATIONS

In sum, I find no persuasive argument for restricting embryo selection (or, similarly, preconception sex selection) as long as there is no empirical evidence of significant social harm from allowing the technology to be freely available. Yet, I would like to press this conclusion in several directions to show what more might be said in defense of sex selection or selecting embryos for other reasons, such as to avoid having a child with a serious genetic disease.

Impact. Significant social harms from resulting gender imbalance in the population would count against allowing access to embryo selection technology. Yet, in an environment resembling contemporary U.S. society, it is hard to imagine that the number of births that employed the technology could be large enough to have a demographic effect. Since the cost, inconvenience, discomfort, risks, and loss of privacy entailed by the procedure would be likely to make embryo selection a rarely employed technology, and since there would be a variety of motivations and procreators, the numbers of individuals produced by the technology in our society (or another that was sufficiently similar to ours) would not be great enough or similar enough to have any significant impact on demographics or on social attitudes towards females or people with disabilities. While studies show that people have preferences about gender and birth order, in actual decisions about using embryo selection those considerations will have to be balanced against the others that mitigate against it. Only those for whom gender or avoiding a genetic disease is extremely important are likely to avail themselves of the technology.

Consequences. Any conclusion about the social impact of a practice has to take all of its effects into account. While my guess is that embryo selection is likely to have only a negligible societal impact, nevertheless, if we were to evaluate that effect we would have to assess all of its consequences, those that count as harms as well as those that count as benefits. Although gender imbalance in the population may turn out to be a harm at some point, other effects of embryo selection are likely to be beneficial. (1) Embryo selection for gender is likely to be used by parents who want an additional child to be of a different gender than other children in the family. Without assisted reproductive technology, "try again" has been the method to achieve that goal. Embryo selection (and preconception sex selection [PSS], if it should be effective) has the social advantage of not adding to society's overpopulation problems. (2) By helping couples achieve the gender balance they want with fewer children, embryo selection (or PSS) can benefit families by easing the economic and human burdens of providing for a large family. Today, when few enjoy the support of an extended family to help with the chores of everyday life and when both parents are typically employed outside the home, additional children tax a family's limited resources. (3) Potential parents, that is, autonomous adults, are in the best position to assess the kind of rearing and companionship experience that would be valuable to them. For those to whom gender or the avoidance of a child with disabilities makes a significant enough difference to justify embryo selection (or PSS), the gender- or genetic-selected child is likely to provide a more rewarding experience. (4) Children produced by embryo selection (or PSS) are also more likely to be attentively reared and to have a good childhood because their parents have chosen the kind of child who they are more likely to nurture well.

Context. Some objectors to embryo selection find the idea of choosing one's offspring, rather that accepting whichever ones happen to arrive, to be immoral *per se* or to support discrimination and therein be immoral. Sympathetic moral imagination can, however, help us to appreciate that embryo selection (or PSS) can be moral or, in some cases, may be obligatory. Consider the hypothetical case of George and Katherine. Many years ago, George had engaged in pederastic behavior. He was apprehended for his assaults on young boys, tried, convicted, and punished for his crimes. After years of psychotherapy he now understands and deeply regrets his previous behavior. He no longer experiences any sexual attraction for young boys. In fact, he has fallen in love with Katherine and they want very much to have a family. After fully discussing George's past and considering their options, they decide that they don't want to chance having a boy. The risk of triggering some old feelings would be far too costly for both George and a son, and George and Katherine would both be very happy as parents to a girl. Because of age-related factors, Katherine needs to use assisted reproductive technology and her obstetrician discusses the option of embryo selection with the couple. They opt for selecting only female embryos for implantation.

As I see it, the behavior of George and Katherine is morally responsible. They consider the value of a child in their lives, the conceivable danger to themselves and their future offspring, and how to minimize the possibility of related harms. Their choice exemplifies far-sighted prudence, appropriate care and concern, and ethical responsibility. It would be immoral for people in their situation to ignore the risks or to eschew embryo selection out of concern for appearing to display sexism. This case makes the point that sex selection is not necessarily immoral and it is not necessarily an act of unacceptable sex discrimination. The circumstances and the reasons for choosing selection can make a significant difference, and there is likely to be a broad array of situations in which embryo selection is ethically acceptable.

Prohibition. Moral imagination can also be used to make a further point. There is a significant difference between judging that a particular act is unethical and deciding that the practice should be legally prohibited. If we could know enough about the situations and reasons involved in other people's procreative decisions, we might decide that some were ethically unacceptable. While that information could be sufficient for our judgment about a particular case, it would not be sufficient to justify legislation that would limit the liberty of everyone. Allowing people to live their lives by their own lights and to make some bad or even unethical decisions is inherent in our valuing liberty. A demonstration of actual overriding harms is the only legitimate justification for constraining liberty.

Selfishness. Finally, we should consider the place of personal satisfaction in moral decisions, particularly in reproductive decisions. The most obvious social problem of serious gender imbalance is that those in the gender majority will be less likely than otherwise of having a heterosexual mating with all its attendant promise of personal satisfaction. And the reason most people want to have children involves the promise of personal satisfaction associated with being a parent. Such pleasures motivate us. They are importantly constitutive of well-being, and the pleasure associated with securing such basic goods is typically taken into account in moral and political philosophy. In the context of recognizing the importance of personal satisfaction as a moral consideration, we should notice that demeaning the pleasure that some people associate with having a child of a particular gender or devaluing the pain that some people associate with having a child with a genetic disease as unethically selfish requires justification. Those who want to decry embryo selection have to explain why the desire to have a child of a particular gender or a child without a genetic disease is unethical while the selfish desire to have any child is ethically acceptable.

WHO MAKES THE CHOICE

My argument, so far, has focused on the unacceptability of government or policy restrictions on embryo selection. The questions that remain involve the proper scope for patient and physician choice. The answers require an understanding of physician professional responsibility and the doctor-patient relationship, subjects that may be even more controversial than the ones addressed so far.

The uncontroversial features of physician professional responsibility involve the doctor's commitment to: (1) using the scientific method and guiding practice by the knowledge provided by science, (2) relying on the cooperative model of practice involving a team of health care providers, and (3) pursuing the moral goal of acting for the patient's good. But, as soon as we recognize that a physician and a patient could have very different views of the good, we confront the controversial problem of whose view of the good should rule? When the doctor cares most about avoiding risks of physical harm and the patient cares more about some other component of her well-being, the doctor's and the patient's values are likely to clash. The issue raised by such conflict involves decisions about the appropriate goals and scope of medicine. These are lofty abstract philosophical questions. But the answers have very practical implications when it comes to embryo selection.

A physician may feel comfortable in going along with some patient requests for embryo selection and also be inclined to refuse the service in other cases. Taking personal comfort as the standard suggests that different obstetricians can each have their own personal standard for providing embryo selection and that there are no professional criteria to be used as a guide in these decisions. While physicians may be comfortable with this Lone Ranger approach to bioethics, recognizing that there are standards for professional behavior points us in another direction.

When we consider a patient's abortion decision or a patient's decision to undergo assisted reproduction with its attendant risks and harms, we can appreciate that a patient's values and goals play an important role and often rightly determine the course of treatment. Some people take a narrow and rigid view of the appropriate goals of medicine as promoting health, curing disease, or preserving life. However, thinking about abortion, assisted reproduction, or even plastic surgery provides a different view of the appropriate goals of medicine, something akin to the use of medicine's special knowledge, skills, and privileges to help promote a set of socially defined goods. This view allows a significant place for the patient's conception of the good in medical decision making. In other words, as long as the treatment requested provides an accepted good, and so long as it is likely to achieve the patient's goals without causing significant harm, the requested treatment should be provided and the patient's view of the good should rule.

Obstetrics has been called upon to promote reproductive choice as a socially accepted good and as an appropriate use of medicine's special knowledge, skills, and privileges. Embryo selection certainly fits within that widely appreciated class of goods. As such, patients should expect access to the technology and cooperation from their physicians in offering and providing the option. Regardless of whether the physician shares the patient's conception of the good and regardless of whether the physician feels comfortable with the decision, the patient's choice should rule, at least in most cases, and the physician would not be justified in withholding the technology.

While the reasons I have offered leave me "comfortable" with this conclusion for cooperating with gender selection and selection against genetic disease, I am inclined to give the opposite answer when it comes to genetic selection for dwarfism or deafness. In those cases, because such disabilities are so widely seen as harms, disabilities, and disadvantages, I think physicians would have good reason for not cooperating with a parental request for embryo selection.

CONCLUSION

In these remarks I have put forward a framework for thinking about the ethics of embryo selection. I have argued that the reasons for restricting the use of the technology are not sufficiently compelling to overcome our commitment to protecting liberty and reproductive liberty in particular. Furthermore, I have urged a view of the doctor-patient relationship that takes the values of patients very seriously and, therefore, accepts patient choice as ruling almost always in reproductive decisions. I suggest that the limitation on this freedom is the traditional stand against doing harm. In the case of embryo selection even though a resulting deaf child or dwarf would not be harmed in the sense that the particular resulting child would not be made worse off, I have broadly interpreted the concept of doing harm to include deliberately selecting a child who is likely to be impaired as creating a harmful outcome.

While a number of my conclusions may invite disagreement, my further agenda in this paper was to suggest that disputes in bioethics are to be settled by giving reasons that other reasonable people could accept. I see this view of morality as preferable to an attitude that accepts moral matters as settled on the grounds of claims about personal comfort or uneasiness. Recalling that the practice of medicine involves the cooperation of a team of physicians and other health care providers, forging a moral consensus among those who will be called upon to act becomes a significant concern. Understanding ethics in terms of reasons invites us to share our concerns and to reason together in defining moral positions in reproductive medicine.

ACKNOWLEDGMENTS

This paper draws on some of my previous work; see Refs. 3–5.

REFERENCES

1. RAMSEY, P. 1968. The morality of abortion. *In* Life or Death: Ethics and Options: 72–73. University of Washington Press. Seattle, WA.
2. MILL, J.S. 1978. On Liberty: 9, 73, 74. Hackett Publishing Co. Indianapolis, IN.
3. RHODES, R. 1995. Clones, Harms, and Rights. Camb. Quart. Healthcare Ethics **4**: 285–290.
4. RHODES, R. 2000. Autonomy, respect, and genetic information policy: a reply to Tuija Takal and Matti Häyry. J. Med. Phil. **25**: 114–120.
5. RHODES, R. 2001. Acceptable sex selection. Am. J. Bioethics **1,1**: 31–32.

Subject Index

Index of Contributors